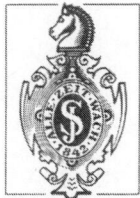

Winifred G. Nayler

Second Generation of Calcium Antagonists

With 81 Figures and 63 Tables

Springer-Verlag Berlin Heidelberg GmbH

Winifred G. Nayler, D.Sc.
The University of Melbourne
Department of Medicine
Austin and Repatriation Hospital
Heidelberg, Victoria, 3084
Australia

ISBN 978-3-540-54215-5   ISBN 978-3-662-02720-2 (eBook)
DOI 10.1007/978-3-662-02720-2

Originally published by Springer-Verlag Berlin Heidelberg New York in 1991.

The use of general descriptive names, trade names, trade marks, etc. in this publication, even if the former are not especially identified, is not to be taken as a sign that such names, as understood by the Trade Marks and Merchandise Marks Act, may accordingly be used freely by anyone.

Product Liability: The publisher can give no guarantee for information about drug dosage and application thereof contained in this book. In every individual case the respective user must check its accuracy by consulting other pharmaceutical literature.

Typesetting: Elsner & Behrens GmbH, 6836 Oftersheim

2127/3140/543210 – Printed on acid-free paper

This book is dedicated to my friend, the Honourable Mr. Justice Crockett O.A., not because of his scholarly approach to the law – which I nevertheless greatly admire – but rather because he taught me to drink Tokay with *ice*.

Foreword

> *"Another damned, thick, square book!*
> *Always scribble, scribble, scribble! Eh!*
> *Mr. Gibbon?"*
> From the Literary Memoirs of Willi-
> am, DUKE OF GLOUCESTER, 1743–1805

The foreword of any book is probably the most difficult to write – not only because it stands at the beginning of an exercise in writing and logic but because it is in this chapter that a reader can expect to find a clear and unambiguous explanation of the author's reason for writing the book and why some subject matter has been included and other subject matter excluded.

Potential readers of this book may not have an inclination to question why some subject matter has been excluded but instead may wonder why another book on calcium antagonists has been published. However, it is arguable with some force that there have been at least three recent developments in the field of calcium antagonism which provide more than adequate support for the view that another book on this topic is warranted. These developments include:

(i)   an improved understanding of the chemical structure, mode of action and architecture of the voltage-activated, calcium antagonist-sensitive calcium channels and their associated calcium-antagonist specific binding sites;

(ii) a more accurate appreciation of how and when the calcium antagonists should be used in the management of a variety of clinical disorders including cerebral ischaemia atherosclerosis, "mild" ischaemic heart disease, ventricular hypertrophy, impaired ventricular relaxation and hypertension (to name but a few), and

(iii) the emergence of a *second generation* of calcium antagonists.

The *"second generation"* calcium antagonists differ from their prototypes – verapamil, diltiazem and nifedipine – not only in terms of their chemistry but also with respect to their tissue selectivity, bio-availability and duration of action. At a time when slow release formulations of the prototype calcium antagonists, or long-acting and sometimes tissue selective second-generation calcium antagonists are being advocated for use on a once-daily basis for the treatment of a variety of clinical conditions, it really is time to dissect out the properties of these new drugs, to consider how they differ from one another and to evaluate their therapeutic usefulness; in short, to ascertain whether these second generation drugs can be expected to fulfil the expectations raised by their protagonists rather than merely replicating the properties of their prototypes. As yet, there is too little information available concerning the clinical expression of the benefits which result from choosing a "second" rather than a "first" generation antagonist for use in the management of most cardiovascular disorders – but there are positive indications that two of the properties which separate the second from the first generation of these drugs are highly desirable. These are the properties of *tissue selectivity* and a *prolonged duration of action*. This book is aimed at exploring why these properties are so advantageous under particular conditions – including stroke, hypertension, atherosclerosis and coronary artery disease.

No attempt has been made here to cover the whole field of calcium antagonism – which, by now, would require several volumes if dealt with properly. Instead it is assumed that the readers already understand the basic mode of action of these drugs at the cellular level (see Nayler, 1988) and that they appreciate their clinical usefulness and limitations (see Opie 1990). In other words, this book is meant to provide an "overview" of the trends in this field, and is written with the hope of imparting some enthusiasm for their expanding use.

Before progressing any further I would like to remind my readers that academic texts are usually conceived with great enthusiasm – and indeed the task of writing such a text gives the author great pleasure. In the background, however, are the "supporting team" – I mean the illustrators, the secretaries, the librarians and those at home who suffer in silence in the hope that one day reason will prevail and a normal orderly life will be restored. Naturally I am deeply and honestly indebted to this "support team" – particularly to my colleague Michael Daly, to Reneé Janssen and Wendy Vanags who have typed this volume, and to Sianna Panagiotopoulos, who, once again, has prepared the illustrations.

So – "another damned, thick, square book".

WINIFRED NAYLER

Contents

Foreword VII

Chapter 1   *The Second Generation of Calcium Antagonists:*
                What Are They?

       – Rationale for the Development of the Second Generation
          Calcium Antagonists: Limitations of the First Generation .   2
       – Are the Second Generation Calcium Antagonists Needed? .   4
       – Summary   7

Chapter 2   *The Chemistry of the Second Generation*
                Calcium Antagonists

       – Derivatives of the Prototype Calcium Antagonists
          Which Interact with The Alpha$_1$ Subunit Binding Sites
          of the L-Type Ca^{2+} Channels   12
       – Other New Calcium Antagonists   19
       – Novel Calcium Antagonists with Additional Antagonist
          Activity   22
       – Summary   23

Chapter 3   *The Molecular Biology of the Voltage-Dependent,*
                Calcium Antagonist-Sensitive Calcium Channels

       – Ca^{2+}-Conducting Channels   26
       – The Voltage-Sensitive Ca^{2+} Channels   26
       – The Molecular Biology of the L-type Ca^{2+} Channel   27
       – The Voltage-Dependent Calcium Antagonist-Sensitive
          Ca^{2+} Channel Complex of *Skeletal Muscle* T-Tubules:
          Subunit Structure and Function   28
       – The Tissue Specificity of the Alpha$_1$ Subunit   34
       – Summary   36

Chapter 4 *Calcium Antagonists and the Calcium Release Channels*
of the Sarcoplasmic Reticulum

- The General Properties of the Sarcoplasmic Reticulum ... 40
- The General Morphology of the Sarcoplasmic
  Reticulum (SR): Evidence of Specialization 41
- The Biochemistry of the Sarcoplasmic Reticulum 43
- The Ultrastructure and Chemistry of the SR Feet
  (The SR Ryanodine Receptor – Ca^{2+} Release Channel) ... 44
- Chemistry 46
- The Intraluminal Contents of the Junctional SR 48
- Characteristics of the SR Ryanodine Receptor –
  Ca^{2+} Release Channel Complex 48
- SR Ca^{2+} Release Channels in Various Pathologies 50
- The Trigger for SR Ca^{2+} Release:
  Differences Between Skeletal and Cardiac Muscle 52
- Calcium Antagonists and SR Ca^{2+} Release 53
- Summary 54

Chapter 5 *"Up" and "Down" Regulation of the Calcium Antagonist*
Binding Sites

- Age-Dependent Changes in Calcium Antagonist
  Binding Site Density 55
- Cardiomyopathies 56
- Ischaemia as a Cause of "Down" Regulation 58
- Effect of Ischaemia on Other Cardiac Receptors 60
- Effect of Drugs and Chemicals on Calcium Antagonist
  Binding Site Density 62
- The Effect of Other Physiological Interventions 65
- Summary 65

Chapter 6 *Oxyradical-Induced Lipid Peroxidation:*
Do Calcium Antagonists Provide Any Protection?

- Chemistry and Production of the Oxyradicals 68
- Sites of Oxyradical Production 70
- Protective Mechanisms 71
- Mode of Action 71
- Evidence of Oxyradical Production in the Heart 73
- Oxyradical-Induced Injury 74
- Oxyradical-Induced Loss of Ca^{2+} Homeostasis 77
- Evidence of Excess Oxyradical Production During
  Myocardial Ischaemia and Post Ischaemic Reperfusion ... 78
- Role of Calcium Antagonists as Protective Agents 79

– Protection Against Oxyradical-Induced Injury:
Are the Calcium Antagonists Effective? 80
– Mode of Action 83
– Summary 83

Chapter 7   Endothelin-1 and the Calcium Antagonists

– The Production of Endothelin-1 86
– Agents and Conditions Which Stimulate Endothelin-1
Production 88
– The Endothelin Receptor 88
– The Endothelin-1 Receptor 89
– Endothelin-1 and the Calcium Antagonists 90
– The Involvement of Endothelin-1 in the Maintenance
of Vascular Tone 93
– Endothelin-1 and the Coronary Circulation:
The Role of the Calcium Antagonists 94
– Endothelin and Hypertension 95
– Endothelin-1 and Atherosclerosis 95
– Summary 95

Chapter 8   Calcium Antagonists and the Stunned Heart

– Stunning, Hibernation or Infarction? 97
– The Clinical Relevance of Myocardial Stunning 98
– Animal Models of Myocardial Stunning 99
– The Electrical, Mechanical, Morphological and Biochemical
Properties of the Pre-Stunned and Stunned Myocardium .. 100
– Possible Mechanisms of Myocardial Stunning 108
– Is Energy Utilization Impaired? 108
– Is the Altered Ultrastructure Responsible? 108
– Is Perfusion Adequate During Reperfusion? 109
– Is There an Abnormal Ca^{2+} Influx? 110
– Do the Myofibrils Become Relatively Insensitive to Ca^{2+}? . 110
– Oxyradical-Mediated Dysfunction: Is this Relevant? 110
– The Sarcoplasmic Reticulum: Is it Involved? 112
– Myocardial Stunning: A Multifactorial Event 112
– Calcium Antagonists and the Stunned Myocardium 114
– Summary 116

Chapter 9   Calcium Antagonists and the Hibernating Myocardium

– The Hibernating Myocardium 118
– Is Myocardial Hibernation an Adaptive Process? 119
– The Identification of the Hibernating Myocardium 119
– The Hibernating Myocardium: It's Clinical Occurrence ... 120

– The Possible Causes of the Depressed Contractile State ... 121
– Effective Remedial Measures 126
– Summary 128

**Chapter 10 Second Generation Calcium Antagonists
and the Ischaemic Myocardium**

– Myocardial Infarction 131
– The Significance of the Early Rise in Cytosolic Ca^{2+} 132
– The Possible Contribution of Endothelin-1
to Ischaemia-Reperfusion Injury 133
– Clinical Evidence of a Protective Role
for the Second Generation Antagonists 135
– Summary 135

**Chapter 11 The Molecular Mechanisms Involved in the
Anti-Atherogenic Effect of the Calcium Antagonists**

– Lesion Formation: Sequence of Events 139
– Factors Concerned with the Initiation of Plaque Formation 140
– The Mechanism Involved in the Macrophage Accumulation
of Low Density Lipoproteins (LDL) 142
– The Progression of the Fatty Streak to the Adult Plaque .. 143
– Calcium-Dependent Processes Which Contribute
to the Formation of Atherosclerotic Lesions 144
– Human Studies Showing an Antiatherosclerotic Effect
of Calcium Antagonist Therapy 145
– Laboratory Studies Relating to the Antiatherosclerotic
Effect of First and Second Generation Calcium Antagonists 146
– The Molecular Mechanisms Involved in the Antiatherogenic
Effect of the Calcium Antagonists 146
– Effect of Calcium Antagonists on Restenosis after PTCA . 149
– Effect of Calcium Antagonists on Coronary Graft Patency . 149
– Endothelial Dysfunction Early in the Atherogenic Process . 150
– Summary 151

**Chapter 12 Second Generation Calcium Antagonists:
Their Use in Congestive Heart Failure**

– The Pathophysiology of Congestive Heart Failure 154
– The Therapeutic Management of the Failing Heart 157
– The Second Generation Calcium Antagonists 158
– Summary 161

Chapter 13 Second Generation Calcium Antagonists
as Blood Pressure Lowering Agents:
The Prevention of Cardiac Hypertrophy

- Calcium and Vascular Smooth Muscle Contraction 163
- The Pathophysiology of Hypertension 165
- Calcium Antagonists as Blood Pressure Lowering Agents . 167
- Mode of Action 170
- Summary 172

Chapter 14 Second Generation Calcium Antagonists
and the Management of Cerebral Ischaemia

- The Ischaemic Brain 173
- Causes of Cerebral Ischaemia 174
- Ischaemic "Stroke" and Subarachnoid Haemorrhage 175
- Aetiology of Acute Cerebral Ischaemia (Stroke)
  and Subarachnoid Haemorrhage 176
- Consequences of Cerebral Ischaemia 177
- Protection of the Ischaemically-Injured Brain 179
- Efficacy of Second Generation Calcium Antagonists
  in the Management of Acute Cerebral Ischaemia 179
- Clinical Data 182
- Mode of Action 182
- Subarachnoid Haemorrhage 183
- Effect of Second Generation Calcium Antagonists
  on Recovery After Subarachnoid Haemorrhage 184
- Summary 184

Chapter 15 Second Generation Calcium Antagonists
and the Coronary Circulation

- Coronary Spasm 187
- Angina Pectoris 188
- Silent Ischaemia 191
- Summary 191

Chapter 16 The Second Generation Calcium Antagonists

- Improved Tissue Selectivity 192
- Relevance of Improved Tissue Selectivity 193
- Duration of Action 194
- Future Directions 195

References 197

Chapter 1

The Second Generation of Calcium Antagonists: What are They?

> "God could cause us considerable embarrassment by revealing all of the secrets of nature to us; we should not know what to do for sheer apathy and boredom".
>
> J.W. GOETHE (1749–1832)

The prototype – or *first generation* – calcium antagonists are verapamil, nifedipine and diltiazem (Fig. 1.1). These are no longer "mystery" drugs. To the contrary, their mode of action has been unravelled (Fleckenstein 1983), their limitations recognized and their efficacy and use in the management of patients with a broad spectrum of cardiovascular and other disorders clearly defined (Nayler 1988; Opie

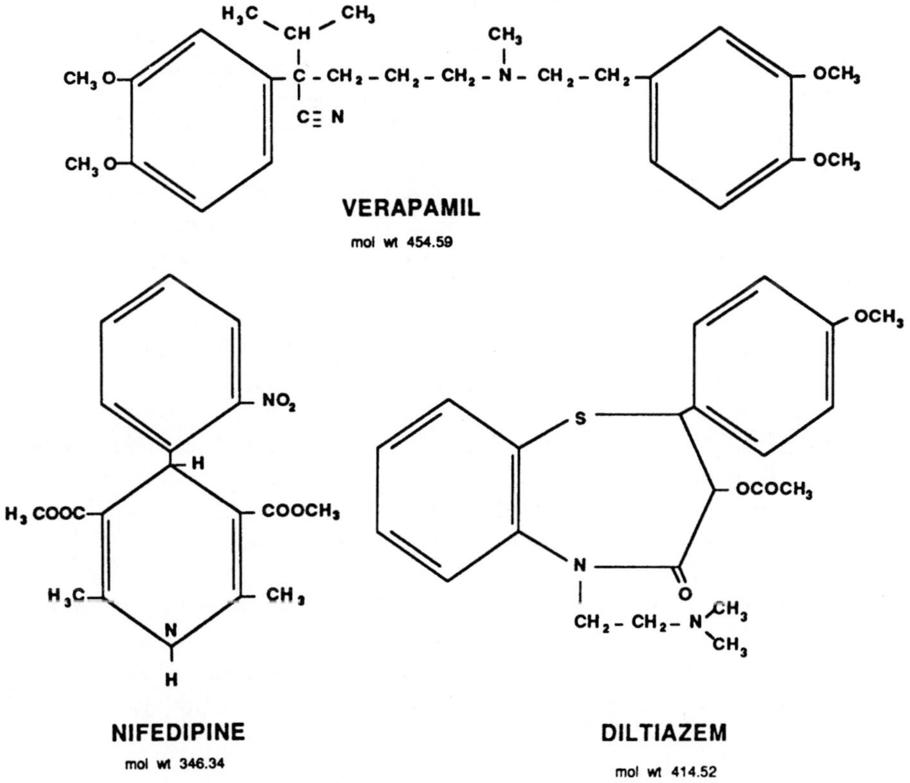

VERAPAMIL

mol wt 454.59

NIFEDIPINE

mol wt 346.34

DILTIAZEM

mol wt 414.52

Fig. 1.1. The chemical formulae of the prototype calcium antagonists – verapamil, nifedipine and diltiazem

1990). These calcium antagonists are here to stay – but to assume that the current state of the art in this particular field has reached its peak is to admit that "sheer apathy and boredom" has invaded this field of pharmacotherapy. This has not happened. Instead, major developments have, and still are taking place, resulting in the emergence of new "second generation" calcium antagonists. This chapter (Chapter 1) outlines why these new calcium antagonists are being developed, and describes some of their advantages. Their chemistry is outlined in the next chapter (Chapter 2).

Rationale for the Development of the Second Generation Calcium Antagonists: Limitations of the First Generation

Perhaps the best way of explaining why a second generation of calcium antagonists even began to be considered is to recall the limitations of the first generation compounds (verapamil, nifedipine and diltiazem). Those limitations are now all too familiar. They include:

(i)   a relatively short duration of action;
(ii) inherent, and usually unwanted negative inotropism;
(iii) in some instances, an inhibitory effect on atrio-ventricular conduction of sufficient intensity as to preclude their use under certain conditions;
(iv) lack of, or inadequate, tissue specificity. For example, nifedipine is a potent but general vasodilator of the arterial system and therefore cannot be used to target a particular vascular bed, such as the coronary or cerebral circulation. Similarly, verapamil does not differentiate between the myocardium, the vasculature and the atrioventricular conducting tissue, and whilst diltiazem is an arterial dilator it also targets both the myocardium *and* the conducting tissue. Moreover,
(v)   there are unwanted, and sometimes troublesome side-effects. Although the particular side-effect depends upon which particular first generation calcium antagonist is being used, the side-effects can be subdivided into two main groups:
(a) secondary, reflex-induced changes – such as reflex tachycardia triggered by the initial vasodilator response to nifedipine, and
(b) trivial, but nevertheless annoying side-effects, including facial flushing, ankle oedema, headaches, dizziness and constipation.

The development of the *second generation calcium antagonists* resulted from the recognition of these limitations which, at the time, seemed to be inherent in the prototypes. In addition, more potent compounds were deemed to be desirable, as were compounds which would easily cross the blood brain barrier. To achieve these aims several different approaches were used. They included (Fig. 1.2):

(i)   the development of potent, tissue specific drugs – for example, nisoldipine (Table 1.1);

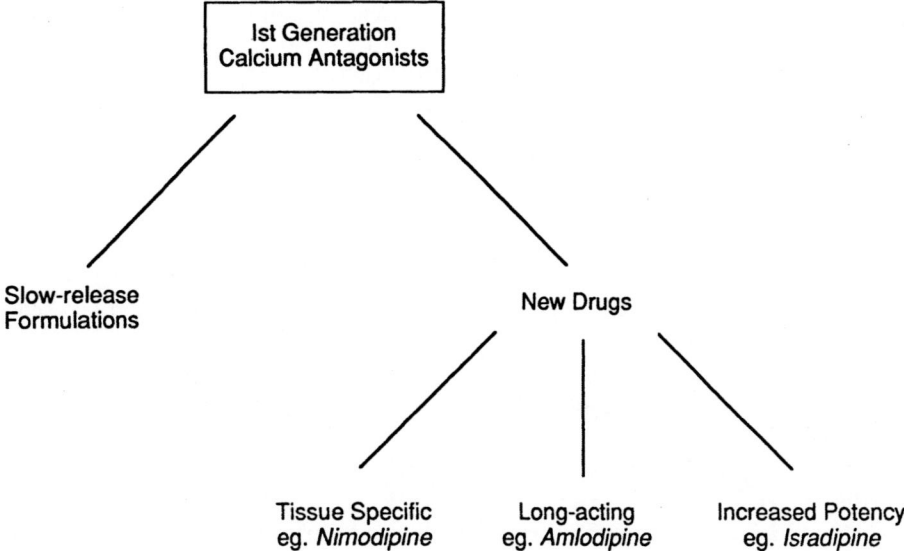

Fig. 1.2. Schematic representation of the evolution of the second generation calcium antagonists

Table 1.1. First and second generation calcium antagonists

Type	Compound
First Generation	Verapamil, nifedipine, diltiazem
Second Generation	
(a) New compounds*	
(i) Tissue specific	Nisoldipine, nimodipine, nitrendipine, isradipine, felodipine, amlodipine, nilvadipine, nicardipine
(ii) Long-acting	Amlodipine, nisoldipine, felodipine, anipamil
(b) New formulations of prototypes	GITS – nifedipine Slow-release (SR) verapamil
(c) Novel compounds*	HOE 166 Fluspirilene (S)-emopamil

This table only contains examples of the calcium antagonists which belong to the various categories. Other examples are given in the next chapter, Chapter 2
* The chemical structure of these and other new compounds are given in the next chapter (Chapter 2)

(ii) the development of longer-acting drugs – for example, amlodipine, isradipine and nisoldipine (Tables 1.1 and 1.2);

(iii) the development of slow release formulations for the prototype drugs – including, the GITS (gastrointestinal therapeutic system) formulation of

Table 1.2. Half-life of some of the second generation calcium antagonists

Drug	T 1/2 (hours)
Amlodipine	35–40
Felodipine	10
Isradipine	8
Nisoldipine	8–11
Nitrendipine	12

T 1/2 refers to the plasma half-life of these second generation calcium antagonists in patients with normal kidney and liver function

    nifedipine and the slow release (SR) formulations of verapamil and felodipine, and

(iv) the development of new compounds, which although chemically unrelated to the prototypes, nevertheless satisfy the criteria for inclusion as calcium antagonists. The compounds HOE 166 and fluspirilene (Glossmann and Striessnig 1990, and Chapter 2) provide examples. Some of these new compounds (e.g. the verapamil-derivative (S)-emopamil) have additional properties such as blockade of the 5-hydroxytryptamine (5-H_2) receptors – at the same concentration as is needed to produce Ca^{2+} channel blockade. In the case of (S)-emopamil this additional property, together with its ability to cross the blood-brain barrier, makes the drug useful in the management of vessel spasm – including cerebral spasm (Defeudis 1989). The possession of additional properties at a therapeutically relevant dose level is not peculiar to the verapamil "daughters" – some of the new dihydropyridine derivatives, for example, also inhibit platelet aggregation (Triggle 1990a).

At the outset, therefore, the rationale which has resulted in the development of the second generation calcium antagonists has been complex and *concept- rather than time*-dependent. For this reason the development of the various slow-release formulations of the existing prototype drugs places these formulations in the second generation category.

Are the Second Generation Calcium Antagonists Needed?

There are several basic reasons why these new drugs (or formulations) are needed. They include:

A. Prolonged Duration of Action: a Prerequisite for Prophylactic Therapy

The need for new long-acting, or slow-release formulations of the existing calcium antagonists was recognized once it was appreciated that these drugs are usually best used prophylactically and, more often than not, on a long term basis.

The problem of developing long-acting calcium antagonists has been approached in two ways:
(i)   the development of new long-acting drugs, and
(ii) the development of slow-release formulations of the prototypes.

Amlodipine (Chapter 2), which owes its long duration action to its slow dissociation from its receptor (Nayler and Gu 1991), fits the first category; the newer formulations of nifedipine (GITS formulation) and verapamil (SR verapamil) belong to the second.

B. Attenuation of Side Effects

The development of the second generation antagonists has provided a secondary benefit, and one which may not have been anticipated. This is because they provide steady plasma levels (Opie 1990) without the peaks and troughs which plagued their forerunners, and presumably because of this the incidence of side-effects has declined dramatically. It is not too difficult to see why this might happen, because many of the side-effects were triggered by the transient but relatively high peak plasma levels that occurred soon after the administration of the standard formulations of the prototypes. Hence, not only has the availability of the second generation calcium antagonists made tissue-selective, prophylactic therapy on a once-a-day basis possible – it has also largely removed the problem of side-effects.

C. Tissue Specificity

The advantages of the second generation calcium antagonists are not limited either to their prolonged duration of action or the abolition or attenuation of their side-effects. The development of tissue specific drugs has represented a major advance, since it means that a particular vascular bed, or organ, can now be targeted. The dihydropyridine derivative, *nimodipine* (Towart 1981) provides a typical example of this development. This particular calcium antagonist is relatively selective for the cerebral vasculature, and readily penetrates the blood brain barrier (Chapter 14). Accordingly it can be used in the management of cerebral ischaemia (Gelmers and Hennerici 1990), without precipitating a marked drop in peripheral vascular resistance, or reflex tachycardia (Gelmers et al. 1988), or negative inotropy.
     Considering all the attempts that have been made to produce tissue specific calcium antagonists three general points emerge:
(i)   the dihydropyridine-based prototype of the first generation calcium antagonists, nifedipine, has more often than not provided the starting point for the second generation compounds;
(ii) tissue specificity has become increasingly targeted – usually in an attempt to provide *vascular selectivity* and thereby reduce the likelihood of unwanted

negative inotropism, or slowed atrio-ventricular conduction, or reflex tachy-cardia.

(iii) As a further, and understandably valuable refinement, specificity within the vasculature has become an identifiable goal. Nimodipine has already been mentioned as belonging to this latter group, because it is relatively selective for the cerebral vasculature (Triggle 1990a; 1990b). Nisoldipine, which is relatively selective for the coronary vasculature, provides another example, and of course there are others.

In many ways increased tissue specificity and a prolonged duration of action were necessary developments in the calcium antagonist field, if the drugs were to achieve their full potential. For example, in the management of patients with hypertrophic cardiomyopathy, the beneficial effect of one of the first generation of antagonists – namely, nifedipine, reflects its efficacy as an arterial vasodilator. However, to achieve the required degree of sustained vasodilation, repetitive dosing throughout the day is required, and such a regime carries with it the risk of producing large swings in blood levels – and indeed, of reaching peak levels of sufficient magnitude as to induce a negative inotropic responses with consequent, but unwanted, reductions in the ejection fraction (Betocchi et al. 1988). Obviously the availability of vascular-specific, long-acting second generation calcium antagonists will remove many of these difficulties.

D. Potency

Improved tissue selectivity, prolonged duration of action and the attenuation of side effects are three of the four properties which distinguish the first and second generation calcium antagonists. The fourth is associated with the enhanced potency which many of these drugs display. For example, isradipine, which, as Figure 1.3 shows, is a dihydropyridine derivative, is considerably more potent than its prototype (Parker et al. 1988). Similarly anipamil (Fig. 1.4) is more potent than its prototype, verapamil (Raschack 1984).

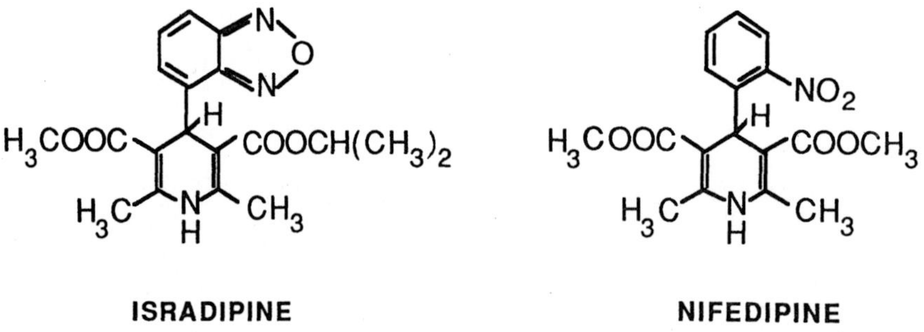

ISRADIPINE   **NIFEDIPINE**

Fig. 1.3. The chemical formula of isradipine, a second generation, dihydropyridine-based calcium antagonist. Note the chemical similarity with nifedipine, a first generation antagonist

Verapamil

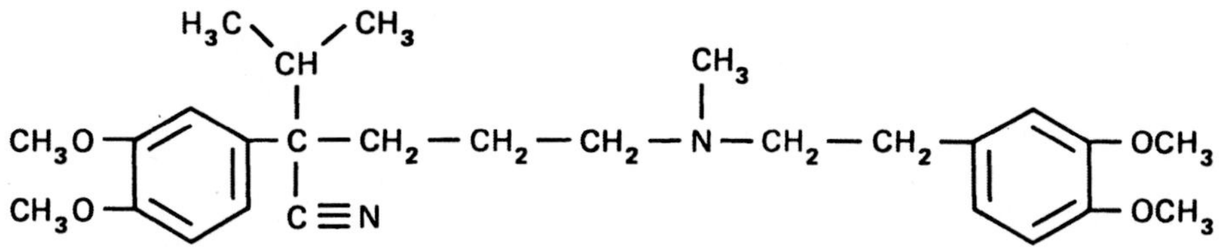

Anipamil

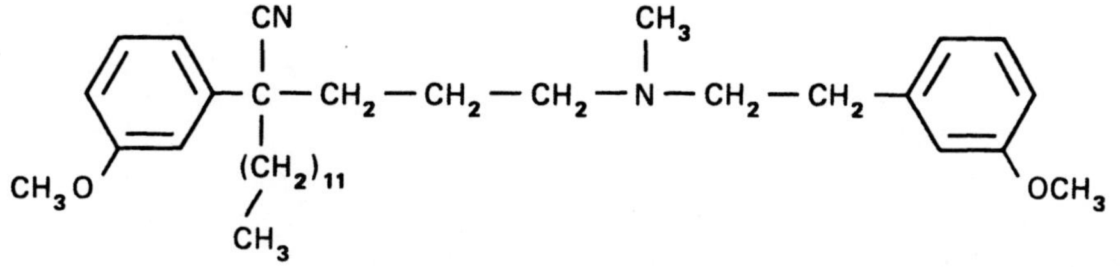

Fig. 1.4. The chemical formula of anipamil, a second generation, phenylalkylamine-based calcium antagonist. Note the chemical similarity with its prototype – verapamil

The following chapters provide a brief account of the chemistry and properties of these second generation antagonists (Chapter 2), an up-to-date account of the molecular biology of the Ca^{2+}-selective channels on which they act, and discussions relating to their clinical efficacy. It will be assumed at the outset that the readers of this book are already familiar with the essential role of Ca^{2+} in excitation-contraction coupling, and with the general mode of action of the calcium antagonists – including their relative selectivity for the L-type Ca^{2+} channels (Nayler 1988). Indeed, it would be almost impossible for clinicians of the nineteen nineties to have escaped having some contact with these drugs – even if that contact has been limited to recommending their use in others!

In Summary

1. The second generation of calcium antagonists were introduced to provide drugs with:
   (i)   a prolonged duration of action.
   (ii) increased tissue selectivity, and
   (iii) increased potency, relative to the first generation, or prototype, drugs.
2. The benefits include:
   (i)   the effective targeting of specific organs and vascular beds;
   (ii) the feasibility of prophylactic therapy;
   (iii) the attenuation of many of the side-effects encountered during the administration of the first generation of antagonists, and

(iv) the introduction of new therapeutically useful calcium antagonists with ancilliary but relevant properties including, in some cases, an antiplatelet aggregating activity and 5-hydroxytryptamine antagonism.

3. The currently available second generation antagonists include:
   (i)   derivatives of the prototype drugs;
   (ii) new, long-acting formulations of the prototypes, and
   (iii) novel drugs, chemically unrelated to the prototypes.

Chapter 2

The Chemistry of the Second Generation Calcium Antagonists

> *"Look back, and smile at perils past."*
> Sir WALTER SCOTT, in the introduction
> to "The Bridal of Triermain".

As discussed in the preceding chapter (Chapter 1), the search for *"second generation"* calcium antagonists began almost as soon as clinicians began using the prototypes, and realized that their therapeutic usefulness was limited by their short duration of action, limited tissue specificity, and unwanted side-effects. From the outset two different approaches were adopted in the search – one aimed at developing new and improved formulations of the prototypes (viz: the controlled release formulation of verapamil (Harder et al. 1991) and the GITS formulation of nifedipine), and the other concentrating on the search for novel compounds with potent calcium antagonist activity. Some of these compounds were derived from the prototypes; others have an entirely different chemistry. Irrespective of which avenue of research was pursued, however, the objective was the same – to develop potent drugs with fewer side effects, a longer duration of action and improved tissue specificity.

This chapter is not intended to provide a detailed account of all of the calcium antagonists which have been developed, or recognized, since the prototypes were invented. Instead it is only intended to provide an account of the chemistry and general properties of some of the more recently discovered antagonists – particularly those which are either more potent, have a longer duration of action, enhanced tissue specificity or an entirely novel chemistry! These compounds will be dealt with in the following order:

(i) derivatives of the prototypes;

(ii) novel compounds, and

(iii) calcium antagonists with additional receptor blocking activity which is expressed over the same dose range as that needed for the expression of the calcium antagonist activity.

Before describing these compounds, however, it may be useful to consider why these drugs are needed at all? There are two answers to this apparently trivial question. Firstly, these drugs, including some of the newer generation, are now being used in the management of a wide range of disorders – including angina (exertional, vasospastic and variant), paroxysmal supraventricular tachyarrhythmias, atrial flutter and fibrillation, hypertension, Raynaud's disease, cerebral vasospasm, myocardial infarction, cardiomyopathies, and adriamycin-induced toxicity and atherosclerosis, *to mention just a few*. Other uses are listed in Table 2.1. Secondly,

Table 2.1. Clinical uses of first and second generation calcium antagonists (after Triggle 1990)

Cardiovascular	Atherosclerosis
	Cerebral ischaemia
	Congestive heart failure
	Hypertrophic cardiomyopathy
	Myocardial infarction
	Peripheral vascular disease
	Hypertension
	Supraventricular tachyarrhythmias
Non-vascular smooth muscle	Achalasia
	Dysmenorrhea
	Eclampsia
	Oesophagial spasm
	Intestinal hypermotility
	Obstructive lung disease
	Premature labour
	Urinary incontinence
Others	Cancer chemotherapy
	Motion sickness
	Epilepsy
	Manic syndrome
	Vertigo
	Tourette's disorder

they are powerful investigative tools – particularly with respect to experiments which are aimed at elucidating the physiological significance of the voltage sensitive Ca^{2+} channels.

The Ca^{2+} channels can be subdivided into two main classes:

(i)   voltage-sensitive channels which are regulated by changes in the transmembrane potential, and

(ii)   receptor-operated channels, which are under ligand control.

The calcium antagonists which are being described here act only on one specific type of voltage-sensitive Ca^{2+} channel – the L-type channel. There are at least two other types of voltage-sensitive Ca^{2+} channels – the T-channels and the N-channels (Bean 1989). As Table 2.2 shows, the L-type Ca^{2+} channel is a large conductance, slowly activating channel – properties which are consistent with its role in excitation-contraction coupling (Triggle 1990b). The transient, small conductance T-channels probably contribute to pacemaker activity, whilst the third type, the N-channels, are primarily confined to neurones.

Associated with the L-class of voltage-dependent channels are the sites at which the three prototype calcium antagonists interact. As described in detail in the next chapter (Chapter 3), these sites are located on a major subunit of the channel, the alpha$_1$ subunit (Triggle et al. 1989 and Chapter 3), which apparently codes for the major properties of the channel – including its electrophysiologic and pharmacological properties (Perez-Reyes et al. 1989).

Table 2.2. Characteristics of voltage-dependent calcium channels

Characteristics	Channel type		
	L	T	N
Conductance (p5)	25	8	12–20
Activator threshold	High	Low	High
Inactivation rate	Slow	Fast	Moderate

Sensitive to
   phenylalkylamines
   benzothiazepines
   dihydropyridines
	Sensitive	Insensitive	Insensitive

The function of the L-type Ca^{2+} channels is to admit Ca^{2+} in a controlled manner for excitation-contraction coupling in cardiac and smooth muscle cells, and for excitation-secretion coupling in some endocrine cells

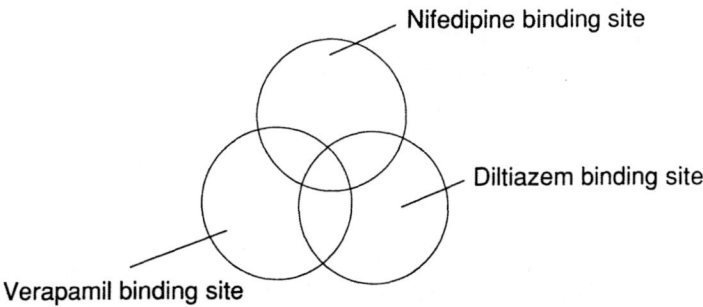

Fig. 2.1. Schematic representation of the binding sites for the three prototype calcium antagonists, derived from phenylalkylamines, benzothiazepines and dihydropyridines. In actual fact it is now reasonably certain that there are other binding sites associated with the L-type Ca^{2+} channel orifice.

Most schematic representations of this subunit depict three binding sites (Fig. 2.1) but as new structural classes of drugs appear it is becoming apparent that this is an oversimplification. Probably there are additional sites of drug interaction, some of which may not even be located on the alpha$_1$ subunit of the channel complex. For example, pimozide (Fig. 2.2) is structurally unrelated to any of the prototype calcium antagonists, but it interacts with a 1:1 stoichiometry with the 1,4 dihydropyridine, benzothiazepine and phenylalkylamine sites – albeit weakly. As Triggle (1990a; 1990b) has suggested, this drug probably also interacts with a fourth but as yet unidentified binding site. There are many other examples of drugs which exhibit the characteristics of L-type Ca^{2+} channel antagonists and yet apparently fail to interact with the three "classical" binding sites on the alpha$_1$ subunit of the channel. HOE 166 (Grassegger et al. 1989) (Fig. 2.2) is another such example. Obviously much remains to be learned about the specific binding sites for the

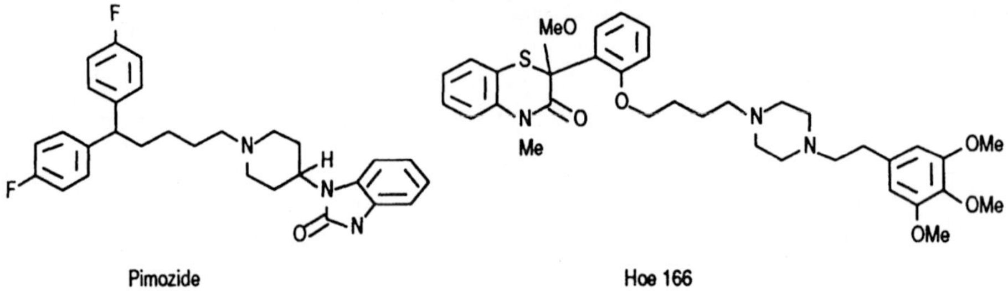

Fig. 2.2. Structural formulae of pimozide and HOE 166 – calcium antagonists which are structurally different from the classical prototypes. Me = CH$_3$

inhibitors of the voltage-sensitive L-type Ca^{2+} channels but as a general rule, the calcium antagonists which are currently in use clinically bind to specific sites associated with the channel.

Derivatives of the Prototype Calcium Antagonists Which Interact with the Alpha$_1$ Subunit Binding Sites of the L-type Ca^{2+} Channels

The Phenylalkylamines

(Prototype, verapamil, 7 – cyano – 1, 7 – bis (3, 4 – dimethoxyphenyl) – 3, 8 – dimethyl – 3 – azanonane).

Second generation members of this group include (Table 2.3) gallopamil (D600), anipamil (Fig. 2.3), falipamil (Fig. 2.4), RO-5967 (Fig. 2.5) and tiapamil. Tiapamil lacks tissue selectivity, is approximately ten times *less* potent than verapamil and therefore need not be mentioned here again. The remaining drugs – gallopamil, anipamil, falipamil and RO-5967 all interact with the verapamil (phenylalkylamine) binding site in the α_1 subunit of the Ca^{2+} channel complex (Chapter 3) but there are interesting and potentially useful differences between them. For example anipamil has a longer duration of action, and is more potent than verapamil, but like verapamil it is equiselective for heart and blood vessels (Table 2.4). Falipamil, however, has an entirely different pharmacological profile in that it "targets" the sinoatrial node – where it slows the rate of depolarization, thereby prolonging the duration of the action potential of the sinoatrial cells (Naudascher et al. 1989). The end-result is a reduction in the I$_f$ component of the pacemaker current – a property which allows this drug to reduce exercise-induced tachycardia without altering blood pressure. Here, then is evidence of tissue selectivity within the drugs which interact with the phenylalkylamine (verapamil) binding sites.

Falipamil is not the only member of this group to exhibit tissue specificity. RO-5967 (Clozel et al. 1989) also interacts with the verapamil binding site but in contrast to verapamil it is only weakly negatively inotropic (Osterrieder and Holck 1989). Instead, it targets the coronary vasculature (Clozel et al. 1989). Some idea of the specificity of this effect can be gained by considering the concentrations of the drug

Table 2.3. Second generation phenylalkylamine-based calcium antagonists

Prototype	Chemistry
dl Verapamil	f- cyano – 1, 7 – bs (3, 4 – dimethoxyphenyl) – 3, 8 – dimethyl – 3 – azanonane
2nd Generation	
Gallopamil (D 600)	f- cyano – 1 – (3, 4 dimethoxyphenyl) – 7 – (3, 4, 5 – trimethoxyphenyl) – 3 – 8 – dimethyl – 3 – azanonane
Anipamil	f – cyano – 1 – 7 – bis (m – methoxyphenyl) – 3 – methyl – 3 – azanonadecane
Falipamil (AQ-A39)	5, 6 – dimethoxy – 2 – (3- [3, 4 – dimethoxy) phenylethyl) methyl-amino propyl) phthalimidine
RO-5967	(1S, 2S) – 2 – [2 – [[3 – (2 – benzimidazolyl) propyl] methylamino] ethyl] – 6 – fluoro – 1, 2, 3, 4 – tetrahydro – 1 – isopropyl – 2 – naphthyl methoxyacetate
Tiapamil (RO 11-1781)	2 – (3, 4 – dimethoxyphenyl) – 2 – [6 – (3, 4 – dimethoxyphenyl) – 4 – methyl – 4 – azahexyl] – 1, 3, dithiane – 1, 1, 3, 3, tetraoxide

These drugs all interact with the verapamil binding site in the Ca^{2+} channel complex. They are all calcium antagonists – as gauged by their ability to inhibit the slow inward Ca^{2+} current associated with L-type channel activation

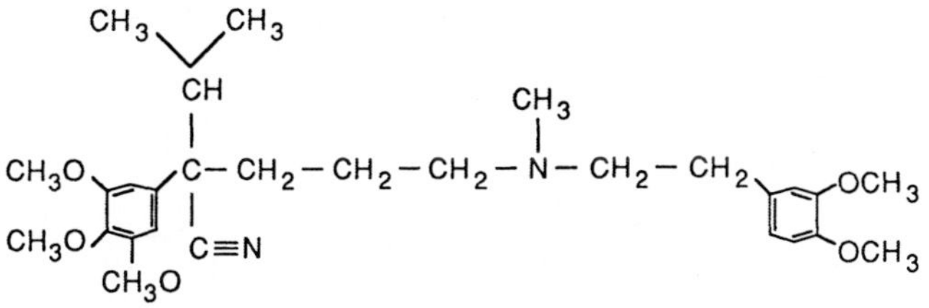

GALLOPAMIL (D600)

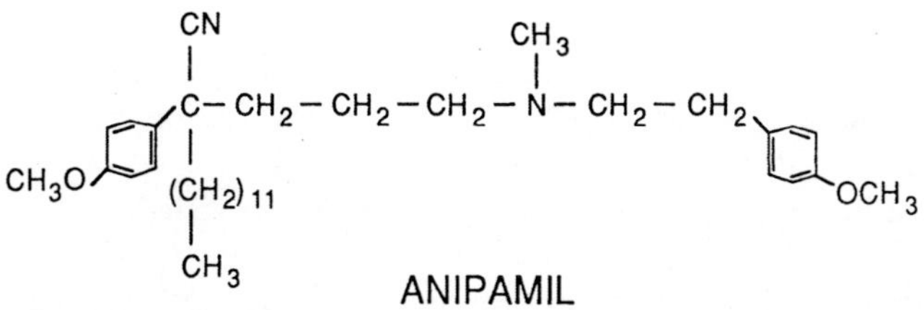

ANIPAMIL

Fig. 2.3. Structural formulae of the second generation phenylalkylamine-based calcium antagonists – gallopamil and anipamil. Gallopamil (D600) is in clinical use

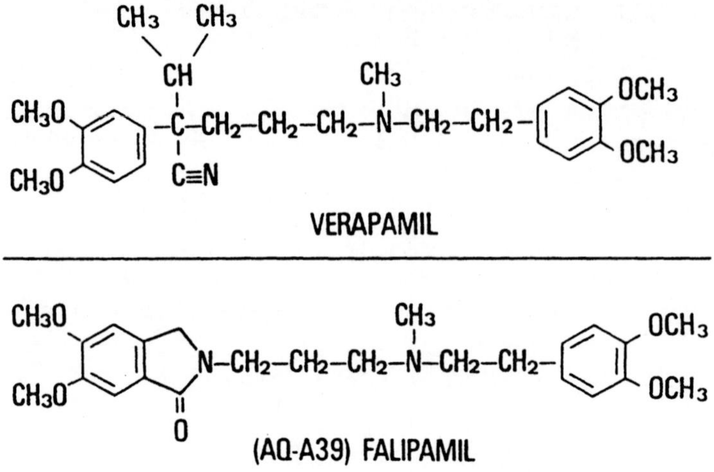

VERAPAMIL

(AQ-A39) FALIPAMIL

Fig. 2.4. Structural formula of falipamil, a second generation phenylalkylamine-based calcium antagonist

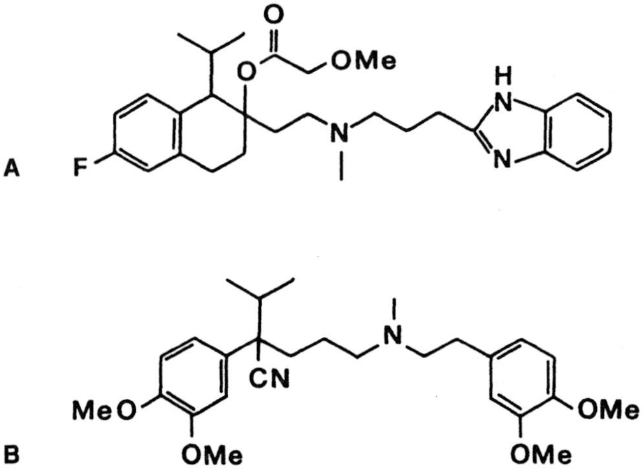

Fig. 2.5. Structure of RO-5967 (A), and verapamil (B)

needed to produce a fifty percent increase in coronary blood flow (EC_{50}), a fifty percent decrease in contractile force (IC_{50}) and a fifty percent reduction in vascular resistance (IC_{50}). These values are listed in Table 2.5 and clearly show the relative selectivity of this calcium antagonist for the coronary vasculature. There is another important difference between verapamil, the prototype, and RO-5967: it concerns its inhibitory effect on gastrointestinal smooth muscle where the effect of verapamil > RO-5967 (Osterrieder and Holck 1989). This

Table 2.4. Relative selectivity of the second generation calcium antagonists which interact with the verapamil binding sites

Calcium antagonist	Tissue			
	Myocardium	Peripheral Vasculature	Coronary Vasculature	Sinoatrial Nodal Tissue/ Atrio-ventricular Conduction
Verapamil	+++	++	++	+++
Gallopamil	+++	++	++	+++
Anipamil	+++	++	++	−
Falipamil	++	++	++	+++++ (sinoatrial)
RO-5967	+	++	+++++++	?

Gallopamil and anipamil are more potent than verapamil. + denotes extent of effect on tissue function

Table 2.5. Relative selectivity of the calcium antagonist RO-5967 for the coronary vasculature

Parameter	nM
Increase in coronary artery blood flow (50%)	$IC_{50} = 54$
Suppression of myocardial contractility (50%)	$IC_{50} = 14000$
Inhibition of aortic constriction (50%)	$IC_{50} = 275$

In terms of tissue selectivity, this means coronary arteries > peripheral vasculature > myocardium. RO-5967 interacts with the verapamil binding site. (Data from Osterrieder and Holck 1989)

may be of importance, because one of the troublesome and persistent side effects of verapamil is constipation.

Falipamil and RO-5967 provide examples of *tissue selectivity* within the second generation of calcium antagonists which bind to the verapamil-phenylalkylamine recognition site on the alpha$_1$ subunit of the channel complex. Gallopamil and anipamil, on the other hand, provide evidence of increased potency (anipamil gallopamil > verapamil), and a longer duration of action (anipamil > verapamil) (Dillon and Nayler 1988). There are other potentially important differences between anipamil and verapamil – as evidenced by the relatively lack of effect of anipamil on atrioventricular conduction.

In general therefore, the "second generation" calcium antagonists which interact with the verapamil binding sites in the L-type Ca^{2+} channel complex show evidence of tissue specificity (Table 2.5), enhanced potency and, in the case of anipamil, a prolonged duration of action, relative to the prototype. It is too early as yet to know whether these "improvements" will enhance the clinical usefulness of this subset of Ca^{2+}-channel antagonists beyond that which is already provided by the slow-release formulation of the prototype. However the relative specificity of RO-5967 for the coronary vasculature, and the specificity of falipamil for sinoatrial nodal tissue provides some interesting alternatives.

The Benzothiazepines

Here the prototype is diltiazem (3 – acetoxy – 2, 3 – dihydro – 5 – (2 – dimethylaminoethyl)– 2 – (p– methoxyphenyl) benzo [b] – (5H) – 1, 5 – thiazepine – 4 – one). As with verapamil, diltiazem lacks vascular selectivity but it is a potent coronary dilator.

"Second generation" benzothiazepine-based calcium antagonists include *KT-362* (Farber and Gross 1989). KT-362 has the following formula: (5– [3– [[2 – 3, 4 – dimethoxyhenyl) – ethyl] amino] – 1 – oxopropyl] – 2, 3, 4, 5, tetrahydro 1, 5 benzothiazepine fumarate). Despite structural similarities between the prototype diltiazem and the "second-generation" KT-362, they have dissimilar modes of action, diltiazem acting as a classical L-type Ca^{2+} channel antagonist, whilst KT-362 acts *intracellularly* – inhibiting intracellular Ca^{2+} release in vascular smooth muscle cells (Eskinder et al. 1989). Unlike diltiazem, KT-362 has only a minimal effect on the coronary circulation. However it may be clinically useful because it decreases heart rate, reduces arterial pressure but *improves collateral* circulation after an acute ischaemic event (Farber and Gross 1989). KT-362, therefore, provides an example of a "second generation" calcium antagonist which closely resembles its prototype as far as its structure is concerned, but which exhibits an entirely different pharmacological profile.

Clentiazem (TA-3090) (+) – (2S – 3S) – 3 acetoxy – 8 – chloro – 5 – (2 – dimethylamino) ethyl) – 2, 3 – dihydro – 2 – (4 – meth – oxyphenyl) – 1, 5 benzothiazepine– 4– (5H) – one maleate (Fig. 2.6) is another "second generation" benzothiazepine derivative (Suzuki et al. 1991). It binds to the classical diltiazem recognition site on the alpha$_1$ subunit but with a greater affinity than its prototype (Suzuki et al. 1991), a property which may explain why it is approximately four times more potent than its prototype (Murata et al. 1988).

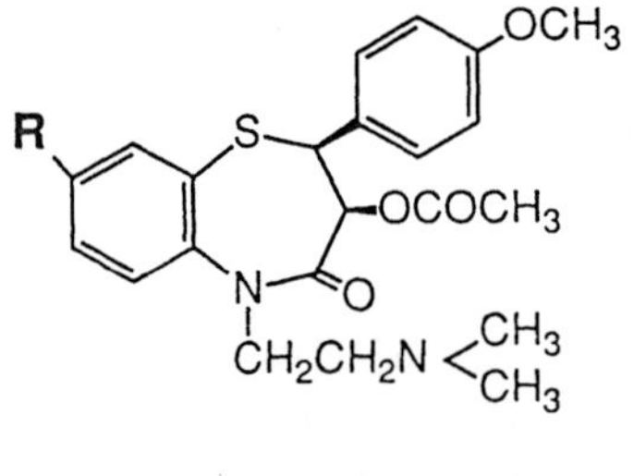

	R	Salt
Clentiazem	Cl	Maleate
Diltiazem	H	HCl

Fig. 2.6. Structure of clentiazem – a "new" calcium antagonist

Hence, as far as the "second generation" diltiazem-type calcium antagonists are concerned, they provide examples of altered tissue specificity, and improved potency.

Table 2.6. Second generation dihydropyridine-based calcium antagonists

Prototype	Chemistry
Nifedipine	1, 4 – dihydro – 2, 6 – dimethyl – 4 (0 – nitrophenyl) pyridine – 3, 5 – dicarboxylic acid dimethyl ester
2nd Generation	
Amlodipine*	2 – (2 – aminoethoxymethyl) – 4 – (0 – chlorophenyl) – 1, 4 – dihydro – 6 – methylpyridine – 3, 5 – dicarboxylic acid 3 – ethyl, 5 – methyl ester maleate
Felodipine*	4 – (2, 3 – dichlorophenyl) – 1, 4 – dihydro – 2, 6 – dimethylpyridine – 3, 5 – dicarboxylic acid 3 – ethyl, 5 – methyl ester
Isradipine*	4 – (benzo – z – oxa – 1, 3 – diazol – 4 – dihydro – 2, 6 – dimethylpyridine – 3, 5 – dicarboxylic acid 3 – isopropyl, 5, methyl ester
Nisoldipine*	1, 4 – dihydro – 2, 6 – dimethyl – 4 – (2 – nitrophenylpyridine) – 3, 5 – dicarboxylic acid diester
Nitrendipine*	1, 4 – dihydro – 2, 6 – dimethyl – 4 – (3 – nitrophenylpyridine –) 3, 5 – dicarboxylic acid 3 – ethyl, 5 – methyl ester
Nimodipine*	1, 4 – dihydro – 2, 6 – dimethyl – 4 – (m – nitrophenyl) pyridine – 3, 5 – dicarboxylic acid 3 – isopropyl, 5 – (2 – methoxyethyl ester)
Nigludipine	1, 4 – dihydro – 2, 6 – dimethyl – 4 – (m – nitrophenyl) pyridine – 3, 5 – dicarboxylic acid 3 – methyl 5 – [3 – 4, 4 – diphenyl – 1 – piperidinyl) propyl] ester
Niludipine	1, 4, dihydro – 2, 6 – dimethyl – 4 – (m – nitrophenyl) pyridine – 3, 5 – dicarboxylic acid bis (2 – propoxyethyl ester)
CD 349	2 – nitratopropyl 3 – nitratopropyl 2, 6 – dimethyl – 4 – (3 – nitrophenyl) – 1, 4 – dihydropyridine – 3, 5 – dicarboxylic acid
Mepirodipine	3 (S) 1 – benzyl – 3 – pyrrolidinyl methyl (4S) – 2, 6 – dimethyl – 4 – (m – nitrophenyl – 1, 4 – dihydropyridine – 3, 5 – dicarboxylate
MDL 72567	5 – (2 – furol) – 1, 4, dihydro – 2, 6 – dimethyl – 4 – (0 – nitrophenyl) pyridine – 3 – carboxylic acid methyl ester
8663S	3 – cyclopentyl – 4, 7 – dihydro – 1, 6 – dimethyl – 4 – (m – nitrophenyl) pyrazolol [3, 4 – b) pyridine – 5 – carboxylic acid methyl ester
Manidipine (CV-4093)	2 – [4 – (diphenyl methyl) – 1 – piperazinyl] ethyl methyl (±) – 1, 4 – dihydro – 2, 6 – dimethyl – 4 – (m – nitrophenyl) – 3, 5 – pyridine dicarboxylate dihydrochloride

This list does not cover all of the nifedipine-derivatives, but it gives some idea of the numerous *modifications which have been made*. * denotes compounds which are already in clinical use

The Dihydropyridines

Here the prototype calcium antagonist is nifedipine (1, 4 – dihydro – 2, 6 – dimethyl – 4 – (δ – nitrophenyl) pyridine – 3, 5 – dicarboxylic acid dimethyl ester). There are more derivatives of this particular prototype than there are of all the others put together. The derivatives include nisoldipine, nimodipine, nitrendipine, nicardipine, amlodipine, felodipine, isradipine, nilvadipine, nigludipine, niludipine, mepirodine, mandipine, CD-349 and many others (Table 2.6). As a general rule these drugs are vascular selective but there are some interesting differences between them – including differences between those which have already been introduced into clinical usage (marked with an asterisk in Table 2.6). For example, amlodipine is a long-acting calcium antagonist. This is due to two factors:

(i)   it has a long plasma half-life (36 hours) (Elliot et al. 1988), and
(ii)   it only slowly dissociates from its receptor (Nayler and Gu 1991).

Amlodipine (Fig. 2.7) also only slowly associates with its receptor, taking several hours to reach asymptote (Nayler and Gu 1991). This may explain why it is relatively free from side effects, because there will be ample time for the baroreceptors to reset.

Nisoldipine (Fig. 2.8) and nimodipine (Fig. 2.9) are also vascular selective but with a difference: nisoldipine specifically targets the coronary vasculature whereas nimodipine preferentially targets the cerebral circulation.

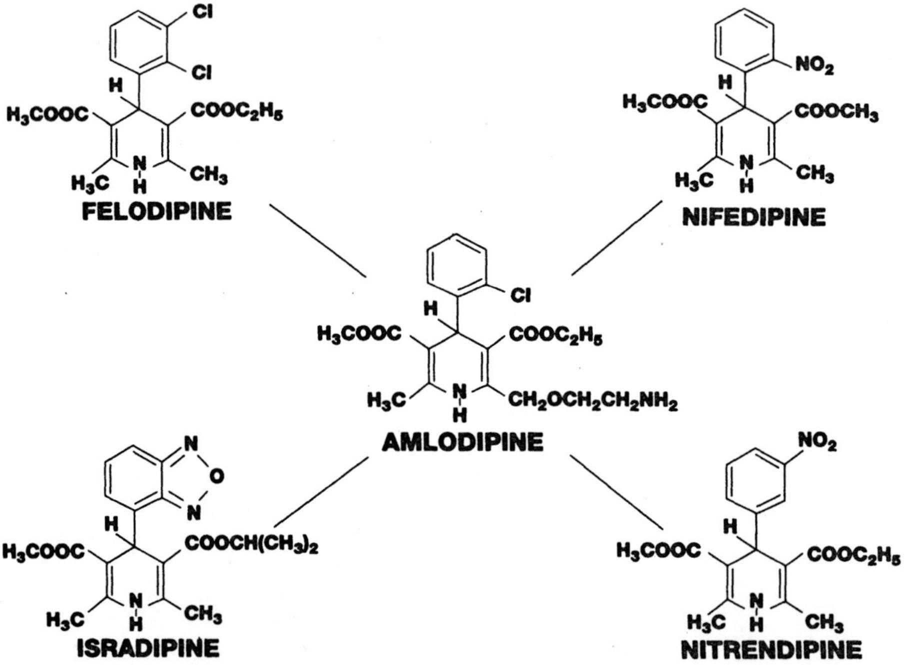

Fig. 2.7. The structure of some "second generation" calcium antagonists and their prototype, nifedipine. Amlodipine is a particularly long acting antagonist, isradipine is highly potent and vascular selective, and felodipine is markedly vasoselective

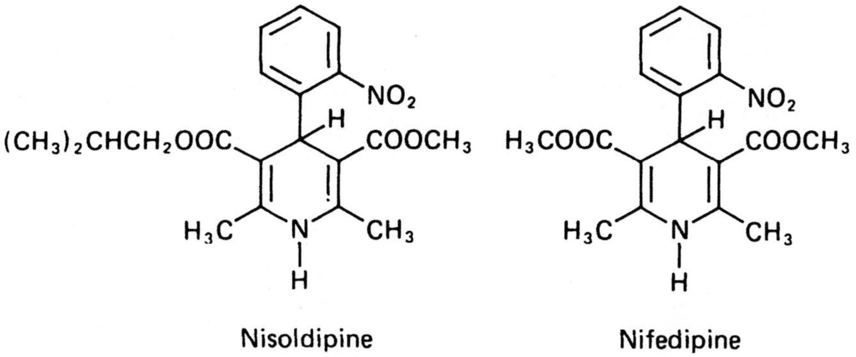

Nisoldipine   Nifedipine

Fig. 2.8. The structure of the "second generation" dihydropyridine-based calcium antagonist, nisoldipine, which is selective for the coronary vasculature

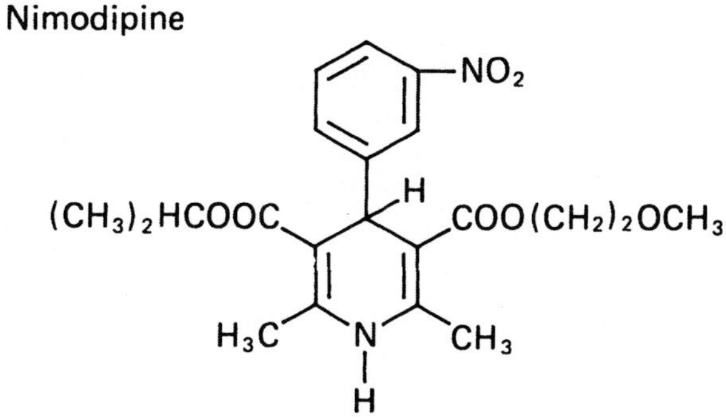

Nimodipine

Fig. 2.9. The second generation dihydropyridine-based calcium antagonist, nimodipine, which is relatively selective for the cerebral circulation

Hence as far as the dihydropyridine-based calcium antagonists are concerned the second generation drugs resemble their prototype in chemical structure, but they are more *vascular* selective, and sometimes, more potent. Furthermore, within the vasculature, some of them target specific vascular beds – an effect which is readily translatable into clinical usage (Table 2.7).

There are many other examples of new dihydropyridine derivatives. One is isradipine (Table 2.6). This is a vascular selective antagonist, but it is far more potent than its prototype (Hof 1987).

Other New Calcium Antagonists

So far mention only has been made of "second generation" members of the phenylalkylamine, benzothiazepine and dihydropyridine-based calcium antagonists. There are, however, many other compounds which might be regarded as being of the "second generation" – because they are either tissue selective or of high potency. For example:

Table 2.7. Clinical usage of "second generation" dihydropyridine-based calcium antagonists

Compound	Plasma half life	Indication	Peculiar property
Amlodipine	36 hr	Hypertension Angina ? Atherosclerosis	Long-duration of action
Isradipine	8 hr	Hypertension Angina ? Atherosclerosis ? Stroke	High Potency Vascular-selective
Felodipine	8 hr	Hypertension Angina	High vascular selectivity
Nisoldipine	8–12 hr	Hypertension Angina	Vascular selective, particularly coronary vessels
Nitrendipine	8 hr	Hypertension	Doubles digoxin availability
Nicardipine	< 12 hr	Hypertension	Vascular-selective
Nimodipine	5 hr	Cerebral spasm Subarachnoid haemorrhage Stroke	Selective for cerebral vessels

The recommended daily dosages for the management of hypertension are as follows:-
    Amlodipine   2.5–10 mg, *once* daily
    Isradipine   2.5–10 mg, twice daily
    Felodipine   7.5–10 mg, twice daily
    Nitredipine   10–20 mg, once-twice daily
    Nicardipine   20–40 mg, three times daily (Opie 1990)
For cerebral spasm: nimodipine: 30–40 mg, three to four times daily
For angina: nisoldipine: 5–20 mg, twice daily
Amlodipine and nicardipine are *light insensitive*

KB-2796

This is a piperazine derivative and therefore partially resembles cinnarizine and flunarizine. The chemical name of KB-2796 is 1 – [bis (4 – fluorophenyl) methyl] – 4 – (2, 3, 4 – trimethoxybenzyl) piperazine (Kanazawa et al. 1990). As is the case for the prototype of this group (cinnarizine), KB-2796 is vasoselective – but more importantly it selectively increases cerebral blood flow. This means that there are now *at least* four calcium antagonists which can be used to target the cerebral circulation: nimodipine (Gaab et al. 1985); nicardipine – although here the effect is less marked (Takenake and Handa 1979), isradipine and KB-2796. In the case of KB-2796 some idea of the magnitude of this specificity can be gained from the fact that the dose of this drug needed to produce a thirty percent increase in cerebral blood flow is some twenty times greater than the amount needed to produce an equivalent increase in vertebral blood flow (Kanazawa et al. 1990).

Diproteverine

This is another relatively newly developed calcium antagonist (Kantelip et al. 1988). It is 1 (3, 4 – diethoxyphenyl) – methyl – 3, 4 – dihydro – 6, 7 bis (1 methyl ethoxy) – isoquinoline. It has little if any effect on peripheral vascular resistance but causes a dose-related depressant effect on sinus node function and atrioventricular conduction, with the greatest effect being on the sinus node. In some ways the effect of diproteverine on sinus node function resembles that of diltiazem – but the peripheral vasodilation of diltiazem is missing.

SD-3211

[(+) (–R) – 3, 4 – dihydro – 2 – [5 – methoxy – 2 – [3 [N – methyl – N – [2 – [(3, 4 – methelene dioxy) phenoxy] ethyl] amino] propoxy] phenyl] – 4 – methyl – 3 – oxo – 2H – 1, 4 benzothiazine] should probably be regarded as a "second generation" diltiazem. However, the effect of this antagonist differs markedly from that of diltiazem, because whereas diltiazem reduces peripheral vascular resistance *and* slows atrioventricular conduction, SD-3211 causes a marked and *sustained* fall in blood *pressure with no* alteration in heart rate (Kageyama et al. 1991). Here then, is an example of a second generation calcium antagonist with increased tissue specificity and a prolonged duration of activity.

As stated at the beginning of this chapter no attempt would be made to list all of the second generation calcium antagonists which have been developed to date. Instead examples have been given to stress the achievements which have been made in the provision of tissue selective, long-acting and highly potent compounds. Probably it is the dihydropyridine group which provide the best examples, because whereas the prototype, nifedipine failed to differentiate between the myocardium and the vasculature, the second generation drugs make this distinction (e.g. nisoldipine and nimodipine) and in some instances (e.g. isradipine) are more potent or (e.g. amlodipine) longer acting, or target a particular vascular bed (e.g. nimodipine). Impressive as these developments might be, they do not exhaust the advances which have been made in this field, because one of the new and quite exciting trends is to develop calcium antagonists which have ancillary receptor blocking activities.

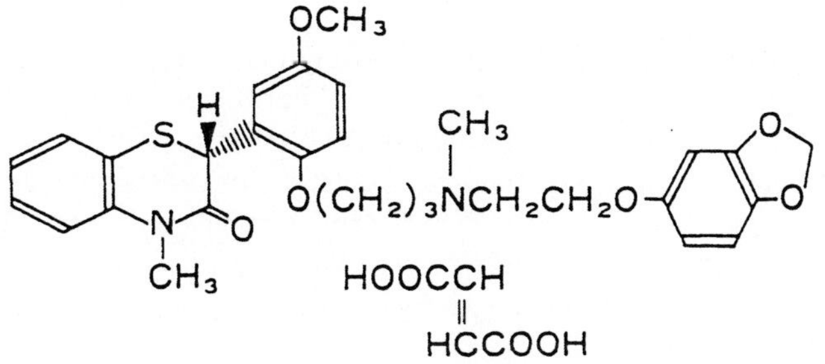

Fig. 2.10. The structural formula of the benzothiazepine second generation derivative, SD-3211

Novel Calcium Antagonists with Additional Antagonist Activity

A relatively new development in the field of calcium antagonism is the deliberate search for compounds which can be used to achieve the simultaneous antagonism of other receptors in addition to the voltage sensitive Ca^{2+} channels, but at the same dose level. Two examples serve to illustrate this trend. The drugs are known as *AHR-16303B* – a joint L-type calcium channel and 5-HT$_2$ receptor antagonist (Barrett et al. 1991a; 1991b), and *naftopidil* – which blocks α_1 adrenoceptors and inhibits Ca^{2+} entry via potential-dependent channels in vascular smooth muscle (Himmel et al. 1991).

AHR-16303B: A Joint 5-HT$_2$ and L- Type Calcium Channel Antagonist

This compound has the following chemical formula: (1 [4 – [3 – [4 – [bis (4 – fluorophenyl) hydroxymethyl] – 1 – piperidinyl] propoxy] phenyl] – 2 – methyl – 1 – propanone ethanedioate (1:1). It produces a concentration-dependent displacement of specifically bound [^{3}H]nimodipine (a vascular selective dihydropyridine-based calcium antagonist), a concentration-dependent inhibition of depolarization-induced influx of calcium into cultured smooth muscle cells and inhibits CaCl$_2$-induced contractions of isolated aortic muscle strips (Barrett et al. 1991a). It therefore *is* a calcium antagonist. Over the same dose range, however, it inhibits 5-hydroxytryptamine-induced vasopressor responses – which makes it a 5H$_2$ receptor antagonist. The logical question to ask is, of course, does this combined receptor antagonism have any possible use, or advantage. With the wealth of evidence which is emerging showing that 5-hydroxytryptamine (serotonin) evokes an exaggerated constrictor response in cerebral and coronary arteries which are either atherosclerotic (Wines et al. 1989; Heistad et al. 1987), have a damaged endothelium or have been subjected to abnormally high perfusion pressures – as in hypertension – (Golino et al. 1989; Lamping and Dole 1987) it seems likely that 5-hydroxytryptamine may be an important mediator of vasospastic or even occlusive events in these blood vessels. Specific antagonism of the 5-hydroxytryptamine receptors, therefore, could easily compliment the antivasospastic and antiatherogenic consequences of calcium channel blockade.

Naftopidil

Naftopidil ((R,S) – 1 – [4 – (2 – methoxyphenyl) – 1 – pi – porazinyl] – 3 – (2 – naphthyloxy) – 2 – propanol) has a pharmacological profile indicative of *combined* α-adrenoceptor and Ca^{2+}-channel blocking activity over the same dose range (Himmel et al. 1991). Evidence of its calcium antagonist activity comes from whole cell patch-clamp studies and from radioligand experiments. Interest in this compound stems, to a large extent, from the idea that combined α-adrenoceptor and Ca^{2+} channel blocking activity could be of use in the management of hypertensive patients.

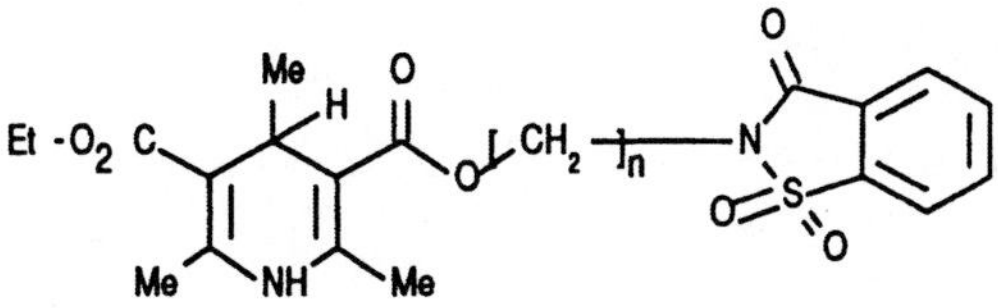

Fig. 2.11. The structural formula of the dihydropyridine-based platelet aggregation inhibitor

There are other examples of drugs which, although developed as potential calcium antagonists in the final analysis have highly significant ancillary properties. One such compound is a nifedipine derivative which lacks the 4-phenyl substituent (Fig. 2.11). This derivative is a potent inhibitor of platelet aggregation at concentrations which seem to have no effect on the cardiovascular system (Sunkel et al. 1988).

In Summary

1. The "second generation" calcium antagonists include:
   (i)   new long-acting formulations of the prototypes;
   (ii) new compounds, some of which are derivatives of the prototypes, and
   (iii) novel compounds, chemically unrelated to the prototypes.
2. The new "second generation" antagonists differ from other prototypes in terms of tissue selectivity, potency and duration of action. For example the duration of action of amlodipine > the prototype, nifedipine; the potency of isradipine > nifedipine, and the selectivity of nisoldipine for the coronary vasculature > the prototype.
3. In addition, there are new compounds, some of which have ancillary receptor blocking activity – for example, some exhibit either α-adrenoceptor or 5-hydroxytryptamine blocking activity at the same dose as that required to achieve Ca^{2+} channel blockade.
4. Some of the differences in tissue selectivity and potency between the second generation calcium antagonists and their prototypes have already found clinical applications.

Appendix to Chapter 2

Table 2.8. Some properties of the second generation calcium antagonists available for clinical use (relative to their prototypes)

Drug	Mol. wt.	Plasma levels (ng/ml) after oral use	% Protein bound
Group 1. Phenylalkylamines			
Prototype			
Verapamil	455.54	80–400	85–90
2nd Generation			
Gallopamil	485.59	25	85–90
Group 2, Dihydropyridines			
Prototype			
Nifedipine	346.75	15–200	95
2nd Generation			
Amlodipine	408.9	2–12	97
Felodipine	384.26	14–115	99
Isradipine	371.4	10	96
Nicardipine	388.42	8–150	99
Nimodipine	418.45	80	95
Nisoldipine	388.42	3–5	99
Nitrendipine	490.55	9–42	98

Chapter 3

The Molecular Biology of the Voltage-Dependent, Calcium Antagonist-Sensitive Calcium Channels

"In this world it is easier for the man who shrinks from being disappointed not to look forward too keenly to moments that promise great pleasure."
"The World of Mr. Mulliner", by P.G. WODEHOUSE, 1935.

Only supreme optimists would be disappointed in the rapidity with which the molecular structure of ion conducting channels (Table 3.1) and some of the ion exchange systems and pumps – for example, the $Na^+ K^+$ ATPase (Shull et al. 1985) and the $Na^+:Ca^{2+}$ exchanger (Nicoll et al. 1990) – have been unravelled. This success is not accidental, and has required the use of increasingly complex techniques – including molecular biology and immunology. The end result, however, is that many of the ion-conducting channels have now been cloned, their aminoacid

Table 3.1. Ion-conducting channels subjected to molecular analysis

Channel type	Reference
Na^+ channels	
Electric eel	Agnew et al. 1978
Electric eel	Noda et al. 1984
Brain	Hartshorne and Catterall 1981
	Noda et al. 1986
Skeletal muscle	Barchi 1983
Cardiac muscle	Lombet and Lazdunski 1984
K^+ channel	
Cardiac muscle	Tseng-Crank et al. 1990
Ca^{2+} channels (Calcium-antagonist sensitive)	
Skeletal muscle	Curtis and Catterall 1984
	Borsotto et al. 1984
	Tanabe et al. 1987
	Leung et al. 1987
	Vaghy et al. 1987a, 1987b
	Nakayama et al. 1987
Cardiac muscle	Cooper at al. 1987
	Mikami et al. 1989
Brain	Curtis and Catterall 1983
	Takahashi and Catterall 1987
Vascular smooth muscle	Koch et al. 1990

sequences determined and in some cases (Yool and Schwartz 1991) their assembly patterns decoded. This chapter is primarily concerned with recent progress which has been made in establishing the molecular structure of the Ca^{2+} channels – or more particularly those voltage-activated Ca^{2+} channels which contain the calcium antagonists binding sites (Striessnig et al. 1990; Vaghy et al. 1987a; 1987b).

Ca^{2+}-Conducting Channels

Ca^{2+}-conducting channels can be divided into two main groups:
(i)   voltage-sensitive channels which permit the influx of extracellular Ca^{2+}, and
(ii) Ca^{2+}-release channels which, depending on the tissue in which they occur, are either voltage- or Ca^{2+}-activated (Chapter 4) but in either case facilitate the exit of intracellularly-stored Ca^{2+} from the sarcoplasmic reticulum to the cytosol.

Only the first of these channel types are relevant to this chapter – and even then it is necessary to be more precise, because not all voltage-activated Ca^{2+} channels are sensitive to the calcium antagonists.

The Voltage-Sensitive Ca^{2+} Channels

Ion-conducting channels which normally admit extracellular Ca^{2+} and which are voltage-sensitive and relatively selective for Ca^{2+} are found in most cells (Bean 1989). By using their biophysical characteristics and pharmacological profiles as a guide, it has been relatively easy to divide these channels into three main categories – designated as L, T and N (Miller 1987). The L-type channels have a large capacitance, a high threshold of activation and *are sensitive to the calcium antagonists* (Table 3.2 and Miller 1987). The N-type channels also have a high threshold of activation but have a lower conductance than the L-channels (Table

Table 3.2. Characteristic properties of the L, N and T-type Ca^{2+} channels

Channel type	L	N	T
Sensitivity to organic calcium antagonists	+	−	−
Channel conductance (picoseimens)	High (25)	Moderate (13)	Low (9)
Activation threshold	Strong depolarization	Strong depolarization	Weak depolarization
Activation voltage	−10 mv	−10 mv	−70 mv

+ denotes the presence, and − the absence of sensitivity to the organic calcium antagonists – such as verapamil, nifedipine or diltiazem

3.2). Moreover, they are *insensitive* to the calcium antagonists, and are predominantly neuronal. The third type of Ca^{2+} channel – the T-channel, activates on weak depolarization, is insensitive to the calcium antagonists and has a lower conductance (Table 3.2) than either the L- or N-type of channel (Hess 1990).

Since this chapter is concerned only with the molecular biology of the calcium antagonist-sensitive Ca^{2+} channels, it follows that it is the L-type Ca^{2+} channel which is most relevant. Within the last few years this channel has been isolated, cloned, it's subunits identified, and its aminoacid composition determined. This is not all – because:

(i)   tissue-specific differences in the composition of some of the subunits have been identified (Koch et al. 1989). This is important, because these differences may contribute to the tissue selectivity displayed by many of the second generation calcium antagonists;

(ii) a dichotomy of function has been recognized for some of the component parts (Tanabe et al. 1987), and

(iii) at least one pathological condition – that of mouse muscular dysgenesis – has been found to involve the absence of one of the major component parts (or subunit as it is usually called) of the channel complex (Beam et al. 1986; Knudson et al. 1989).

Irrespective of where they occur, however, the L-type Ca^{2+} channels are easy to identify, because an integral part of one of their subunits (the α_1 subunit) contains the specific, high affinity binding sites for the calcium antagonists (Curtis and Catterall 1984). Because of this, and because dihydropyridine-based (DHP) calcium antagonists are usually used as markers for these binding sites, the whole channel complex, or sometimes just the α_1 subunit of that complex, is often referred to as "the DHP receptor".

The Molecular Biology of the L-type Ca^{2+} Channel

Given that cardiac and smooth muscle cells are far more sensitive to the calcium antagonists than their skeletal muscle counterparts it might have been assumed that studies on the molecular composition and subunit structure of the Ca^{2+} channel complex and its associated calcium-antagonist binding domains would have started with membranes prepared from either smooth or cardiac muscle cells. This did not happen, however. Instead skeletal muscle membranes were used (Glossmann et al. 1983; Fosset et al. 1983). The reason for this is now abundantly clear, since although excitation-contraction coupling in skeletal muscle is not directly dependent on the transsarcolemmal influx of Ca^{2+}, skeletal muscle myocytes have substantial voltage-activated Ca^{2+}-dependent currents (Sanchez and Stefani 1978). These currents are calcium antagonist-sensitive and originate from the transverse tubular system – that is, from the areas where the sarcolemma invaginates into the cytosol. These transverse tubular membranes (or T-tubules) are continuous with the sarcolemma and at one stage were regarded simply as being pure sarcolemma. *However, antibodies raised against purified skeletal muscle T-tubular membrane*

Table 3.3. Comparison between the cardiac and skeletal muscle calcium antagonist-sensitive calcium channels

Property	Cardiac muscle	Skeletal muscle
Mg^{2+} permeability	−	+
Mean Open Time	Short	Long
Activation kinetics	Fast	Slow
Conductance to 110 Mm Ba^{2+}	22–7 ps	10.6 ps
Sensitivity to divalent blockers	$Ca^{2+} > Co^{2+}$	$Ca^{2+} \sim Co^{2+}$
Activity at −100 V	−	+

Data from McKenna et al. 1990
− denotes "No" and + "Yes"; ps = picoseimens

react only with T-tubules (Rosemblat et al. 1981) and not with the adjacent sarcolemma or the sarcoplasmic reticulum (an intracellular network of tubules which becomes specialized whenever it approaches the T-tubules, Chapter 4). Since the assembly of subunits which constitute these Ca^{2+} channels also contain the high affinity binding sites for the calcium antagonists, many investigators have used radioactively labelled dihydropyridines as markers for these channel complexes. One of the surprising findings is that the density of these binding sites in purified skeletal muscle transverse tubules is at least tenfold (Catterall et al. 1989) and possibly fifty to one hundred times greater (Fosset et al. 1983; Glossmann et al. 1983) than in any other tissue. Obviously, therefore, this was a reasonable starting point for studies which were aimed at elucidating the molecular biology of the channel and its associated calcium antagonist binding sites. With the benefit of hindsight however, some caution should have been exerted before the results obtained for the skeletal muscle membranes were regarded as being universal. This is because:

(i)   there are tissue specific differences in the molecular structure of some of the channel subunits (Slish et al. 1989);

(ii) there are tissue-dependent functional differences in the electrophysiological properties of the channels (Table 3.3), and

(iii) only a small proportion (about 5 percent) of the calcium antagonist (DHP) binding sites are associated with functional voltage-activated Ca^{2+} conducting channels (Schwartz et al. 1985).

The Voltage-Dependent Calcium Antagonist-Sensitive Ca^{2+} Channel Complex of Skeletal Muscle T-Tubules: Subunit Structure and Function

The voltage-dependent, calcium-antagonist-sensitive Ca^{2+} channel of skeletal muscle is an oligomeric structure consisting of five putative subunits – designated α_1, α_2, β, γ and δ (Catterall et al. 1989). Precisely how these subunits fit together so as to

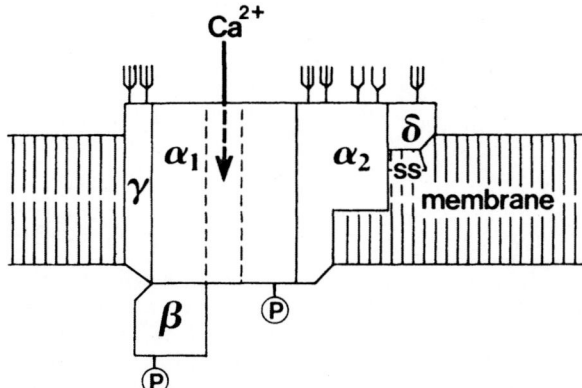

Fig. 3.1. Schematic representation of the manner in which
the various subunits of an
L-type Ca^{2+} channel are assembled, providing a central
pore. P = phosphorylation site
(after Catterall et al. 1989, with
permission)

form a Ca^{2+}-selective, voltage-sensitive L-type channel is still a subject of debate, but the cartoon shown in Figure 3.1 indicates one possible method of assembly (Fig. 3.1 and Catterall et al. 1989). Of all the subunits the α_1 unit is probably the most important because:

(i)   it contains the binding sites for the prototype calcium antagonists (Vaghy et al. 1987a; 1987b; Striessnig et al. 1988; 1990);

(ii) when incorporated into planar lipid bilayers (Flockerzi et al. 1986; Curtis and Catterall 1986; Smith et al. 1989), or microinjected into cells which lack an endogenous α_1 subunit (Knudson et al. 1989) it functions as a calcium-antagonist sensitive Ca^{2+} channel, and

(iii) it almost certainly contains the voltage sensor (Tanabe et al. 1990).

The Chemistry of the Skeletal Muscle α_1 Subunit

When isolated by classical chromatographic techniques, the α_1 subunit appears as a 175 kDa protein. It is not extensively glycosylated (Takahashi et al. 1987) and is substantially hydrophobic. Molecular biological studies have established its primary aminoacid sequence (Tanabe et al. 1987; Ellis et al. 1988). There are 1873 aminoacids (Tanabe et al. 1987), the nucleotide sequences of which are 55 percent homologous with those of the Na$^+$ channel (Noda et al. 1984; 1986). This homology with the Na$^+$ channel extends well beyond the aminoacid composition of the subunits, however, because in both instances the aminoacids are arranged in four repeating hydrophobic motifs, each of which contains six membrane-spanning segments (Fig. 3.2). Presumably these membrane-spanning segments are arranged in an α helical manner. Five of the segments (S1, S2, S3, S5 and S6) are hydrophobic but S4 is positively charged. Segment S4 is also different in that it contains an arginine or lysine residue at every third or fourth position. The aminoacid sequence of the S4 region appears to be a highly conserved sequence – it is conserved in all Na$^+$ channels (from the eel to rat brain) and is present in all Ca^{2+} channel α_1 subunits so far examined. For some years investigators have believed that this S4 segment forms part of – or is – the voltage sensor but recently, evidence obtained from using

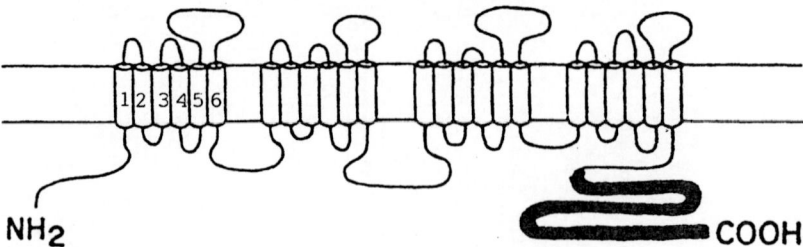

Fig. 3.2. Schematic representation of the organization of the DHP receptor as it occurs in cardiac and skeletal muscle. The heavily shaded area denotes the long carboxy terminus. This probably contains binding sites for regulatory agents. Note that there are four homologous units, each of which contains six putative transmembrane segments (S1–6, from left to right) (after Tanabe et al. 1990)

chimaeric (or modified) α_1 isoforms has shown that the voltage sensing component of the α_1 subunit is not restricted to the transmembranous regions of the skeletal muscle subunit but may also involve the cytoplasmic region between (Fig. 3.2) repeats 2 and 3 (Tanabe et al. 1990). As if the structure and chemical composition of the α_1 subunit of the Ca^{2+} channel complex is not complicated enough, a relatively new finding implies that there are further complications ahead – due to the presence of a hitherto unrecognized "extension" of the 175 kDa fraction which is normally lost during the isolation procedures. Evidence of this missing component has been obtained during recent studies on the chemistry of the cloned form of this α_1 subunit, which now appears to be a 212 kDa protein – and not, as the previous studies would suggest, a 175 kDa protein (de Jongh et al. 1989). It seems that the α_1 subunit probably consists of *two* components both of which are encoded by the same gene (de Jongh et al. 1989). The whole subunit is the 212 kDa fraction. Removal of the terminal ~320 aminoacids from this 212 kDa protein yields the 175 unit (which has been known, until now, as the α_1 subunit), together with a much smaller unit. The smaller component (terminal 320 aminoacid fraction) of the 212 kDa α_1 subunit contains several potential sites for cAMP-dependent phosphorylation – and therefore almost certainly has a regulatory role.

Discovery of this previously missing subunit of the α_1 subunit may help to resolve why it is that the isolated 175 kDa subunit requires additional cAMP-dependent phosphorylation for maximum activation – probably its main potential sites for phosphorylation are missing (Hymel et al. 1988b)!

In Summary

1. The α_1 subunit of the skeletal muscle Ca^{2+} channel is an oligomeric structure with membrane spanning and cytoplasmic domains. When cloned, a 212 kDa unit is obtained. When isolated chromatographically only a 175 kDa fraction is retained. Insertion of this 175 kDa unit into planar lipid bilayers evokes calcium antagonist-sensitive slow Ca^{2+} channel activity. The fundamental

Table 3.4. Biochemical properties of the calcium-antagonist receptor complex

Property	Subunit				
	α_1	α_2	β	γ	δ
Calcium antagonist binding sites	Yes	No	No	No	No
Glycosylation sites	No	Yes	No	Yes	Yes
Hydrophobic domains	Strong	Weak	N.D.	N.D.	N.D.
Transmembrane domains	24	1	0	4	?
Molecular Weights (kDa)	175 + 37 (212)	140–150	55	32	24 + 27
Subunits	Yes (2)	0	0	0	Yes (2)

N.D. Not detectable
Data from Schwartz et al. 1988; Ruth et al. 1989; Jay et al. 1989. The α_1 subunit consists of two subunits: the main unit has a m.w. of 175 kDa and is associated with a much smaller (?) regulatory unit of 37 kDa. The total molecular weight, therefore, is 212 kDa

component of the Ca^{2+} channel and its associated calcium antagonist binding sites must therefore reside within the 175 kDa fraction. Presumably the remainder of the 212 kDa unit (the last ~320 aminoacids of the C terminal) have a regulatory function and are needed for regulated channel activity.

2.   The 175 kDa fraction of the Ca^{2+} channel α_1 subunit is homologous with a subunit of the Na^+ channel. In both cases, the subunit is arranged so as to form four repeating motifs, each one of which contains six membrane spanning units – making a total of twenty four (Table 3.4).

The α_2 subunit

This component of the DHP-receptor channel complex is almost as large as the α_1 subunit and together they account for the major part of the 400 kDa channel complex. The α_2 subunit (Fig. 3.1) contains 1106 aminoacids and, depending upon the precise biochemical conditions used for its isolation, has a molecular weight of between 167 and 175 kDa. There are at least two cAMP-dependent phosphorylation sites but perhaps the most striking feature is the presence of as many as eighteen potential glycosylation sites. It can be assumed with a fair degree of certainty, therefore, that this particular subunit is heavily glycosylated.

In contrast to the α_1 subunit (Fig. 3.1) the α_2 subunit:

(i)   lacks any calcium antagonist binding sites;
(ii)   lacks any appreciable homology with any other known aminoacid sequence;
(iii) possesses relatively few (probably no more than three) transmembrane domains, and
(iv)   is substantially hydrophobic (Ellis et al. 1988).

To some extent the characteristics of the α_2 subunit of the Ca^{2+} channel complex can be likened to those of the β-subunit of the $Na^+ K^+$ ATPase enzyme. Both are heavily glycosylated, and both probably play an important structural role in ensuring that the closely associated α_1 subunit is correctly inserted in the membrane. As far as the Ca^{2+} channel complex is concerned, if the α_2 subunit controls, or regulates, the way in which the α_1 subunit is orientated in the membrane, and if the correct orientation of the α_1 complex is important or contributes to the proper function of the α_1 complex as a calcium antagonist sensitive, Ca^{2+}-conducting channel, it is not surprising to find that the Ca^{2+}-conducting capacity of isolated α_1 complexes which have been inserted into lipid bilayers are enhanced when α_2 subunits are added (Mikami et al. 1989), even though the α_2 subunit does not function as an ion-conducting channel. Observations such as these have given rise to the idea that although the α_1 subunit alone is capable of functioning as a Ca^{2+} channel, under normal conditions its Ca^{2+} conducting activity is influenced by the attendant subunits – including the heavily glycosylated, relatively large α_2 subunit.

The δ Subunit

Compared to the α_1 and α_2 subunits, the δ subunit is small. In fact it accounts for as little as six percent of the total mass (400 kDa) of the channel complex.

The properties of this δ subunit (Fig. 3.1) can be summarized as follows:
(i)   it is almost certainly not a single glycoprotein. Instead it probably is a complex of two glycoproteins – one with a molecular weight of 27 kDa and the other 24 kDa (de Jongh et al. 1990). In addition,
(ii)   it, like the α_2 subunit, is heavily glycosylated;
(iii) it is disulphide-linked to the α_2 subunit (Fig. 3.1); and
(iv)   in contrast to the α_1 subunit, it, and the associated α_2 subunit, are resistant to proteolysis. This subunit,
(v)   resembles the α_2 subunit in being devoid of any calcium antagonist binding activity, and
(vi)   is encoded by the same gene as the α_2 subunit (de Jongh et al. 1990).

Some readers may question whether the α_2-δ complex should even be considered as being a part of the Ca^{2+} channel complex. After all, it could just be associated with the α_1 complex by chance, or as a secondary consequence of the biochemical techniques used in the isolation procedures. There are several reasons for rejecting such a negative approach:
(i)   the α_1 and the α_2-δ subunits co-sediment on sucrose gradients;
(ii)   antibodies which are specific for the α_1 subunit immunoprecipitate with the α_2-δ complex, and
(iii) antibodies against α_2 immunoprecipitate α_1.

The α_2-δ complex is a well preserved complex. Certainly it is not peculiar to skeletal muscle, because similar disulphide-linked complexes have been detected and identified in Ca^{2+} channel preparations derived from a variety of tissues, including the heart, brain and vascular smooth muscle.

The γ Subunit

This, like the δ subunit, is a relatively minor component of the channel complex – at least as far as its size is concerned. It is a 32 kDa protein, and seems to contain only 222 aminoacids (Jay et al. 1989). It's major properties are as follows:
(i)   like the $α_2$-δ complex, it is heavily glycosylated;
(ii) it has four potential membrane spanning segments, and
(iii) it has two potential glycosylation sites and at least six sites suitable for phosphorylation.
(iv) Undoubtedly the most *unusual feature of this subunit is that it contains ten cysteine residues.*

The β Subunit

As with the δ and γ subunit components of the skeletal muscle Ca^{2+} channel complex, the β subunit (Fig. 3.1) is a relatively small component part. It contains only 524 aminoacids, and has a molecular weight of 58 kDa (Ruth et al. 1989). Relatively little information is available concerning the structure of this subunit, other than that it is:
(i)   hydrophilic, and probably associated with the intracellular domain of the $α_1$ subunit; that
(ii) it lacks typical membrane spanning regions; but
(iii) contains sites suitable for phosphorylation. Moreover,
(iv) it lacks calcium antagonist binding activity, and
(v)   lacks homology with any other known aminoacid sequence. Nevertheless polypeptides of similar size are known to be associated with other ion-conducting channels – including the Na^+ and K^+ channels.

Assembly of the $α_1$, $α_2$, δ, γ and β Components of the Channel Complex

Dissecting out the various component parts of the Ca^{2+} channel complex provided the rationale for assuming that the DHP-receptor Ca^{2+} channel complex of skeletal muscle is a composite structure which, when assembled as shown in Figure 3.1, can function as a voltage-sensitive, cation-selective channel. Although complex, the model is quite logical: it assumes that the $α_1$ subunit is the component which functions as an ion-selective channel, is voltage-sensitive and contains the specific, high affinity binding sites for the prototype calcium antagonists. According to this model, this central $α_1$ component is surrounded by the other subunits ($α_2$, δ, β and γ), some of which are regulatory (by way of phosphorylation) whilst others contribute to the physical stabilization of the $α_1$ complex in the membrane. Because of its phosphorylation sites and lack of hydrophobicity, it is reasonable to assume that the β subunit of the complex attaches itself to the cytoplasmic side of the α_1 unit (Fig. 3.1). The δ subunit, however, which is known to be disulphide-linked to the α_2 subunit, must surely extend to the extracellular surface, because of its potential for glycosylation.

The Tissue Specificity of the Alpha$_1$ Subunit

Arguments supporting the hypothesis of *tissue specificity* with respect to the α_1 subunit component of the DHP-receptor Ca^{2+} channel complex are steadily gaining ground. The arguments are based on the following observations:

(i)   Mice born with the genetically determined and fatal condition of muscular dysgenesis lack functional α_1 receptors in their skeletal but not in their cardiac calcium channel complexes (Pincon-Raymond et al. 1985; Beam et al. 1986; Mikami et al. 1989), indicating that different genes code for these subunits in the two tissues (cardiac and skeletal muscle).

(ii)   mRNA blot analysis with probes for the α_1 subunit show the expected band for skeletal muscle, but only a weak hybridizing signal for the DNA from cardiac muscle, and absolutely no signal for ileal or brain tissue (Ellis et al. 1988);

(iii) the functional characteristics of the skeletal muscle Ca^{2+} channels are quite different from those of similar channels in other tissues. Examples of these differences include the fact that:

(a)   the unitary conductance of the skeletal muscle channels is smaller, and

(b)   their gating is ten times slower than that obtained for cardiac muscle Ca^{2+} channels (Hess 1990); and

(iv)   the injection of cDNA plasmids coding for *cardiac* α_1 subunits into skeletal muscle myotubules obtained from the dysgenic mice which lack functional endogenous α_1 subunits results in the restoration of α_1 subunit activity (as indicated by the restoration of Ca^{2+} currents) in the dysgenic skeletal tissue, but the Ca^{2+} currents are now of the cardiac type and depend upon the presence of extracellular Ca^{2+} to evoke excitation-contraction coupling (Mikami et al. 1989). By contrast, the injection of an expressed plasmid carrying the skeletal muscle DHP-receptor – α_1 subunit complementary DNA – restores excitation-contraction coupling and L-type Ca^{2+} current but in this case the resultant excitation-contraction coupling process is now of the skeletal muscle type, in that it does not require extracellular Ca^{2+} (Tanabe et al. 1988).

(v)   Cloning and subsequent aminoacid sequencing of the various tissue types of α_1 subunits (cardiac, skeletal and smooth muscle) have revealed differences in their biochemical composition. In the case of cardiac and aortic smooth muscle cells there is a close similarity in composition (93 percent homology, Table 3.5), indicating that these units are probably encoded by the same gene. Brain α_1 subunits also closely resemble, but are not totally homologous (Table 3.5) with their cardiac muscle equivalents. By contrast the aortic, cardiac and brain α_1 subunits are only 66, 64.7 and 75 percent homologous respectively with their skeletal muscle equivalents (Table 3.5, and Koch et al. 1989; 1990). Presumably

Table 3.5. Tissue specificity of the α_1 subunit of the Ca^{2+} channel – DHP-receptor complex

Origin of the α_1 subunit	% homology relative to	
	Cardiac α_1	Skeletal α_1
Skeletal muscle	65	
Cardiac muscle		65
Aortic smooth muscle	93	66
Brain		75

Data from Koch et al. 1990; Slish et al. 1989; Koch et al. 1989.
% Homology refers to homology with respect to their aminoacid composition

the skeletal muscle subunit is encoded by an entirely different gene – hence its very different aminoacid composition.

Although it is well beyond the scope of this book to set out in detail the precise differences in the aminoacid composition of the α_1 subunits as they occur in the different tissues there are some general guide lines which can be summarised as follows:
(i)   the membrane spanning units (Fig. 3.2) are, in the main, well conserved, although there are some minor differences;
(ii) the S4 voltage-sensor component of each motif is preserved, irrespective of tissue and contains positively charged residues at every third or fourth aminoacid position;
(iii) the majority of changes involve either:
      (a) the intracellular and extracellular loops connecting the various components of each motif, and between the motifs, and
      (b) the carboxy tail (Fig. 3.2).

As far as the *cardiac* α_1 subunit component of the DHP-receptor Ca^{2+} channel complex is concerned:
(i)   the intracellular loops connecting segments S3 and S4 of motif 4 differ from that of skeletal muscle, even to the extent of there being eight fewer aminoacids;
(ii) segment 3 of motif 4 (Fig. 3.2) differs in its aminoacid composition from that found for the same segment of the same motif in skeletal muscle (Slish et al. 1989; Koch et al. 1990);
(iii) the number and location of sites which are suitable for phosphorylation differ from those found in skeletal muscle α_1 subunits, and
(iv) the carboxy (or C) terminus of the cardiac α_1 complex contains seventy three more aminoacids than its skeletal muscle counterpart (Slish et al. 1989).

In Aortic Smooth Muscle

(i)   Segment 3 of motif 4 (Fig. 3.2) closely resembles the cardiac and not the skeletal muscle prototype (Koch et al. 1990), and

(ii) the aminoacid composition of the terminal intracellular carboxy tail is different. However,

(iii) the S4 transmembrane domain in each of the four motifs (Fig. 3.2) is preserved exactly as it occurs in the cardiac and skeletal muscle subunits.

In Brain (Koch et al. 1989):

(i)   the S4 transmembrane domain of each motif is preserved;

(ii) the S3 segment of motif 4 differs from its skeletal muscle counterpart, and

(iii) there is a difference in the aminoacid sequence of the cytoplasmic loop which precedes the well preserved S4 domain of motif 4.

In general, therefore, although the essential structure consisting of the four repeating motifs each of which contains six transmembrane domains is perfectly preserved in cardiac, skeletal, brain and aortic Ca^{2+} channel α_1 subunit complexes, there are subtle tissue-specific differences which seem to centre around:

(i)   the transmembrane segment 3 of motif 4;

(ii) the relatively long carboxy tail;

(iii) the distribution of potential phosphorylation sites, and

(iv) the cytoplasmic loop connecting segments 3 and 4 of motif 4.

The Component of the Skeletal Muscle Alpha$_1$ Subunit Which Dictates the Ability of Skeletal Muscle to Accomplish Excitation-Contraction Coupling in the Absence of Extracellular Ca^{2+}

If, as outlined in the preceding sections of this chapter, the main differences between the α_1 subunits (the DHP-receptor) of the skeletal and cardiac muscle Ca^{2+} channel complexes involve the carboxy terminal region of the complex as well as the cytoplasmic loops connecting the repeat motifs, the question naturally arises as to which of these differences determines the need for extracellular Ca^{2+} to facilitate excitation-contraction coupling. Chimaeric manipulations of the complex have recently revealed that it is the cytoplasmic link that connects motifs 2 and 3 of the α_1 complex (Fig. 3.2) which holds the key (Tanabe et al. 1990).

In Summary

1. During the past two or three years considerable progress has been made in establishing the molecular structure of the calcium antagonist sensitive, voltage activated L-type Ca^{2+} channels.

2. Irrespective of tissue type the complex consists of at least five subunits designated, for convenience, as α_1, α_2, β, γ and δ (Fig. 3.1).

3. The α_2, β, γ and δ components of this complex provide sites for phosphorylation and glycosylation, and therefore may be important for physically stabilizing the α_1 subunit in the membrane, as well as providing possible sites for regulation.

4. The α_1 subunit provides two major functions:
   (i) it is the Ca^{2+} channel, and
   (ii) it contains specific high affinity binding sites for the calcium antagonists.

5. This α_1 subunit has a complex ultrastructure. Irrespective of tissue type it consists of four repeat motifs each of which contains six transmembrane (S1 – S6) domains. In addition there is a long carboxy terminus, and cytoplasmic loops connecting the various segments, and domains (Fig. 3.2).

6. Of these transmembrane domains, S4, is perfectly conserved in all species and tissues so far examined. This segment contains charged aminoacid residues at every third or fourth position in the aminoacid sequence, and largely because of this it is believed to be *"the voltage sensor"*.

7. Tissue dependent differences in the composition of the α_1 subunit include:
   (i)   differences in the aminoacid composition of the S3 segment of motif 4;
   (ii) differences in the aminoacid composition and length of the carboxy terminus, and
   (iii) variations in the length and aminoacid composition of the various cytoplasmic loops connecting individual segments within each motif, or between successive motifs. The loop which precedes the S4 domain of motif 4 appears to be of particular importance.

8. These tissue-dependent differences in the composition of the α_1 subunit of the channel complex probably contribute to the tissue specificity which some of the calcium antagonists display, since they interact with this α_1 subunit.

Chapter 4

Calcium Antagonists and the Calcium Release Channels of the Sarcoplasmic Reticulum

"Houses are built to live in and not to look on; therefore, let use be preferred before uniformity – except where both may be had."
FRANCIS BACON (1561 – 1626)

Mammalian, cardiac and skeletal muscle cells contain an intricate intracellular network of tubules known as the sarcoplasmic reticulum (SR). This tubular network:

(i)   actively accumulates Ca^{2+} from the cytosol, thereby allowing relaxation to occur (Schwartz 1971), and

(ii) releases Ca^{2+} for excitation-contraction coupling (Fig. 4.1) (Fabiato 1985).

The second of these functions – the release of Ca^{2+} – involves the opening of specific ion-conducting channels located in "feet-like" connections which bridge the narrow gap between the sarcolemma and the SR both at the periphery of the cell and at the sarcolemmal invaginations which form the transverse tubular system. A general impression of the appearance and spacing of these bridge-like structures can be gained from the electron micrograph reproduced as Fig. 4.2, which shows a section through a typical *junctional region* (a region where the electron dense "feet" intervene between the sarcoplasmic reticulum and the sarcolemma) of the SR in heart muscle, in this case rat ventricular muscle. However it is not the physical appearance of these projections which is of paramount importance; rather it is the fact that these projections contain the exit channels which allow Ca^{2+} ions to move from the intraluminal SR storage sites into the adjacent cytosol.

The real purpose of this chapter is to describe how calcium antagonists can *indirectly* influence the signal transduction pathways responsible for activating these Ca^{2+} release channels because such an effect may contribute to their ability to improve diastolic function under certain conditions (Walsh 1989). At the outset, however, it should be noted that the structure and function of these channels differs markedly from that of the sarcolemmal L-type Ca^{2+} channels described in the previous chapter (Chapter 3) – although both are large conductance channels. Nor should it be imagined that a *direct* effect of the calcium antagonists is being considered, because the SR lacks high affinity calcium antagonist binding sites. This does not mean, however, that therapeutically relevant concentrations of calcium antagonists could not *indirectly* influence the Ca^{2+} release process. Any explanation of how this could happen, however, requires an understanding of the general properties of the SR and the morphology of it's bridging structures.

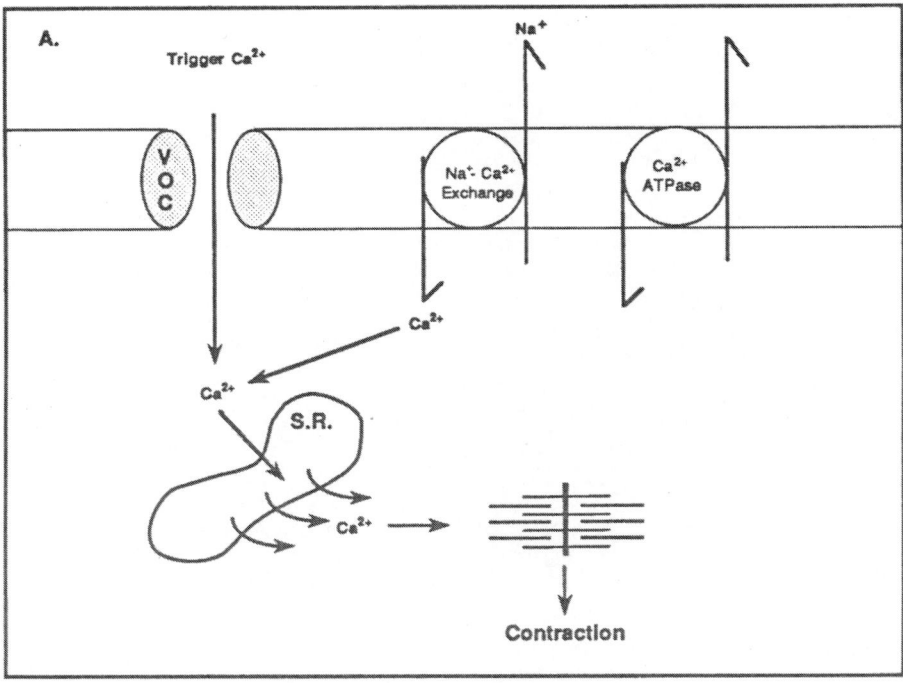

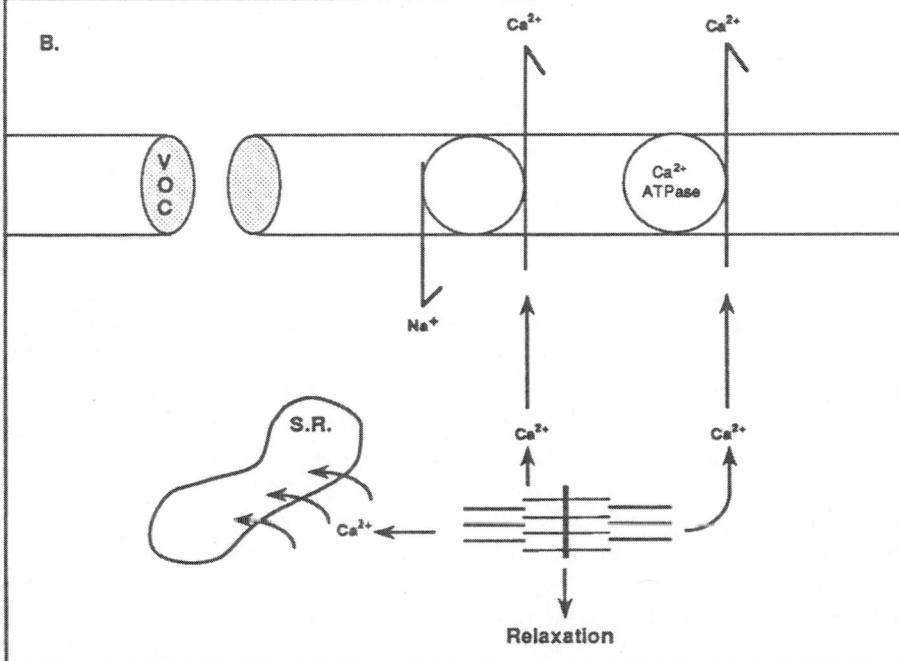

Fig. 4.1. Schematic representation of the involvement of Ca^{2+} in excitation-contraction coupling. A: *Contraction*. B: *Relaxation*

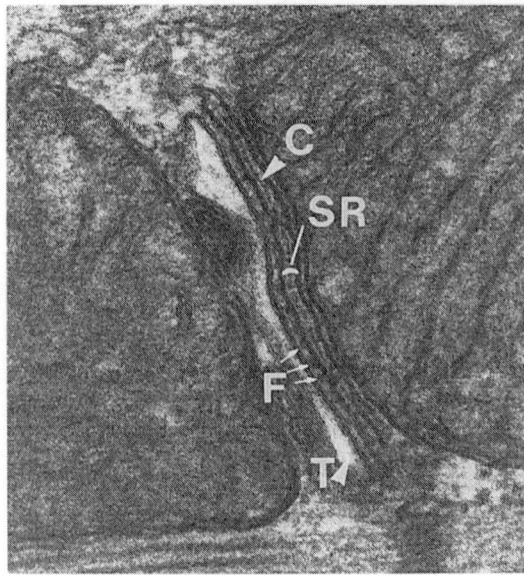

Fig. 4.2. Electronmicrograph of the specialized region which forms whenever the sarcolemma (SR) approaches the sarcolemma, particularly where the sarcolemma forms a transverse tubule (T). Note the narrow gap separating the SR from the T-tubule, the feet-like protrusions which bridge the gap (F) and the intraluminal densities (C) in the SR. This density is due to the presence of calsequestrin, a Ca^{2+} binding protein. Mag. ×93,500. The section is of rat ventricular muscle, and was kindly supplied by Dr. N. Severs

The General Properties of the Sarcoplasmic Reticulum

The SR is a relatively complex organelle; far more complex than was imagined when it was first isolated in the late sixties and early seventies (Schwartz 1971). However it is now known that the main functions of the SR can be divided into three distinct categories:

(i) Ca^{2+} retrieval;
(ii) Ca^{2+} storage, and
(iii) Ca^{2+} release.

The Ca^{2+} retrieval process is well characterized (de Meis and Inesi 1982) and involves the activation of an endogenous SR $Ca^{2+}Mg^{2+}$ ATPase enzyme, resulting in the hydrolysis of adenosine triphosphate (ATP) and the subsequent release of sufficient energy to pump Ca^{2+} back into the SR against the prevailing concentration gradient (de Meis and Inesi 1982). The major events involved in this process (a process which holds the key to the mechanisms involved in the transition from systole to diastole in the heart, and from contraction to relaxation in skeletal muscle) were established in the seventies (Schwartz 1971) but it was not until the mid nineteen eighties that the aminoacid sequence of the relevant ATPase enzyme was determined (Maclennan et al. 1985). By this time interest was beginning to develop in the mechanism which enable the SR to release, as well as retrieve, Ca^{2+}. Obviously a release mechanism must exist, since both cardiac and skeletal muscle utilize Ca^{2+} from the SR during excitation-contraction coupling (Fabiato 1985).

The question which needed to be answered was deceptively simple ... how did excitation at the sarcolemma affect the functioning of the SR so that instead of Ca^{2+}

being accumulated it was now released? The "feet-like" structures bridging the 10 –
20nm gap between the sarcolemma and the reticulum (Fig. 4.2) held the answer to
this puzzle because they:

(i)   sense excitation-induced changes in the functioning of the sarcolemma and
      then signal the adjacent SR, across the intervening "junctional" gap (Fig. 4.2),
      (Dulhuntly 1989; Agnew 1989), and

(ii) contain or constitute channels through which Ca^{2+} ions can pass (Wagen-
      knecht et al. 1989).

The General Morphology of the Sarcoplasmic Reticulum (SR): Evidence of Specialization

Not so long ago it was considered adequate to describe the SR as a "lace-like"
network of tubules which occasionally approach the sarcolemma but which also
traverse the cytosol and envelop the myofibrils. The micro-anatomists first
described the SR in this way and such a description agrees well with the impression
gained from the early electron micrographs. Such a description is totally inadequate, however, because whilst it accurately describes the great bulk of the SR, it
fails to draw attention to the areas of marked and intricate specialisation which have
already been mentioned (Fig. 4.2) and which occur whenever the SR approaches the
sarcolemma and its invaginations (Franzini-Armstrong and Wunzi 1983). These
specialized regions – the *"terminal"* or *"junctional"* cisternae – are contiguous with
the remainder of the SR which, more often than not, is known as *"longitudinal SR"*
(Table 4.1). The "feet-like" structures which span the junctional gap are remarkably
uniform in appearance, with little inter-species variation (Franzini-Armstrong
1970; Franzini-Armstrong and Wunzi 1983; Dulhuntly 1989). The average spacing
between them is around 30nm (Franzini-Armstrong 1970; Somlyo 1979) – a spacing

Table 4.1. Characterization of the light and heavy components of the cardiac sarcoplasmic
reticulum (SR)

Property	"Light" Fraction (longitudinal SR)	"Heavy" Fraction (junctional SR)
Calcium loading rate ($\mu mol \cdot mg^{-1} min^{-1}$)	0.93 ± 0.08	0.16 ± 0.02
Density of [^{3}H]ryanodine binding sites (pmol · mg protein^{-1})	1.67 ± 0.33	8.78 ± 1.87
Calsequestrin (M.W. 60 kDa)	+	++++++
Ca^{2+} release rate	slow	fast
Percentage of membrane protein $Ca^{2+} - Mg^{2+}$ ATPase	90	60

Data from Lai and Meissner 1989; Glossmann and Striessnig 1990; Dulhunty 1989; Inui et al. 1988.
+ denotes the amount of calsequestrin which is present

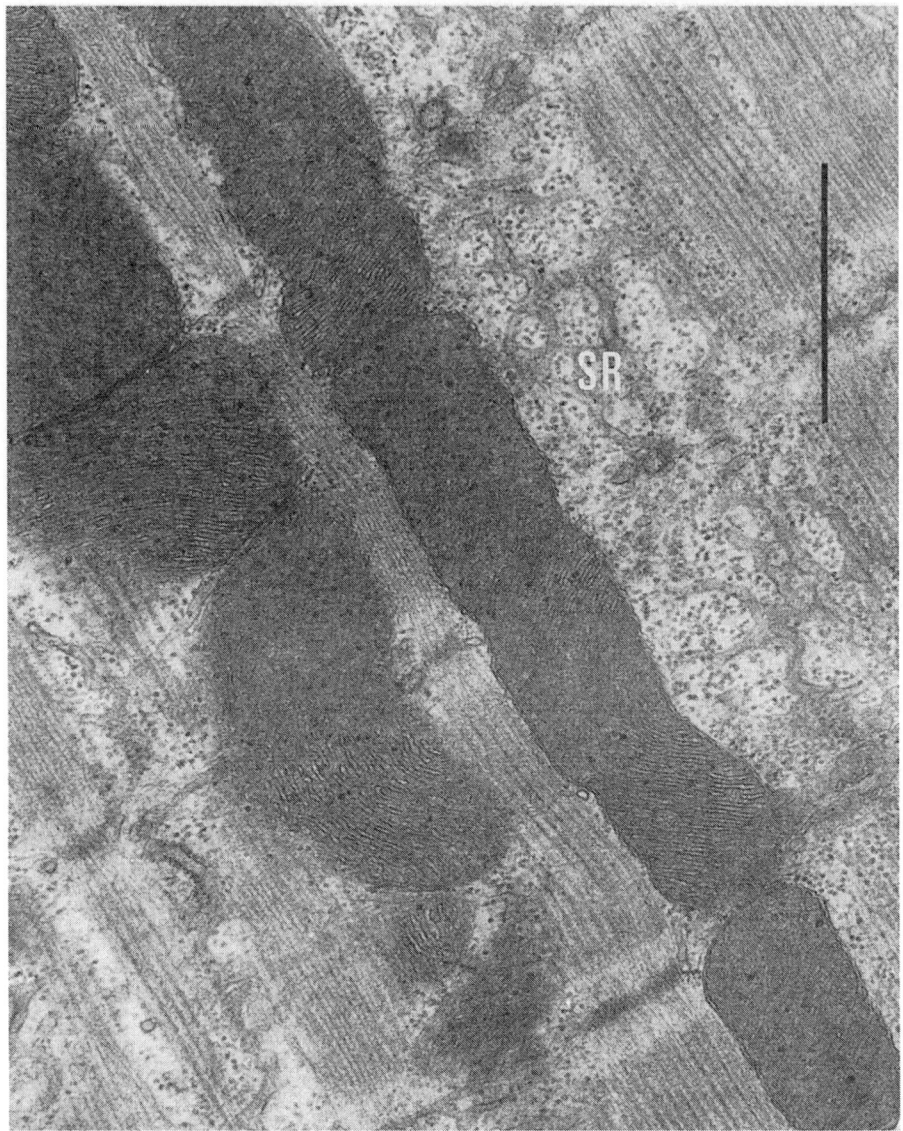

Fig. 4.3. The non-specialized regions of the SR. Note that this part of the SR encircles the myofibrils and courses through the cytosol. It's location, therefore, is ideally suited for the task it performs – that of retrieving Ca^{2+}. Mag. $\times 135,000$

which meshes perfectly with that of small "tuft-like" protrusions, or "tethers", which protrude from the cytosolic face of the sarcolemmal T-tubular invaginations (Dulhuntly 1989).

On the basis of its morphology, therefore, the SR can be subdivided into the following regions:

(i)   a lace-like network of interconnecting tubules which encircle the myofilaments and traverse the cytosol (Fig. 4.3), and

(ii) specialized areas which occur when the SR and the sarcolemma closely approach one another, and which are characterized by:

(a)   junctional bridges (or "feet"), and

(b)   intraluminal densities (Fig. 4.2).

The Biochemistry of the Sarcoplasmic Reticulum

The SR is also biochemically heterogeneous. Evidence of this heterogeneity is easily obtained by fragmenting and then centrifuging the SR. This yields two subcellular fractions – one *"light"*, the other *"heavy"*. The biochemical profiles of these two fractions are quite dissimilar. The "light" fraction (Table 4.1):

(i)   accumulates Ca^{2+} rapidly;

(ii) contains little (if any) of calsequestrin (Fig. 4.2) – the 60 kDa Ca^{2+}-storage protein, despite the fact that the SR is known to contain large amounts of this particular protein (Maclennan and Holland 1975);

(iii) has relatively few ryanodine binding sites (ryanodine is a plant alkaloid which binds specifically to the junctional feet (Lai and Meissner 1989)). In addition,

(iv) approximately 90 percent of the "light" membrane fraction protein occurs as the 110 kDa $Ca^{2+}Mg^{2+}$ ATPase enzyme – the enzyme which is responsible for pumping the Ca^{2+} back into the SR, to facilitate relaxation (Meissner 1975).

By contrast (Table 4.1) the "heavy" fraction:

(i)   accumulates Ca^{2+} slowly;

(ii) contains an abundance of calsequestrin;

(iii) is rich in ryanodine binding sites;

(iv) has only 60 percent of its protein as the $Ca^{2+} Mg^{2+}$ ATPase enzyme (Lai and Meissner 1989);

(v)   contains a large (400 kDa) protein which is immunologically-related to the junctional "feet" (Kawamoto et al. 1986), and

(vi) in contrast to the "light" fraction, releases Ca^{2+} at a relatively rapid rate.

Presumably the "light" fraction contains membranes which originate from that part of the SR which is predominantly concerned with Ca^{2+} retrieval whereas the "heavy" fraction originates from those specialized regions which contain the junctional feet and the Ca^{2+}-storing protein, calsequestrin.

Mention has already been made of the fact that *ryanodine* binding sites are prevalent in the transjunctional foot structures. Ryanodine is an alkaloid derived from the plant *Ryania Speciosa Vahl*. Although initially developed for use as an insecticide its toxicity – which results in irreversible skeletal muscle contracture and flaccid paralysis of the heart (Fill and Coronado 1988) – prevents its use for this purpose. The reason for mentioning it here is not only because it binds to specific, high affinity 400 kDa binding sites in the "feet" structures of the SR – but also because when isolated and inserted into artificial lipid bilayers these ryanodine-

Table 4.2. Tissue distribution of specific binding sites for [^{3}H]ryanodine in junctional "feet" processes

Tissue	Species	Reference
Skeletal Muscle	Rabbit	Inui et al. 1987
	Rabbit	Lai et al. 1988
	Human	Zorzato et al. 1990
	Rabbit	Zorzato et al. 1990
Cardiac Muscle	Rabbit	Rardon et al. 1989
	Dog ventricle	Inui et al. 1988
Brain	Rabbit	McPherson and Campbell 1990

specific 400 kDa binding sites (which are synonymous with the "feet" structures) function as Ca^{2+}-release channels (Lai and Meissner 1989; Nagasaki and Fleischer 1988; Holmberg and Williams 1989; Rardon et al. 1989).

The chemistry of the ryanodine binding sites and the ion-conducting and electrical properties of the channels which are associated with them will be described later in this chapter. For the moment, however, it is sufficient to note that:
(i)   the 400 kDa ryanodine binding protein which forms part of the SR junctional feet processes can also function as an ion-conducting channel;
(ii) this 400 kDa protein is not restricted to the SR junctional "feet" processes of cardiac and skeletal muscle: it occurs in other tissue, including the brain (Table 4.2).

The Ultrastructure and Chemistry of the SR Feet (the SR Ryanodine Receptor – Ca^{2+} Release Channel)

Reconstituted, three dimensional images of the junctional SR "bridges" (or "feet") have revealed the presence of a squarish structure, the volume of which slightly exceeds 3,800nm^3 (Wagenknecht et al. 1989; Agnew 1989). Each foot process seems to connect with, or sit on, a 4nm thick, 14nm wide base-plate which inserts into the SR membrane and which seems to contain a central pore. It is this pore which almost certainly is the orifice of the Ca^{2+} exit channel! Sitting astride the base-plate and extending into the junctional gap area are four copies of the 400 kDa ryanodine binding polypeptide, the four copies being arranged in a left-handed quadrafoil manner. At their distant ends these 400 kDa polypeptide structures make direct contact with regularly-spaced, tuft-like ovoid shaped discs which are arranged on the cytosolic face of the sarcolemmal membrane in the form of tetramers. The spacing of these tetramers is such that they occur with a periodicity of around 30nm (Dulhuntly 1989) – a periodicity which exactly matches that of the bridge complexes which extend from the apposing surface of the SR. These ovoid-shaped disc-like structures are believed to be DHP receptors (some of which are present in the α$_1$ subunit of the L-type slow Ca^{2+} channels described in the last chapter). If this is true,

Table 4.3. Properties of SR ryanodine receptor – Ca^{2+} channel release complex

Composition	Tetrameric: four polypeptides with M.W. 400 kDa

Conductance*
 (i) Skeletal 100 pS
(ii) Cardiac 80 pS
Duration of opening 60–100 µsec

Activators	mM Caffeine
(increase in P_0)	mM ATP
	$Ca^{2+} > \mu M$
	Ryanodine (low µM)
	Annexin VI
	Sulmazole
	Doxorubicin (µM short exposure)
Inhibitors	µM Ruthenium red
(decrease in P_0)	µM Doxorubicin (prolonged exposure)
	> 300 µM ryanodine

* Conductance measured in the presence of 50 mM Ca^{2+} P_0 – probability of the channel being it its open state
(Data from Williams and Ashley 1989; Holmberg and Williams 1989; Ondrias et al. 1990; Diaz-Monez et al. 1990; Nagasaki and Fleischer 1988)

then there is no reason to doubt that a direct pathway exists whereby a signal can be transmitted from the DHP receptor (Knudson et al. 1988), to the specialized junctional regions of the SR – hence to the regions where the Ca^{2+}-storing protein, calsequestrin, is concentrated. The situation is further complicated by the fact of the DHP receptors having a dual function – they can act as slow L-type Ca^{2+} channels *and* as voltage sensors (Tanabe et al. 1988). This dual mode of action may help to explain why excitation at the cell surface can directly trigger SR Ca^{2+} release in skeletal muscle, without involving extracellular Ca^{2+}, whereas in cardiac muscle the presence of extracellular Ca^{2+} is essential. In skeletal muscle the SR release channel (the foot or ryanodine receptor) responds directly to membrane depolarization, the voltage charge being relayed directly to it through the DHP receptors, which are acting as voltage sensors (Rios and Brum 1987; Schneider and Chandler 1973). By contrast, in cardiac muscle the DHP receptors function mainly as Ca^{2+} channels, allowing Ca^{2+} to enter to provoke a Ca^{2+}-induced activation (Table 4.3) of the SR Ca^{2+} release channels (Fabiato and Fabiato 1979; Valdeolmillos et al. 1989; Kentish et al. 1990). In both cases the end result is the same, with the DHP receptors at the cell surface signalling the SR Ca^{2+} release process.

In summary, therefore, the bridge (ryanodine receptor) which spans the SR junctional gap has the following distinctive properties:
(i)   at the SR surface it is attached to a base plate which has a central pore;
(ii) the bulk of the bridge consists of four repeats of a 400 kDa polypeptide arranged in a quadrafoil manner, and
(iii) the whole structure is aligned and makes contact with regularly spaced "tuft"-like ovoid discs which extend outwards from the apposing surface of the

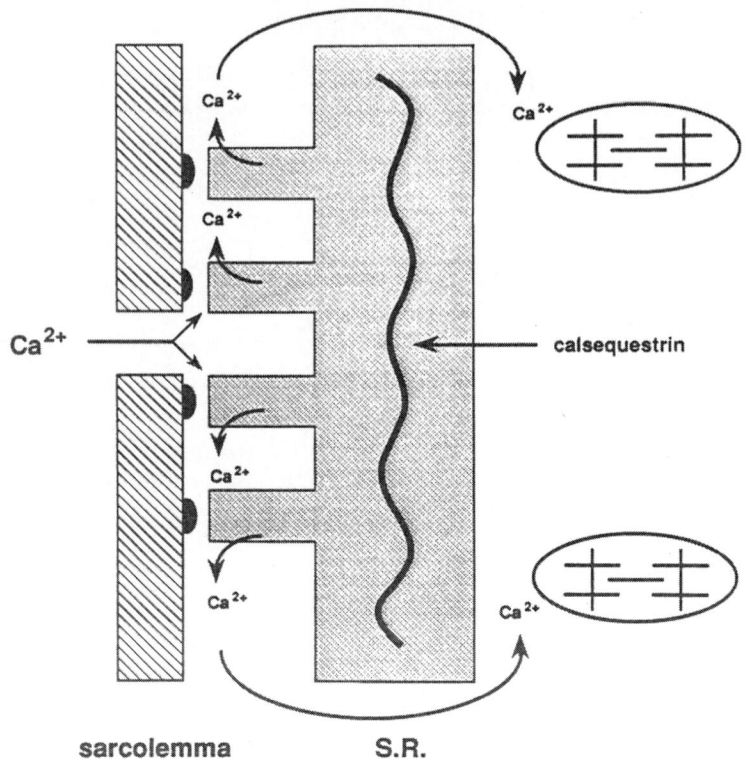

Fig. 4.4. Diagramatic representation of the interrelationship- between the DHP receptors in the sarcolemma and the bridges (ryanodine receptors, SR Ca^{2+} release channels) which span the junctional gap. (After Glossmann and Striessnig 1990)

sarcolemma (Fig. 4.4). These sarcolemmal protuberances are almost certainly DHP receptor binding sites, and they can function either as voltage sensors or as Ca^{2+} ion-conducting channels (Fill et al. 1989). In addition,

(iv) whereas in skeletal muscle the link between the sarcolemmal voltage sensor (the DHP receptor) and the SR release mechanism is direct, in cardiac muscle the SR release process is activated by Ca^{2+} entering the junctional gap by way of the voltage-sensitive L-type Ca^{2+} channel (Cleemann and Morad 1991; Nabauer and Morad 1990; Wibo et al. 1991).

Chemistry

The junctional bridge or foot process is synonymous with the ryanodine receptor – a fact which has made the isolation and purification of the foot structure relatively easy, because radioactively labelled ryanodine can be used as a marker. The receptor has been cloned (Agnew 1989; Takeshima et al. 1989; Zorzato et al. 1990) and sequenced. For rabbit skeletal muscle the structure contains 5,037 aminoacid

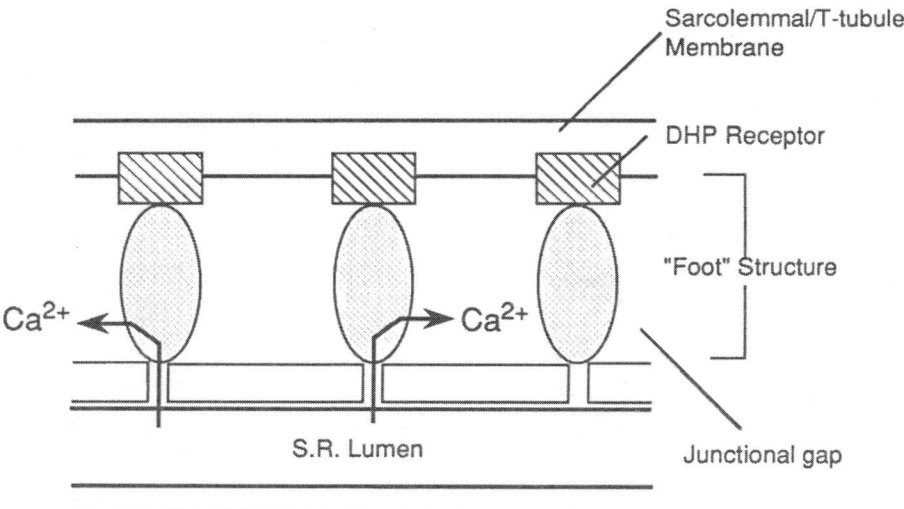

Sarcolemmal/T-tubule Membrane

DHP Receptor

"Foot" Structure

Ca^{2+}

Ca^{2+}

S.R. Lumen

Junctional gap

Fig. 4.5. Diagramatic representation of the possible insertion of the hydrophobic tail of the ryanodine receptor into transjunctional regions of the SR. Note that there appear to be sites for the binding of regulatory complexes close to these transjunctional regions. (From Takeshima et al. (1989) with permission)

residues, arranged with a carboxy but without a NH_2 terminus (Takeshima et al. 1989). At the carboxyterminus there seems to be a hydrophobic tail containing around 500 aminoacid residues. Probably this portion of the sequence is normally inserted into the SR membrane – possibly so as to form a series of transmembrane segments. According to Takeshima and his colleagues (Takeshima et al. 1989) there are four such transmembrane segments, but others argue that they may be as many as ten or twelve. No matter how they are organised, however these transmembranous segments must align themselves so as to form a central pore – the Ca^{2+} exit pore or channel.

Close to the transmembrane sequence there are aminoacids which could be expected to provide suitable binding sites for some of the SR channel modulators (Table 3.3), including, Ca^{2+}, calmodulin and adenine nucleotides (Williams and Ashley 1989; Zorzato et al. 1990). The remainder, and therefore by far the greatest part of the aminoacid sequence, is highly hydrophilic. In all probability this is the part of the ryanodine receptor complex (or bridge) which extends out into the cytosol-filled junctional gap (Fig. 4.5).

When taken together, therefore, data obtained from studies relating to both the ultrastructure and chemistry of the bridge complex supports the idea of these structures being divided into three sections:

(i)   a *transmembranous* region – containing around 500 predominantly hydrophobic residues;

(ii)   a short *regulatory* section, located adjacent to the transmembranous units, and

(iii) a bulky hydrophilic component containing around 45,000 aminoacid residues and constituting that part of the bridge complex which extends into the cytosol to approach the apposing membrane of the sarcolemma (or T tubule).

Before describing how this bridge-like ryanodine binding complex functions as an ion-conducting channel, and its probable role in excitation-contraction coupling, some attention should be given to the intraluminal composition of the SR as it occurs in the junctional regions. After all, it is here that the Ca^{2+} which has been retrieved by the longitudinal regions of the SR is collected and stored for subsequent release in response to a signal delivered by way of the bridge-like structures which have just been described.

The Intraluminal Contents of the Junctional SR

The electronmicrograph shown as Figure 4.2 indicates quite clearly the presence of electron dense material in the lumen of the junctional SR. This is due to the presence of strands of calsequestrin – the Ca^{2+}-storing protein. Generally the strands form a diffuse network, but near the "feet" they orientate themselves in register with the "feet". This structural relationship between the "feet" traversing the junctional gap and the intraluminal Ca^{2+} storage system fits well with the notion that Ca^{2+} which has been stored in the SR can be made available for release through a process which involves the feet-like structures of the junctional SR.

Characteristics of the SR Ryanodine Receptor – Ca^{2+} Release Channel Complex

When isolated, purified and inserted into a planar lipid bilayer the 400 kDa ryanodine receptor (which is synonymous with the junctional "feet" or bridge-structure, Fig. 4.2) functions as an ion conducting channel, irrespective of whether the receptor is harvested from skeletal (Smith et al. 1986; Imagawa et al. 1987; Hymel et al. 1988a; Lai et al. 1988; Fill et al. 1989), or cardiac muscle (Rousseau et al. 1986; Rardon et al. 1989; Williams and Ashley 1989; Holmberg and Williams 1989). Single channel recordings of these channels show that they have a relatively high conductance for divalent cations, including Ca^{2+} (80-100 pS in 50nM Ca^{2+}, Lai et al. 1988), that the probability of their being in the "open" state increases as the applied potential becomes more positive, and that they can remain open for as long as 100μseconds (Table 4.3). A fairly typical tracing of the electrical activity recorded from such a channel -in this particular case the channel was isolated from the SR of human heart muscle – is shown in the left hand panel of Figure 4.6. Now, assuming that these channels provide the pathway for SR Ca^{2+} release, it would be reasonable to assume that substances which stimulate (Ca^{2+}, adenine nucleotides and caffeine) or inhibit (magnesium, and ruthenium red) Ca^{2+} release from isolated SR vesicles in which the release channels are still intact and in situ in their native membranes

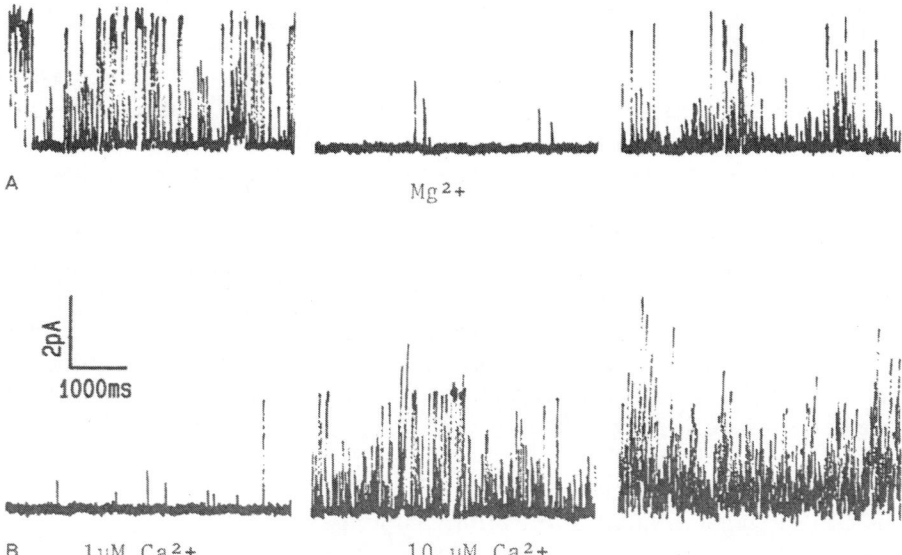

Fig. 4.6. Current fluctuations in a bilayer into which SR Ca^{2+} channels from human heart muscle have been inserted. *Upper tracing* Recording A: in the presence of 10μM Ca^{2+} and 1mM Mg^{2+} (note the inhibitory effect of Mg^{2+}). Recording B: in the presence of 1μM Ca^{2+}, and then following the addition of 10μM Ca^{2+} this data was kindly provided by Dr. A.J. Williams

(Meissner, 1986) would have a similar effect on the isolated channels. This is exactly what has been found. For example, the middle panel of the recording shown in Figure 4.6 shows the inhibitory effect of 1mM Mg^{2+} on channel activity. In the second series of tracings shown in this figure (Fig. 4.6) the first panel (left hand panel) shows a relatively quiescent pattern of activity. This is because the Ca^{2+} concentration has been reduced to the low (1μM) micromolar level. The second panel shows the effect of adding more Ca^{2+} (10μM). Other activators (Table 4.3) include millimolar concentrations of ATP, of caffeine (Holmberg and Williams 1989) and of the cardiotoxic benzimidazole derivative, sulmazole (Williams and Ashley 1989). Inhibitors include ruthenium red, calmodulin, and millimolar concentrations of either ryanodine (Meissner 1986) or Mg^{2+} (Holmberg and Williams 1989). The SR even seems to generate its own endogenous regulators. There is for example the 67 kDa protein, annexin VI which binds phospholipids in a Ca^{2+}-dependent manner and which immunolocalization studies have shown to be present in the intraluminal space of the junctional (or "heavy") SR (Diaz-Munoz et al. 1990). This endogenous protein activates the Ca^{2+} release channels, by increasing the probability (P_0) of their being in an open state (Diaz-Munoz et al. 1990).

Annexin VI is not the only naturally occurring protein which modifies the gating behaviour of the SR release channels. For example, when calmodulin is added to the cis (myoplasmic) side of the channel it *decreases* the probability of the channel being *in its open state, without altering the conductance of the channel* (Smith et al. 1989).

There may indeed be a "yin-yan" situation here, with myoplasmic calmodulin acting to reduce (Table 4.3) and intraluminal annexin VI tending to increase the probability of the channels being open. Of course the same "yin-yan" situation exists for Ca^{2+} and Mg^{2+}, with Ca^{2+} increasing and Mg^{2+} decreasing the likelihood of the channels being in their open state (Fig. 4.6).

Some compounds have a dose- or time-dependent effect on these channels. Take ryanodine for example. In low micromolar concentrations it increases the probability (P_0) of the channel being open, whereas at higher concentrations (e.g. $30.0\mu M$) it reduces P_0 (Nagasaki and Fleischer 1988; Rardon et al. 1989). Doxorubicin, a drug which is widely used in chemotherapy but which can be cardiotoxic, also has a biphasic effect on the channels but here the effect is *time-dependent*. When first added it activates the channels, increasing their mean open time (Ondrias et al. 1990) but more prolonged exposure causes channel inactivation, an effect which probably contributes to the drugs cardiotoxicity.

SR Ca^{2+} Release Channels in Various Pathologies

Cardiac SR

The effect of various pathological conditions on the functioning of these SR release channels is just beginning to be investigated. Already there is some evidence which suggests that ischaemia may increase the time the cardiac SR channels remain in their open state (Feher et al. 1989). This is an interesting and perhaps unexpected finding, because during ischaemia the tissue reserves of ATP are rapidly depleted, and since ATP increases the probability of these channels being in their open state (Holmberg and Williams 1989) it might have been anticipated that the ischaemia-induced decline in tissue ATP would entice the channels to remain closed. Indeed if the SR channels were behaving logically this is how they should function, because a rise in cytosolic Ca^{2+} such as that which must occur if the SR Ca^{2+} release channels remain in their open state will only hasten cell death and tissue necrosis (Chapter 10).

The cause of this ischaemia-induced increase in the "open" time of the SR Ca^{2+} release channels has probably just been identified. It seems to involve the activation of the Ca^{2+}-dependent cytoplasmic protease enzyme, calpain II. Cardiac muscle contains an abundance of this enzyme. When activated it selectively degrades the SR feet structures (Rardon et al. 1990) and in so doing impairs the functioning of the Ca^{2+} release channels they contain, leaving their unitary conductance unchanged but increasing the open time probability very substantially. It is not too difficult to imagine how the prolonged opening times of these Ca^{2+} release channels could mediate Ca^{2+} overload (Fig. 4.7).

Although ischaemia causes the SR to "leak" Ca^{2+} into the cytosol, and that "leak" involves a ryanodine-sensitive pathway (Feher et al. 1989) cardiac failure seems to have no *direct* effect on the functioning of isolated individual channels (Holmberg and Williams 1989). However, under in vivo conditions there are various ways in which the functioning of these channels could be *indirectly* affected and

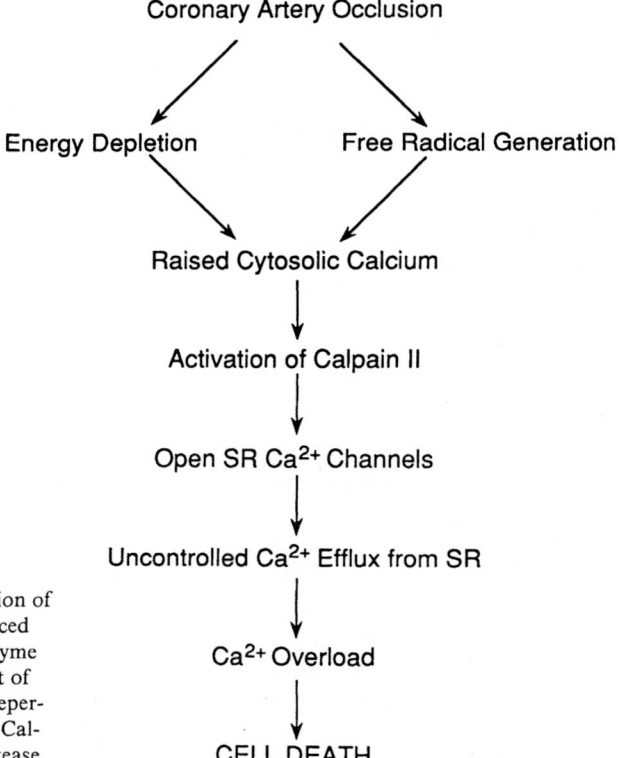

Coronary Artery Occlusion

Energy Depletion   Free Radical Generation

Raised Cytosolic Calcium

Activation of Calpain II

Open SR Ca²⁺ Channels

Uncontrolled Ca²⁺ Efflux from SR

Ca²⁺ Overload

CELL DEATH

Fig. 4.7. Schematic representation of the consequences of Ca^{2+}-induced activation of the calpain II enzyme with respect to the involvement of SR Ca^{2+} release in ischaemia-reperfusion induced Ca^{2+} overload. Calpain II is a Ca^{2+}-activated protease

which would not be detected on the basis of single channel recordings obtained from reconstituted isolated channels. Thus:

(i)   channel density may be altered;
(ii) the intraluminal Ca^{2+} storage capacity may change, or
(iii) the concentration of inhibitory ligands (Mg^{2+}, calmodulin) relative to the availability of activating ligands (annexin VI, Ca^{2+}, ATP) may alter.

Skeletal Muscle SR

Although the structure of the skeletal muscle SR Ca^{2+} release channel has been particularly well studied, the possibility of its holding the key to skeletal muscle pathologies has not yet been explored to any great depth. This is perhaps understandable, because after all, these Ca^{2+} release channels have only just been characterized. As far as skeletal muscle is concerned, it has been established that the gene which encodes the receptor is located on the proximal long arm of chromosome 19 (Zorzato et al. 1990). The defective functioning of this gene does *not* cause myotonic dystrophy. It is, however, associated with malignant hyperthermia (Zorzato et al. 1990) – a condition which is sometimes triggered by halothane or succinylcholine and which is characterized by hypermetabolism, skeletal muscle stiffness, and a raised myoplasmic Ca^{2+} (Iaizzo et al. 1988). Of course the fault may not always lie with the SR Ca^{2+} release channel. There is, for example, a strain of transgenic mice which die at birth due to respiratory paralysis. These mice lack the genetic coding for the all-important voltage sensor of the system – the DHP receptor (Tanabe et al. 1988).

The Trigger for SR Ca^{2+} Release: Differences Between Skeletal and Cardiac Muscle

Basic Machinery of the Release Mechanism

Even though the structural components of the transduction pathway involved in the triggering of SR Ca^{2+} release in cardiac and skeletal muscle are similar – the sarcolemmal DHP receptor (or α_1 subunit of the slow Ca^{2+} channel), the SR ryanodine receptor (or junctional foot process), and the base-plate insertion into the SR membrane – they are not identical because:

(i)   in cardiac muscle the junctional bridge processes, contain *two* types of ryanodine specific binding sites – a *high affinity* site, with a K_D approaching $1\mu M$, and a low affinity site (Inui et al. 1988). By contrast skeletal muscle only seems to contain one class of ryanodine binding site, and here the K_D is around $50 nM$ (K_D is the concentration of the ligand – in this case ^3H-ryanodine – needed to occupy half of the binding sites). In addition,

(ii) there are fewer ryanodine binding sites (Ca^{2+} release channels) in cardiac muscle. For dog heart, for example, the density of these sites is 5.1 pmol per mg protein^{-1} compared with 20 pmol per mg^{-1} for skeletal muscle (Inui et al. 1988). Despite these differences, the basic structural components are the same in both tissues – which is more than can be said for the trigger mechanism of the release process, which seems to differ between the two tissues.

In *skeletal muscle* the signal which is relayed to the SR to evoke Ca^{2+} release is the voltage-dependent intramembranous charge movement which is sensed by the DHP receptor and transferred directly to the SR, by way of the junctional "feet" (Fig. 4.2) (Nabauer et al. 1989) – as if a physical link is involved.

   In *cardiac muscle* a different system applies, because here it is the *voltage-induced influx of Ca^{2+}* ions which provides the trigger (Nabauer et al. 1989; Nabauer and Morad 1990; Cleemann and Morad 1991). There are at least three lines of evidence which support this claim for cardiac muscle:

(i)   when Ba^{2+} ions are substituted as the charge carrier for the slow Ca^{2+} channel they are effectively transported through the channel and function as charge carriers but they do not initiate SR Ca^{2+} release (Nabauer et al. 1989);

(ii) converting the predominantly Ca^{2+}-conducting channel into a Na^+-conducting channel (by exposing the tissue to the chelator, ethylenediaminetetraacetic acid, EDTA), so that Na^+ ions now function as the charge carrier, does not result in SR Ca^{2+} release, and

(iii) removing extracellular Ca^{2+} under conditions in which other charge carriers, including K$^+$ and Mg^{2+}, pass through the channel fails to promote SR Ca^{2+} release (Nabauer et al. 1989).

It seems, therefore, that, as Nabauer et al (1989) have already claimed *"the influx of calcium through the calcium channel is a mandatory link in the processes that couple membrane depolarization to the release of calcium"* in cardiac muscle. By contrast, in skeletal muscle the process is not cation specific but instead is *charge* sensitive.

Calcium Antagonists and SR Ca^{2+} Release

The SR Ca^{2+} release channel (the ryanodine receptor) is quite unlike the sarcolemmal L-type slow Ca^{2+} channel in that:
(i)   it lacks specific high affinity binding sites for calcium antagonists, and
(ii) it is not highly selective for Ca^{2+} ions.

Nevertheless, because the DHP receptor (alpha$_1$ subunit of the calcium channel) in cardiac muscle forms an integral part of the transduction pathway whereby membrane depolarization promotes an influx of Ca^{2+} across the junctional gap to the vicinity of the SR Ca^{2+} storage and release machinery, and because the Ca^{2+} release mechanism is triggered by the arrival of that Ca^{2+}, it would be surprising if the calcium antagonists did not have an effect on the whole process. In fact, these drugs do interfere with excitation-contraction coupling, and hence indirectly with the process of SR Ca^{2+} release (Wier and Yue 1985). This inhibitory effect is not on the SR Ca^{2+} release channel, but rather on its activating mechanism. In cardiac muscle this involves a reduction in the number of Ca^{2+} ions which reach the SR to promote Ca^{2+} release (Fig. 4.8), an effect which must contribute to their negative inotropy and perhaps even to their effect on diastolic relaxation.

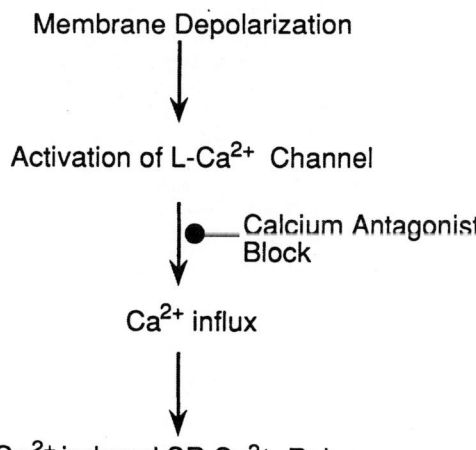

Fig. 4.8. Schematic representation of the possible interaction of calcium antagonists with the mechanisms involved in the release of Ca^{2+} from cardiac SR

In Summary

1. The sarcoplasmic reticulum (SR) is morphologically and biochemically hetero-geneous.
2. It's morphological heterogeneity involves regions which are involved primarily in Ca^{2+} retrieval from the cytosol, and others which modulate Ca^{2+} release.
3. These SR Ca^{2+} release complexes involve:
   (i)   sarcolemmal-located DHP receptors;
   (ii) a junctional process bridging the gap between the sarcolemma and the SR, and
   (iii) an anchor point with a central pore in the SR membrane.
4. In skeletal muscle activation of the Ca^{2+} release channels in the SR involves the direct transduction of the excitatory signal from the DHP receptor (which functions as a voltage sensor) to the "release machinery" of the SR.
5. In cardiac muscle the DHP receptor complex associated with the L-type Ca^{2+} channels allows Ca^{2+} to enter in response to membrane depolarization, and this Ca^{2+} then serves as the "trigger" for the SR Ca^{2+}-release machinery.
6. During ischaemia the cardiac SR Ca^{2+} channels have a high probability of remaining in their open state, possibly because of calpain II activation.
7. In cardiac muscle the Ca^{2+} antagonists indirectly influence the SR Ca^{2+} release by reducing the availability of the trigger Ca^{2+}.

Chapter 5

"Up" and "Down" Regulation
of the Calcium Antagonist Binding Sites

> *"I spent the afternoon musing on Life. If
> you come to think of it, what a queer
> thing Life is! So unlike anything else."*
> P.G. WODEHOUSE, in "Rallying Round
> Old George"

The location of the high affinity calcium antagonist binding sites in the alpha$_1$ subunit of the L-type calcium channel was described in Chapter 3. The radioactive labelling of calcium antagonists has simplified the task of identifying their binding sites. If the "binders and grinders" are at work they will homogenize the relevant tissue, harvest the membranes and then, using the appropriately labelled calcium antagonist, proceed to determine the density (B_{max}), affinity (K_D) and specificity of the sites. The other approach – and one which is popular at the moment – involves whole tissue autoradiography. In some ways this is preferable, because it avoids using homogenized tissue which necessarily contains broken cells. Irrespective of which approach is adopted it soon becomes apparent that as far as the calcium antagonist binding sites are concerned they, like other receptors "up" and "down" regulate. For example, age affects their density (Marangos et al. 1984; Dillon et al. 1989). Some drugs, including ethanol, cause "up regulation" (increase in binding site density) (Brennan et al. 1989) others – including prolonged phenylephrine administration (Gengo et al. 1988a) and calcium antagonist therapy (Panza et al. 1985), can cause "down" regulation (decrease in binding site density). This chapter outlines some of the conditions which either "up" or "down" regulate the calcium antagonist binding sites. Discussion of this topic is highly relevant at the moment, because the use of the long-acting second generation calcium antagonists might be expected to cause receptor down-regulation – and hence tachyphylaxis. As yet, however, there is no evidence of tachyphylaxis being a problem with the use of the newer, longer acting antagonists.

Age-Dependent Changes in Calcium Antagonist Binding Site Density

A precedent has already been set for an effect of age – or more accurately development – on cardiac receptors, because experiments which were carried out some time ago showed that although rabbit cardiac β_1 adrenoceptors are readily identifiable by the twenty first day of gestation and hence approximately ten days before birth, during the last ten days of foetal development their density progressively increases. Even so, at birth the levels are only approximately half that found in adults (Hatjis and McLaughlin 1982, and Table 5.1). A similar situation

Table 5.1. Effect of development on the density (B_{max}) of cardiac beta$_1$-adrenoceptor and calcium antagonist binding sites

Age	B_{max} (fmol · mg protein^{-1})	
	β_1-adrenoceptors	Calcium antagonist
Foetus (days)		
17	22 ± 2**	12†
Neonate (days)		
3–4	42 ± 12**	75†
15		176 ± 15†
Adult		
9 weeks	22 ± 4**	207 ± 9++
25 weeks		254 ± 10++

β-adrenoceptor data taken from (**) Komjima et al. 1990 and relates to specific [^{3}H]-dihydroalprenolol binding to rat cardiac membranes. Calcium antagonist binding data taken from Kazazoglou et al. (1983) (†) and from Dillon et al. 1989 (++) respectively, who used tritiated nitrendipine and tritiated isradipine respectively as Ca^{2+}-binding ligands

seems to exist for the cardiac calcium antagonist binding sites, the levels in rat cardiac cell membranes almost doubling between four and forty days after birth (Kazazoglou et al. 1983, and Table 5.1). After that time the levels seem to remain steady (Dillon et al. 1989). This early post natal increase in calcium antagonist binding site density is not peculiar to the heart. Brain, cerebellum and skeletal muscle all show a similar increase (Kazazoglou et al. 1983), but whether the increase involves the externalization of pre-existing binding sites, or de novo synthesis is a question waiting to be answered.

Calcium antagonist and β-adrenoceptor binding sites are not the only sites which show age-dependent changes in density. The density of cardiac muscarinic cholinergic receptors (labelled with [^{3}H]quinuclidinyl benzilate (QNB)) for example, decreases during neonatal development (Kojima et al. 1990).

Cardiomyopathies

Hypertrophied left ventricles are richly endowed with voltage-sensitive Ca^{2+} channels, (Mayoux et al. 1988) and an unusually large Ca^{2+}-current (Keung 1989). It should not be too surprising to find, therefore, that the density of the calcium antagonist binding sites is enhanced under these conditions (Table 5.2). There are, however, some exceptions. For example, hearts from young (about two months old) cardiomyopathic hamsters exhibit a relatively normal binding site density, but by the time these animals are four to six months old (Table 5.2) the levels have increased, sometimes quite dramatically. In adult cardiomyopathic patients the levels are also relatively high (Table 5.2), but whether this is causally related to the development of the myopathy, or an innocent consequence, is unknown.

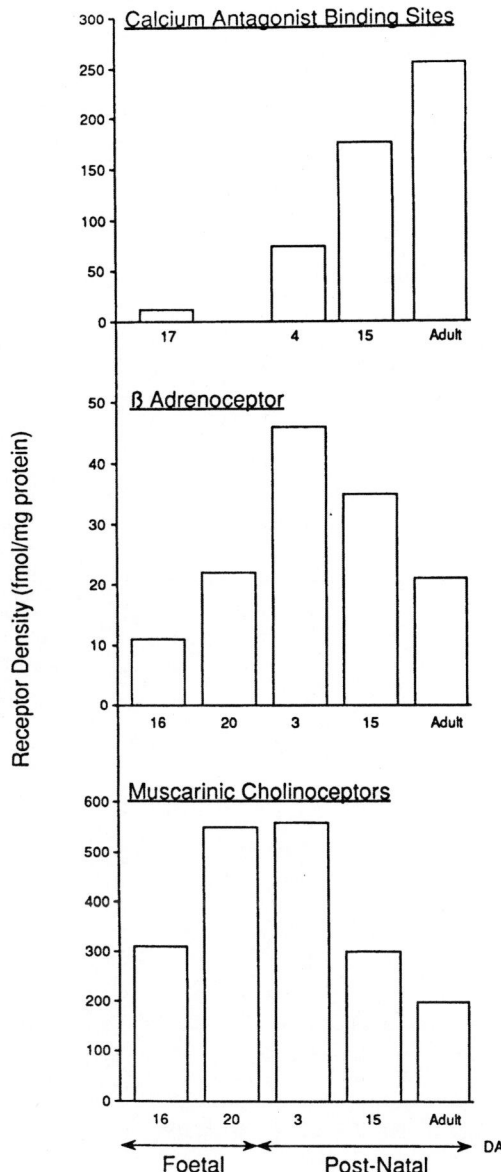

Fig. 5.1. Effect of development on the density of cardiac calcium antagonist binding sites, and β-adrenoceptor (labelled with [³H]-dihydroalprenolol), and muscarinic (labelled with [³H]-quinuclidinyl benzilate) receptors in rat cardiac cell membranes. (Data for β-adrenoceptor and muscarinic receptors from Kojima et al. 1990.)

Hence, *age*, and *cardiomyopathies* provide two examples of conditions which result in, or are associated with, "up" regulation of the cardiac calcium antagonist binding sites. However, the reverse phenomenon – viz, *"down"* regulation – also occurs; ischaemia is one of the causes.

Table 5.2. Calcium antagonist binding site density in cardiomyopathic hearts

Model	Percentage increase (relative to control)	Reference
Cardiomyopathic Hamster		
Age: 50–60 days	No change	Howlett and Gordon 1987
4 months	50%	Finkel et al. 1987a, 1987b
4–6 months	50%	Finkel et al. 1987a, 1987b
Human		
Adult	162%	Finkel et al. 1988
Adult	33%	Wagner et al. 1989

Table 5.3. Effect of ischaemia and hypoxia on cardiac and brain calcium antagonist binding site density

Tissue	Condition	Percentage change in binding site density	Reference
Cardiac			
Rat heart	Global ischaemia	↓83%	Dillon and Nayler 1987
	Hypoxia	↓52%	Nayler et al. 1985
Guinea pig heart	Hypoxia	↓73%	Matucci et al. 1987
Brain			
Rat hippocampus	Ischaemia	↑62%	Magnoni et al. 1988
Gerbil frontal cortex	Ischaemia	↓63%	Kenny et a. 1986

↑ denotes an increase, and ↓ a decrease, relative to control

Ischaemia as a Cause of "Down" Regulation

Data relating to the effect of ischaemia on the density of cardiac and other calcium antagonist binding sites is summarized in Table 5.3. Brain and cortex, and cardiac myocytes respond in the same way – by "down" regulating their binding sites. The hippocampus, (Table 5.3), however, responds in the opposite manner. Obviously, therefore, there is some degree of tissue specificity in the response (Ferrante and Triggle 1990).

The ischaemia-induced decrease in cardiac calcium antagonist binding site density reaches significant proportions within twenty five minutes of ischaemia, rapidly reaches asymptote, persists (Fig. 5.2) and is not accompanied by any change

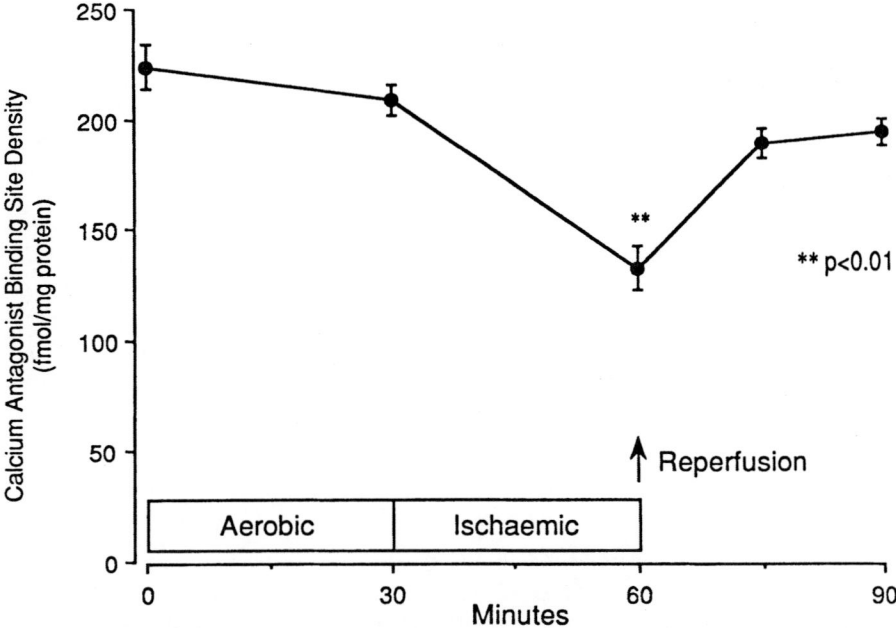

Fig. 5.2. Effect of global ischaemia on the density of rat cardiac calcium antagonist binding sites – using [^{3}H]-PN200-100 (Isradipine) as a marker. Note that upon reperfusion the density of binding returned towards more normal values

in selectivity (Nayler et al. 1985). The rapidity with which this "down" regulation occurs makes it difficult to account for in terms other than receptor internalization. Under physiological conditions about three quarters of the high affinity calcium antagonist binding sites (receptors) are located in the plasma membrane. The remainder are associated with a so-called "light membrane fraction" – an intracellular pool of membranes which lack the classical membrane markers. Presumably ischaemic conditions disturb the balance between the plasma membrane and the light-membrane content of these binding sites, favouring their retention in the light fraction (Fig. 5.3). Reperfusion (Fig. 5.2) seems to rectify this situation.

Why ischaemia alters calcium antagonist binding sites density is unclear at the moment. Certainly such an effect could not have been anticipated, because other receptors (β-adrenoceptors, α-adrenoceptors and endothelin-1 binding sites) move in the opposite direction, as described below. Acidosis and energy depletion have been shown *not* to be responsible (Gu et al. 1989a), and since reperfusion results in the rapid recovery of a normal binding site density oxyradicals are probably not involved. If this had been the case then reperfusion should have exacerbated the problem, because it is accompanied by a burst of oxyradical production (Zweier et al. 1987a). Whatever the cause, the end-result is an ischaemia-induced reduction in available calcium antagonist binding sites. This does not necessarily mean that the *number of calcium channels* has been reduced because, as described in Chapter 3,

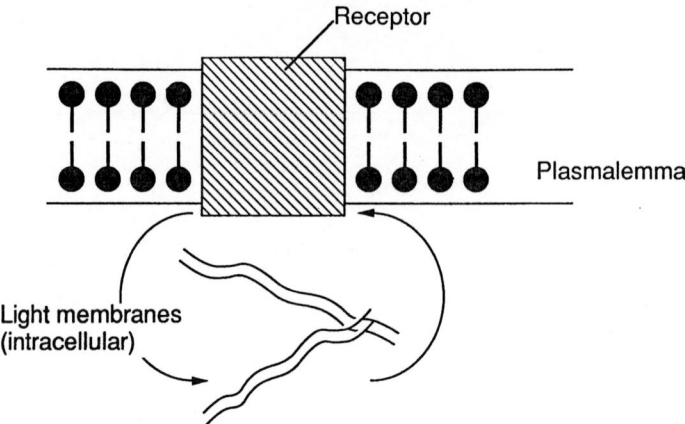

Fig. 5.3. Schematic representation of the events involved in receptor externalization and internalization

not all of the calcium antagonist binding sites are associated with the $alpha_1$ subunits of the channel complex. Some seem to be located in other parts of the membrane where, as described in Chapter 4, they apparently function as voltage sensors, relaying information to the junctional feet of the sarcoplasmic reticulum. Maybe it is these receptors, and not those which are housed in the $alpha_1$ subunit of the channel complex which "down-regulate".

Effect of Ischaemia on Other Cardiac Receptors

Adrenergic Receptors

Myocardial ischaemia induces the release of considerable quantities of endogenous catecholamines – mainly noradrenaline (Schomig 1990) – an effect which theoretically should result in the desensitization and internalization of the adrenoceptors (Strasser et al. 1990). This does not happen, however. Despite extracellular concentrations of noradrenaline reaching levels one hundred to one thousand times greater than normal (Schomig 1990) ischaemia causes a gradual *increase* in cardiac β- (Strasser et al. 1990; Thandroyen et al. 1990) and α- (Corr et al. 1981) adrenoceptor density. Once again, this increase reflects a redistribution of receptors between the plasma membrane and the intracellular light-membrane fraction and *not* de novo synthesis (Maisel et al. 1986). As far as the β-adrenoceptors are concerned the externalization process is blunted by propranolol.

Endothelin-1 Binding Sites (Receptors)

Cardiac cell membranes contain specific high affinity binding sites for the polypeptide, endothelin-1 (Nayler 1990). The physiological and pharmacological

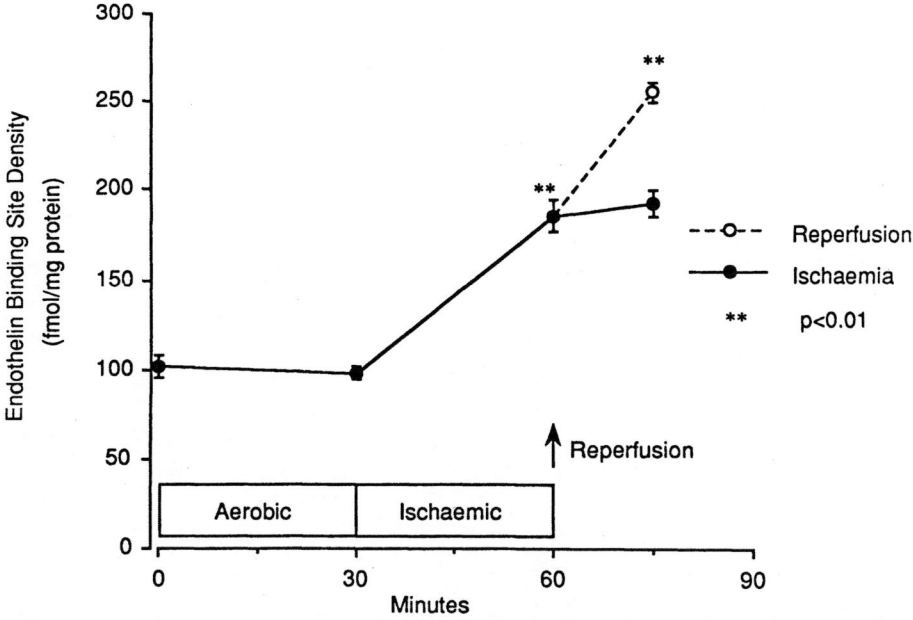

Fig. 5.4. Effect of global ischaemia, at 37 °C, and subsequent reperfusion, on the density of cardiac endothelin-1 binding sites. Note that whereas ischaemia caused an increase in the density of the endothelin-1 binding sites (Liu et al. 1990), the density of the calcium antagonist binding sites declines (Fig. 5.2) – as if there is a "push-pull" or yin-yan system in operation

properties of this polypeptide are described in Chapter 7. The topic is mentioned here only to provide another example of a membrane-located receptor which becomes externalized during ischaemia. In many ways the response resembles that of the adrenoceptors, in that it is triggered by relatively short periods of ischaemia and involves externalization rather than de novo synthesis (Liu et al. 1990; Nayler et al. 1990a; 1990b). There are some differences, however, because whereas reperfusion results in the prompt restoration of normal α- and β-adrenoceptor density at the cell surface, in the case of the endothelin-1 receptor there is a further externalization (Fig. 5.4). Curiously, both the ischaemia and reperfusion-induced externalization of the endothelin-1 receptor is markedly attenuated by calcium antagonist pretreatment (Chapter 7) – an effect which may contribute to the cardioprotective effect of these drugs.

In general, therefore, and as Figure 5.5 shows, although the density of cardiac β- and α-adrenoceptors, and endothelin-1 receptors *increases* during ischaemia, calcium antagonist binding sites behave in the opposite manner, with a *reduction* in density. The failure of the β-adrenoceptors to internalize in response to ischaemia – and therefore to mimic the behaviour of the calcium antagonist binding sites in this respect – cannot be explained in terms of an inability to internalize, because this is exactly what happens when a cholesterol-rich diet is consumed (Tsuji et al. 1987), or the receptors are persistently stimulated (Chuang et al. 1980).

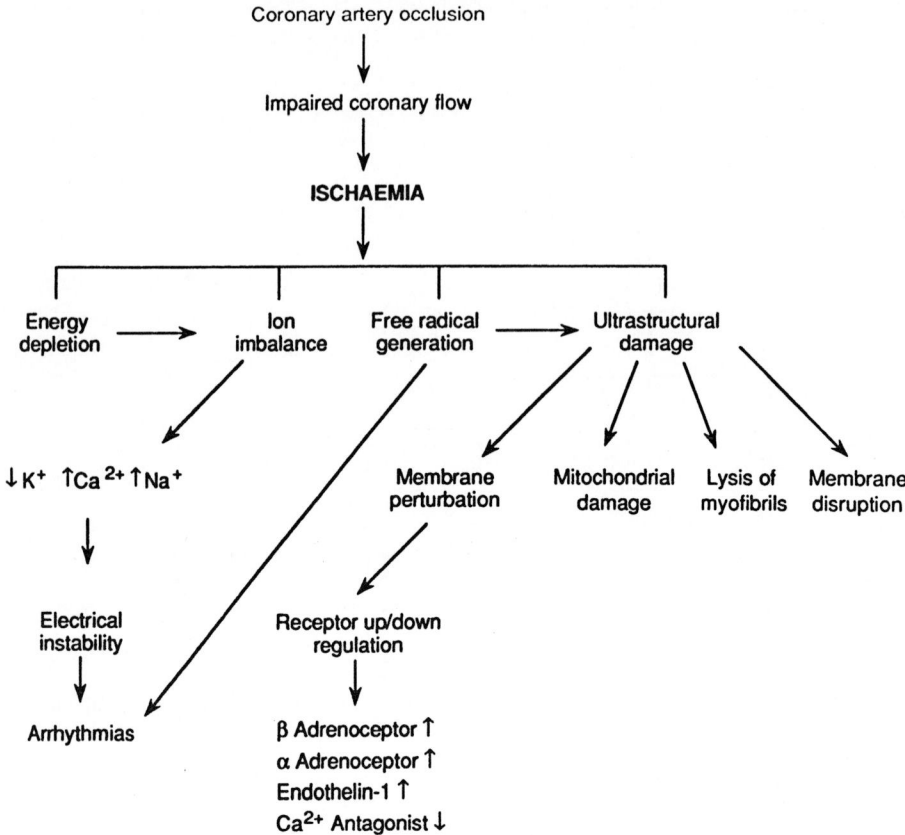

Fig. 5.5. Schematic representation of the consequences of inadequate coronary perfusion, including the resultant changes in cardiac receptor density. ↑ denotes an increase, and ↓ a decrease, relative to controls

Effect of Drugs and Chemicals
on Calcium Antagonist Binding Site Density

Physiological changes and pathological conditions are not the only factors which modulate calcium antagonist binding site density. Some drugs, including morphine, alcohol, reserpine and 6-hydroxydopamine have such an effect.

Morphine

Prolonged treatment with morphine increases the dihydropyridine binding site density in some areas of the brain (Ramkumar and El-Fakahany 1984; 1988) but in others, such as the cortex and cerebellum (Pillai and Ross 1987), the levels fall.

Alcohol (Ethanol)

Chronic alcohol consumption "up" regulates the calcium antagonist binding sites (Brennan et al. 1989) and, as can be seen from Figure 5.6, it is not only the brain which is affected!

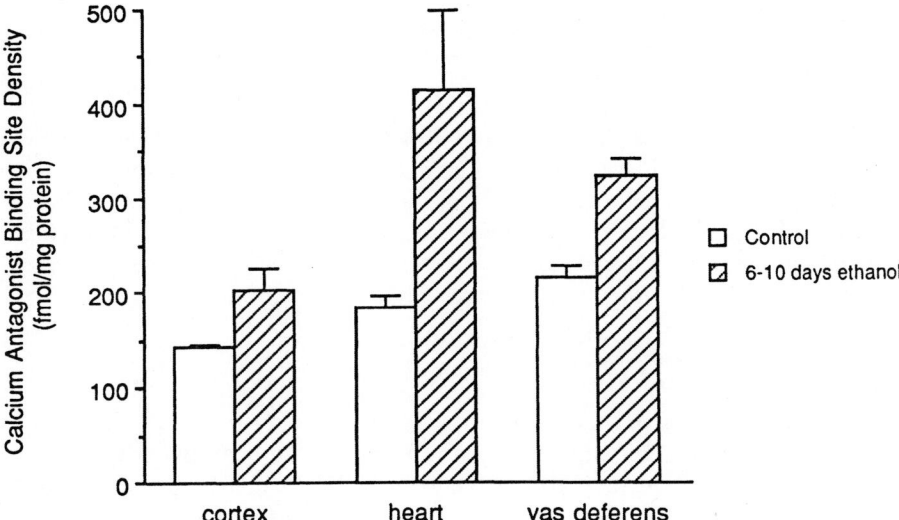

Fig. 5.6. Effect of orally administered alcohol on calcium antagonist binding site density (using tritiated nitrendipine as a marker) in rat cortical, heart and vas deferens membranes. (Data from Brennan et al. 1989.)

Table 5.4. Effect of alcohol on density (B_{max}) of calcium antagonist binding sites in the brain

Treatment regime	Tissue	% change (↑) in B_{max}	Reference
7 days alcohol	Rat brain	↑50%	Dolin et al. 1987
25 days alcohol	Rat brain	↑55%	Lucchi et al. 1985
40 min alcohol	Rat cortex,	↑36%	Rius et al. 1987b
	hippocampus and	↑33%	Rius et al. 1987b
	striatum	↑52%	Rius et al. 1987b

Radioactively labelled nitrendipine and nimodipine were used to establish the density of the calcium antagonist binding sites. The alcohol-induced increase in binding site density was abolished upon alcohol withdrawal, the levels returning to control values. Ca^{2+}-uptake studies showed that the newly externalized receptors were functional. Where ↑ denotes an increase relative to control rats maintained on a normal diet

Reserpine

Chronic reserpine administration (3–5 days) causes a small decrease (22 percent) in cardiac dihydropyridine binding site density (labelled with tagged nimodipine), at a time when β-adrenoceptor density is enhanced (Ramkumar and El-Fakahany 1986). Here, then is another example of a situation in which the cardiac calcium antagonist binding sites and β-adrenoceptors move in opposite directions – the one internalizing whilst the other externalizes.

6-Hydroxydopamine

This agent is often used experimentally to deplete the endogenous catecholamines. Whether this effect is a direct or indirect consequence of its administration has yet to be determined, but the same concentrations that are used to catecholamine deplete also increase the dihydropyridine binding site density (labelled with radioactive nitrendipine) in both brain (Sanna et al. 1986; Bolger et al. 1987) and cardiac (Renaud et al. 1984; Skattebol and Triggle 1986) cell membranes.

Calcium antagonists

Prolonged intravenous nifedipine can "down" regulate dihydropyridine binding sites in rat heart and brain membranes (Gengo et al. 1988b) but the specificity of the effect must be questioned, because other membrane-located receptors also down regulate (Gengo et al. 1988b). There is other evidence which supports the notion that prolonged calcium antagonist therapy (dihydropyridine- or phenylalkylamine-based antagonists) may cause some "down" regulation – at least in the brain (Panza et al. 1985). The lack of any significant tachyphylaxis as far as the cardiovascular system is concerned probably reflects the existence of "spare" receptors – or a tissue specific response – because "down" regulation is usually associated with loss of sensitivity. Since the use of long-acting calcium antagonists means that the calcium antagonist binding sites will be continuously "bombarded" by these drugs the absence of marked tachyphylaxis is surprising, but important, the more so because of the need to use these drugs long-term (as in the management of hypertension) and sometimes prophylactically – as in the management of patients with coronary artery disease.

Lead

Chronic lead exposure "up" regulates the density of the calcium antagonist binding sites, particularly in the brain (cortex and striatum), where increases of approximately fifty percent occur (Rius et al. 1986; 1987a). One wonders what this might do to brain function!

Table 5.5. Conditions which "up" and "down" regulate calcium antagonist binding site density

Condition	Change in binding site density	Reference
Ischaemia	↓	Nayler et al. 1985
Hypertension	↑	Sharma et al. 1986
Cardiomyopathy	↑	Wagner et al. 1986
Denervation	↑	Schmid et al. 1984
Hypothyroidism	↓	Hawthorn et al. 1988
Hyperthyroidism	↑	Hawthorn et al. 1988
Lead intoxication	↑	Rius et al. 1987a
Reserpine	↓	Ramkumar and El-Fakahany 1986
6-Hydroxydopamine	↑	Skattebol and Triggle 1986
Chronic calcium antagonist therapy	↓	Gengo et al. 1988b

Where ↑ denotes an increase and ↓ a decrease in the high affinity binding site density. As a general rule these changes occurred without significant changes in affinity or selectivity

The Effect of Other Physiological Interventions

The examples of drug-induced "up" and "down" regulation of calcium antagonist binding sites which have been given so far should be sufficient proof of the fact that these binding sites resemble other receptors in undergoing "up" and "down" regulation. The only physiological intervention which has been mentioned so far, however, is that of ischaemia – which causes "down" regulation. Other interventions are just as effective. For example, thyroxine-induced hypothyroidism "down" regulates, and propylthiouracil-induced hyperthyroidism "up" regulates these binding sites in cardiac and vascular smooth muscle cells (Hawthorn et al. 1988). Denervation causes "up" regulation (Schmid et al. 1984) – at least in skeletal muscle. Persistent hypertension acts in the same way, causing "up" regulation in the brain and the heart (Chatelain et al. 1984; Sharma et al. 1986; Ishi et al. 1986, and Table 5.5).

In Summary

1. Calcium antagonist binding sites (high affinity and therefore physiologically significant) resemble other receptors in exhibiting reversible "up" and "down" regulation.
2. Conditions which cause "up" regulation include hypertension, cardiomyopathy, denervation, hyperthyroidism, lead intoxication, alcohol and 6-hydroxydopamine.
3. Conditions which cause "down" regulation include ischaemia, hypothyroidism, reserpine and chronic calcium antagonist therapy.

4. The rapidity with which these changes take place, and their rapid reversibility, indicate that only a proportion of the tissue's total store of calcium antagonist binding sites are available at the cell surface at any one time.

5. Since tachyphylaxis is not encountered to any significant extent during long-term use of the first or second generation calcium antagonists, some of the receptors which "down" regulate when exposed to calcium antagonists must be either "spare" receptors, or receptors which are not housed in the alpha$_1$ subunit of the calcium channel complex.

Chapter 6

Oxyradical-Induced Lipid Peroxidation:
Do Calcium Antagonists Provide any Protection?

"They make it a wilderness, and call it peace"
from "Agricola", by TACITUS, 98 A.D.

Oxyradicals are highly reactive metabolites of molecular oxygen (O_2) which, if allowed to accumulate, cause havoc. It is now widely believed that they contribute to the aetiology of a variety of cardiovascular disorders – including reperfusion-induced arrhythmias (Bernier and Hearse 1988), post-ischaemic reperfusion injury (Meerson et al. 1982; McCord 1985; Thompson and Hess 1986; Simpson and Lucchesi 1987; Henry et al. 1990b), myocardial stunning (Bolli 1990), as well as inflammation (Thompson and Hess 1986), atherosclerosis (Southorn and Powis 1988) and even anthracycline drug-induced toxicity (Milei et al. 1986). Needless to say they are also implicated in the aetiology of other disorders not directly associated with the cardiovascular system – disorders which range from general inflammatory responses (McCord 1983) to fibroplasia in neonates (Feher et al. 1987) to drug and alcohol-induced hepatotoxicity (Shaw et al. 1981; Ryle 1984), and even to skeletal muscle injury caused by sustained tetanic contraction (Zebra et al. 1990). Even the central nervous system does not escape (Demopoulos et al. 1980). However, irrespective of the nature of the target organ (heart, blood vessels, brain, liver etc.), oxyradicals provoke irreversible injury because they cause peroxidation of lipid-containing membranes, and proteins. As far as the lipid-containing membranes are concerned, peroxidation of their lipids results in increased membrane fluidity resulting, in turn, in increased permeability and loss of integrity – both of which are undesirable end-points. Proteins are likewise affected, and the results are just as undesirable, particularly if an enzyme is involved – because it results in their partial or complete inactivation.

During the past decade, and probably once it became evident that oxyradicals are implicated in so many clinical disorders (Thompson and Hess 1986; Lucchesi 1990; Bolli 1990), there has been an escalation of interest in them, particularly with respect to:
(i)   their chemistry;
(ii) where they are produced;
(iii) the nature of the injury they cause, and
(iv) the identification and mode of action of agents which, for whatever reason, attenuate the damage they induce.

Chemistry and Production of the Oxyradicals

As stated at the beginning of this chapter, oxyradicals are reactive molecules derived by the univalent reduction of molecular oxygen (McCord 1985). Members of the group include:
(i)   the superoxide anion $.O_2^-$;
(ii) an intermediary, H_2O_2, and
(iii) the hydroxyl radical, $.OH$;

Because the $.OH$ and $.O_2^-$ radicals both have unpaired electrons in their orbits they are highly reactive. As far as their relative toxicities are concerned $.OH > .O_2^- >> H_2O_2$.

The Superoxide Anion, $.O_2^-$

This is produced by the univalent reduction of molecular oxygen (O_2), as follows:

$$O_2 \xrightarrow{\ e^- \ } .O_2^-,$$

with the superoxide anion $(.O_2^-)$ being formed with the acceptance of the first electron (e^-). The $.O_2^-$ radical is then free to act as either a reducing or an oxidizing agent – an aqueous environment favours a reducing action but under hydrophobic conditions – such as occurs in cell membranes – an oxidizing activity is preferred.

Hydrogen Peroxide

Dismutation of the superoxide anion $(.O_2^-)$ produces another reactive oxygen species, H_2O_2. The reaction involves the enzyme superoxide dismutase (SOD) as follows:

$$.O_2^- + .O_2^- + 2H^+ \xrightarrow{\ SOD \ } H_2O_2 + O_2.$$

Under normal physiological conditions H_2O_2 is seldom left to accumulate. Instead it is reduced to water by reactions involving either catalase or glutathione peroxidase, as follows:

$$2H_2O_2 \xrightarrow{\ catalase \ } 2H_2O + O_2,$$

or

$$H_2O_2 \xrightarrow{\ glutathione\ peroxidase \ } \text{oxidized glutathione} + 2H_2O.$$

Under some pathological conditions, however, this safety net fails – mainly because the tissue supplies of the catalase and peroxidase enzymes have been depleted. This happens, for example, during prolonged episodes of ischaemia.

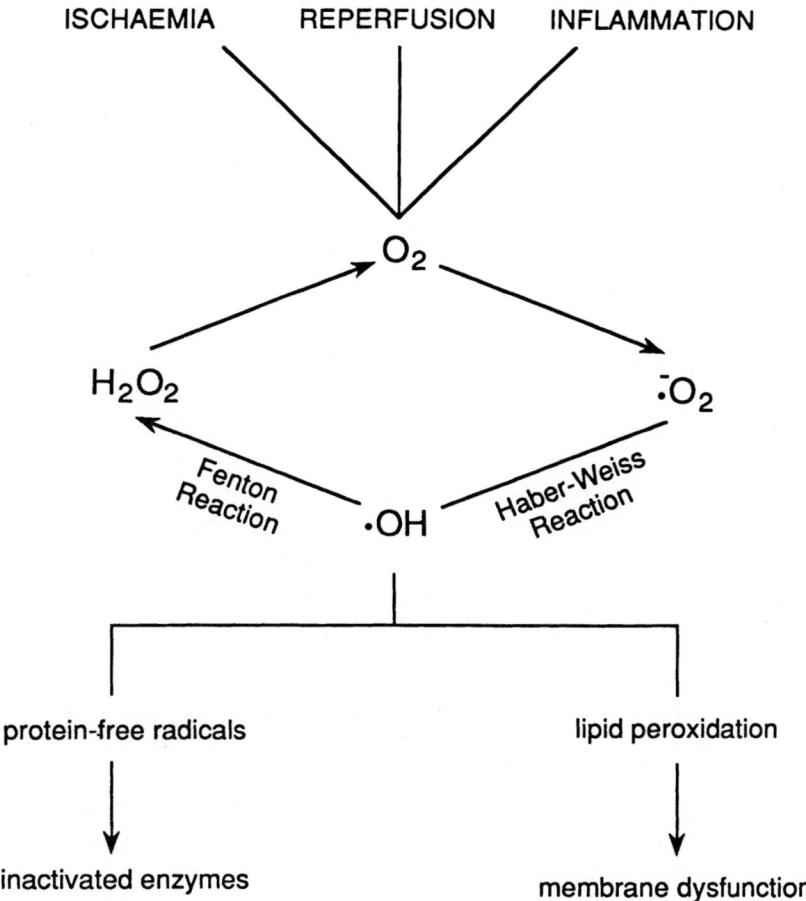

Fig. 6.1. Schematic representation of the events involved in and the consequences of uncontrolled oxyradical production

The Hydroxyl Radical (.OH)

The major danger associated with the accumulation of H_2O_2 is that it can be metabolized to yield the highly reactive and unstable .OH radical. This can occur in two ways – by the Haber-Weiss reaction, involving a metal chelate as follows:

$$Me^{n+} \text{ chelate} + .O_2^- \rightarrow Me^{(n-1)} \text{ chelate} + O_2$$

$$Me^{(n-1)} \text{ chelate} + H_2O_2 \rightarrow Me^{n+} \text{ chelate} + OH^- + .OH, \text{ or}$$

the Fenton reaction. This is iron dependent, and proceeds as follows:

$$Fe^{3+} + H_2O_2 \rightarrow Fe^{2+} + OH^- + .OH.$$

The .OH radicals which are formed in this way are particularly toxic, because they are destructive radicals which abstract hydrogen ions from unsaturated fatty acid side chains and from proteins, and in so doing initiate reactions which terminate in lipid peroxidation, protein degradation (Fig. 6.1) and cell death.

Sites of Oxyradical Production

As far as the heart is concerned there are a multiplicity of sites at which oxyradicals are produced. They include:
(i)   the sarcoplasmic reticulum (Hess et al. 1981);
(ii)   the mitochondria, particularly if the intramitochondrial electron transport system is deranged – as happens during ischaemia, and post-ischaemic reperfusion, for example (Nohl 1987), or during hypoxia;
(iii) aggregating neutrophils (Lucchesi 1990). It may be of interest to note that nicotine potentiates $.O_2^-$ production by neutrophils (Jay et al. 1986), even at concentrations equivalent to that found in blood plasma of smokers! Maybe this is why smoking is a risk factor as far as the cardiovascular system is concerned. Returning to sites of oxyradical production there are other sites of production, including
(iv)   sites which favour the autoxidation of catecholamines, and
(v)   the endothelium (Lucchesi 1990). Here oxyradical production may involve:
       (a) arachidonic acid metabolism, and
       (b) a xanthine oxidase induced catabolism of hypoxanthine – as shown in Figure 6.2. This method of production may not be very relevant to the human heart, however, because the human heart only contains extraordinarily small amounts of xanthine oxidase (Grum et al. 1989).

Oxyradicals, therefore are widely produced, both intracellularly and extracellularly.

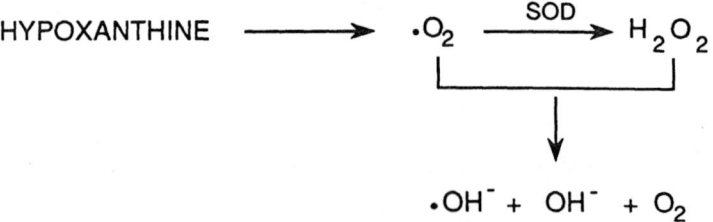

Fig. 6.2. The production of $.O_2^-$, $.H_2O_2$ and .OH from hypoxanthine. $.O_2^-$ and H_2O_2 interact, in the presence of catalytic iron, to generate .OH by way of the Haber Weiss reaction. $.O_2^-$(superoxide anion), .OH(hydroxyl radical), H_2O_2(hydrogen peroxide)

Table 6.1. Mechanisms normally involved in controlling oxyradical accumulation

1. *Degradative enzymes*
   e.g.   superoxide dismutase $(.O_2^- \rightarrow H_2O_2 + O_2)$
           catalase $(H_2O_2 \rightarrow H_2O + 1/2\,O_2)$
           glutathione peroxidase $(H_2O_2 \rightarrow 2H_2O)$

2. *Antioxidants*
   e.g.   ascorbic acid (vitamin C)
           vitamins E, K
           thiols
           ubiquinone (coenzyme Q – a constituent of the mitochondrial respiratory chain)

3. *Scavengers*
   e.g.   glucose
           mannitol
           vitamin E

Protective Mechanisms

If oxyradicals are so widely produced, and are such reactive molecules (McCord 1985) then it could have been anticipated that tissues which are capable of generating them would contain systems geared towards controlling their production, or reducing their toxicity. Under normal physiological conditions such systems do exist. They can be divided into three main categories – *degradative enzymes*, *antioxidants*, and *scavengers*.

1. *Degradative enzymes.* These include the *superoxide dismutase* (SOD) enzyme, the enzyme which catalyzes the dismutation of $.O_2^-$ to H_2O_2 $(2.O_2^- + 2H^+ \rightarrow O_2 + H_2O_2)$, and the *catalase* (CAT) and *glutathione peroxidase* enzymes, both of which degrade H_2O_2 to $H_2O + O_2$ (Table 6.1).

2. *Antioxidants* (Table 6.1). Members of this group protect against the toxicity caused by the interaction of the oxyradicals and their intermediaries with other systems, including lipid-containing membranes. Vitamins E and K, and the ubiquinones belong here.

3. *Scavengers* – so called because they "disarm" the oxyradicals by interacting with them. Examples include (Table 6.1) mannitol and glucose (both of which scavenge .OH) and vitamin E – a natural scavenger for $.O_2^-$.

Mode of Action

Because oxygen-centred free radicals contain an unpaired electron they react with almost all tissues – and particularly if SH-containing aminoacids or unsaturated fatty acids are present. The consequences include:

(i)   peroxidation of membrane phospholipids – a process which renders normally impermeable membranes freely permeable and fragile;

(ii) denaturation of proteins – with a resultant loss of structure and inactivation of enzymes (Fig. 6.3, and Table 6.2);

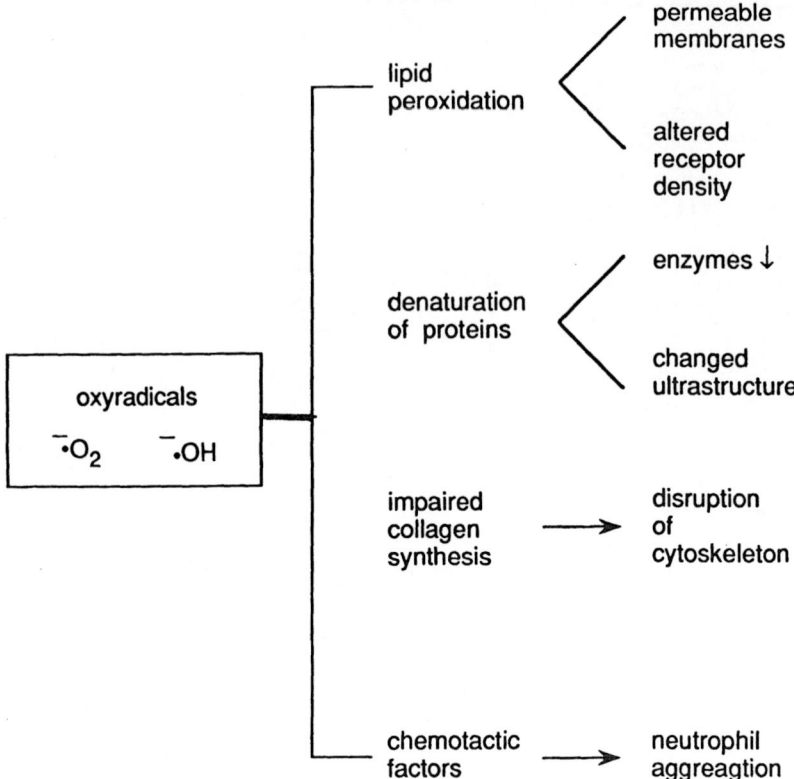

Fig. 6.3. Schematic representation of some of the consequences of oxyradical activity

Table 6.2. Cellular actions of oxyradicals

Cardiac tissue	Response	Reference
Proteins	Denatured	Davies 1987
Collagen synthesis	Slowed	Davies 1987
Membranes	Made hyperpermeable by lipid peroxidation	Thompson and Hess 1986 Yamada et al. 1990
Cardiac enzymes and exchangers		
Sarcolemmal		
(i) Na^+-K^{++} ATPase	Activity diminished	Kramer et al. 1984
(ii) Ca^{2+} ATPase	Activity diminished	Kaneko et al. 1989
(iii) Na^+:Ca^{2+} exchanger	Activity increased	Reeves et al. 1986
Cardiac sarcoplasmic reticulum		
(i) Ca^{2+} uptake	Slowed	Rowe et al. 1983 Thompson and Hess 1986
(ii) Ca^{2+} Mg^{2+} ATPase activity	Reduced	Thompson and Hess 1986
Cardiac Myofibrils		
Ca^{2+} sensitivity	Reduced	Przyklenk et al. 1990

(iii) impaired collagen synthesis – resulting in disruption of the cytoskeleton (Davies 1987), and

(iv) the generation of chemotactic factors, some of which encourage neutrophils to adhere to sites of vessel wall injury (Lucchesi 1990). These adhering neutrophils then proceed to invade the underlying tissue where they contribute to the processes involved in the formation of atherosclerotic lesions (Chapter 11). They themselves release cytotoxins – some of which are oxyradicals. Even under the best of circumstances, therefore, the adherence of neutrophils to the vessel wall is likely to be hazardous (Jackson et al. 1986) and to result, in the short term, in injury, and in the long term, contribute to the factors which are involved in the generation of atherosclerotic lesions (Chapter 11).

Evidence of Oxyradical Production in the Heart

Under certain circumstances, and particularly during ischaemia (Rao et al. 1983) and post-ischaemic reperfusion (Garlick et al. 1987; Bolli 1990; Ferrari et al. 1990), the heart is an avid producer of oxyradicals – and the human heart is no exception! There are several different ways of monitoring oxyradical production – one direct, others indirect. The direct method involves using electron paramagnetic resonance spectroscopy (EPR) together with a spin trap agent – such as α phenyl N-tert-butylnitrone (PBN). Bolli and his colleagues (Bolli et al. 1988; 1989) used this technique when they were monitoring the production of oxyradicals during myocardial ischaemia, and the rapid burst of production which occurs upon reperfusion. The other methods involve monitoring the production of one of the products of lipid peroxidation – usually malondialdehyde (MDA), a peroxidation product of polyunsaturated fatty acids. Some investigators use chemical assays to monitor malondialdehyde production; others use chemiluminescent techniques (Henry et al. 1990a; 1990b).

In hearts which contain xanthine oxidase it is relatively easy to see why the catabolism of hypoxanthine provides an important source of oxyradicals during conditions of impaired perfusion, because:

(i)   ischaemia (or hypoxia) favours the conversion of a relatively inactive xanthine dehydrogenase enzyme to the active xanthine oxidase form (Fig. 6.4);

(ii)   *secondly*, a xanthine-based substrate is needed and under ischaemic conditions this is provided by the catabolism of adenosine triphosphate and its subsequent degradation to inosine and hypoxanthine, as shown in Fig. 6.4;

(iii) *thirdly*, the intracellular defence mechanisms – including superoxide dismutase – and glutathione peroxidase – are massively depleted during ischaemia (Ferrari et al. 1985).

Since the human heart is relatively deficient in xanthine oxidase alternative sources of oxyfree radical production must be activated to generate the free radicals which accumulate during ischaemia, and upon reperfusion. Probably the autoxidation of the released catecholamines (Schomig 1990), and disturbances of the mitochondrial *electron transport chain* assume a more significant role. Irrespective of where they

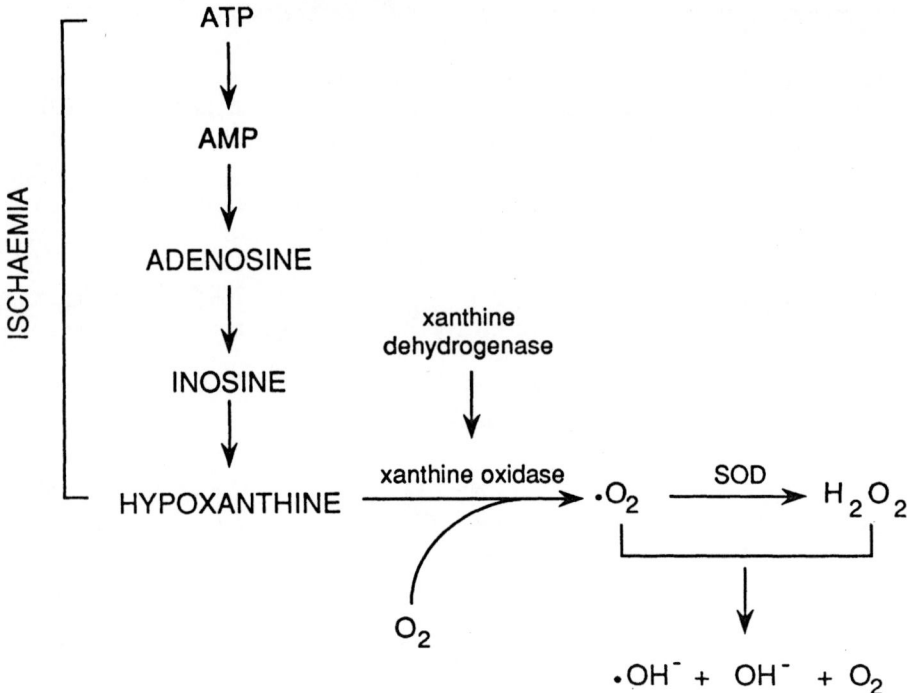

Fig. 6.4. Schematic representation of the production of .OH and .O$_2^-$ from hypoxanthine during ischaemia and postischaemic reperfusion. During ischaemia the adenine nucleotides are degraded to hypoxanthine and if the tissue contains xanthine oxidase the hypoxanthine is usually rapidly degraded to .O$_2^-$. In some species, but not in man, xanthine oxidase is concentrated in the endothelial cells

are produced, however, there is no longer any doubt concerning the ability of in situ hearts to generate oxyfree radicals during conditions of oxidative stress (Ferrari et al. 1990). Nor is there any lingering doubt concerning their ability to provoke lethal injury.

Oxyradical-Induced Injury

At the cellular level activated oxygen species (oxyradicals) are capable of causing widespread havoc, mainly because they:
(i)   cause lipid peroxidation (oxidative deterioration of the polyunsaturated fatty acid components of membranes) (Thompson and Hess 1986);
(ii) denature proteins (Davies 1987);
(iii) inactivate enzymes (Davies 1987);
(iv) slow collagen synthesis (Davies 1987), and
(v)   either increase (as is the case for the endothelin-1 receptor in cardiac muscle cell membranes (Fig. 6.5)) or decrease (as is the case for β-adrenoceptors (Kramer et al. 1986)) the availability of membrane-located receptors.

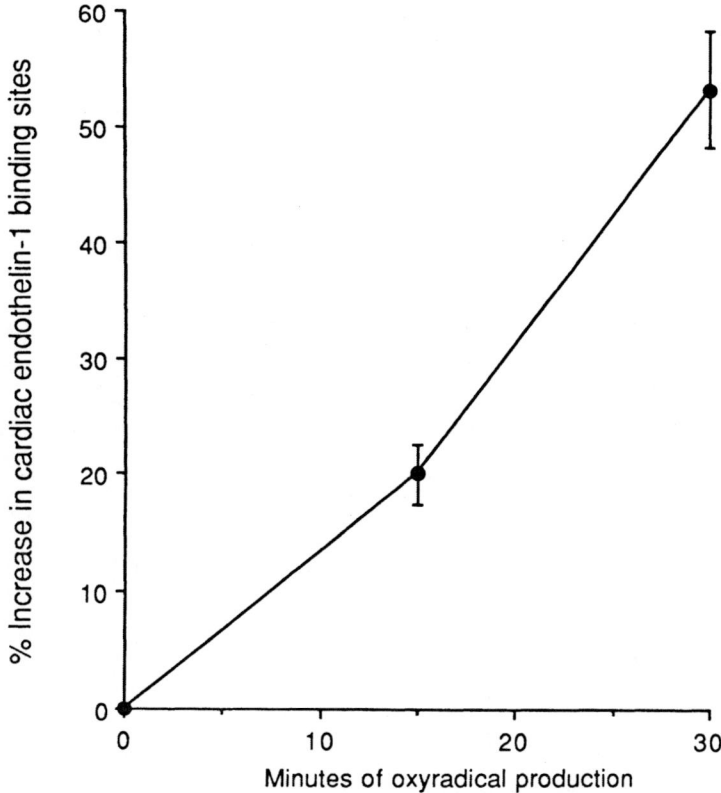

Fig. 6.5. Effect of oxyradical generation (from purine base plus xanthine oxidase) on endothelin-1 binding sites on rat cardiac cell membranes. The xanthine oxidase (0.01 units/ml) and purine substrate (2.3mM purine) were added to the coronary perfusion circuit 15 or 30 minutes before the membranes were harvested and assayed for high affinity ^{125}1-endothelin binding site density. (Data provided by Dr. J. Liu, University of Melbourne.)

As far as the myocardium is concerned the consequences of uncontrolled oxyradical formation and accumulation can be quite devastating. The sarcolemma becomes hyperpermeable, and in addition exhibits a slowed $Na^+ K^+$ ATPase (Kramer et al. 1984), a slowed Ca^{2+}-activated ATPase (Kaneko et al. 1989) and an enhanced $Na^+:Ca^{2+}$ exchange activity (Reeves et al. 1986). As Figure 6.6 shows these changes alone could cause excessive Ca^{2+} accumulation, and more so, if they are parallelled by a reduced availability of energy (as ATP). Moreover, since the $Ca^{2+}Mg^{2+}$ ATPase and Ca^{2+} accumulating activity of the sarcoplasmic reticulum is reduced (Thompson and Hess 1986; Rowe et al. 1983) the excess Ca^{2+} is likely to remain in the cytosol where presumably it is free to activate any Ca^{2+}-sensitive proteases and phospholipases which are still functional. Even this is not the end of the story, however, since either because of a direct consequence of being exposed to oxyradicals (Przyklenk et al. 1990) or because of their denaturation by the Ca^{2+}-activated proteases, or simply *because they will have been exposed to excess* Ca^{2+} (Kitakaze et al. 1987) the

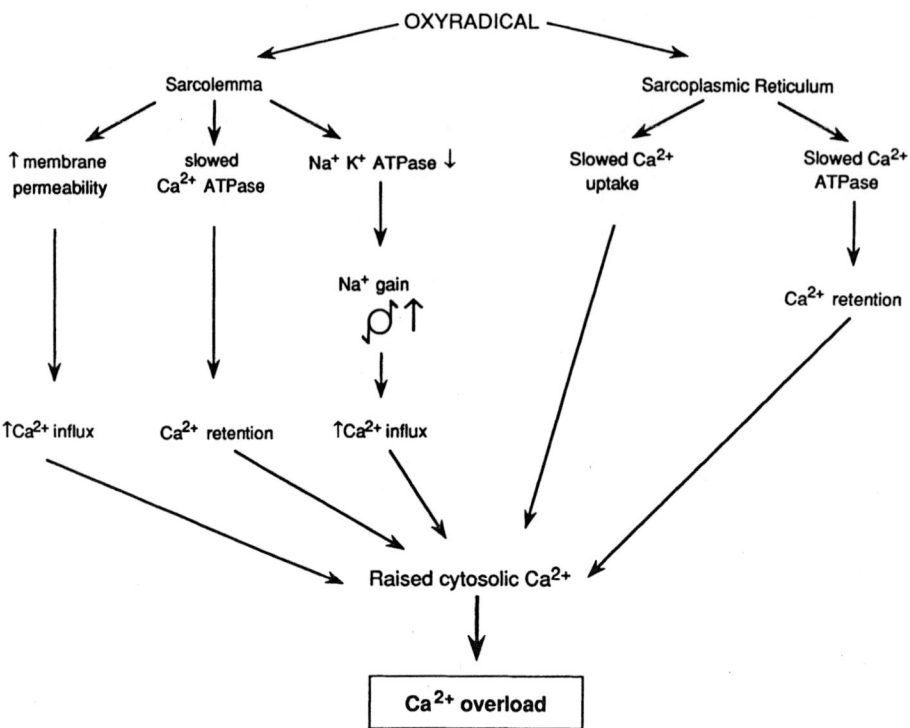

Fig. 6.6. Effect of oxyradicals on mechanisms responsible for maintaining Ca^{2+} homeostasis in cardiac myocytes. ↑ denotes an increase, and ↓ a decrease

contractile activity of the myofibrils declines, and they lose their sensitivity to Ca^{2+}. Other changes occur. For example, arrhythmias develop (Bernier and Hearse 1988) and the mitochondria become damaged – presumably as a direct result of lipid peroxidation. Nor does the vasculature escape injury. It's endothelium becomes hyperpermeable (Korthius et al. 1985; Yamada et al. 1990), neutrophil adhesion occurs (Lewis et al. 1988) – this may be an important event with regard to the initiation of atherogenic plaque formation – and the ability of the endothelial cells to generate prostacyclin is impaired (Whorton et al. 1985). Of equal importance is the change in shape of the endothelial cells (Hinshaw et al. 1989) – changing from flat, sheet-like layers of cells to cells which are "up-ended" – so that they protrude into the lumen of the associated blood vessel – or lymphatic.

In summary, therefore, and as summarized in Table 6.2 and Figure 6.6, the devastating effects of uncontrolled oxyradical generation and accumulation are such that it is difficult to see how affected cells can escape losing homeostasis with respect to Ca^{2+}. In many ways the situation resembles that of the proverbial "dog chasing its tail" – because calcium actually potentiates oxyradical-induced injury (Malis and Bonventre 1986)!

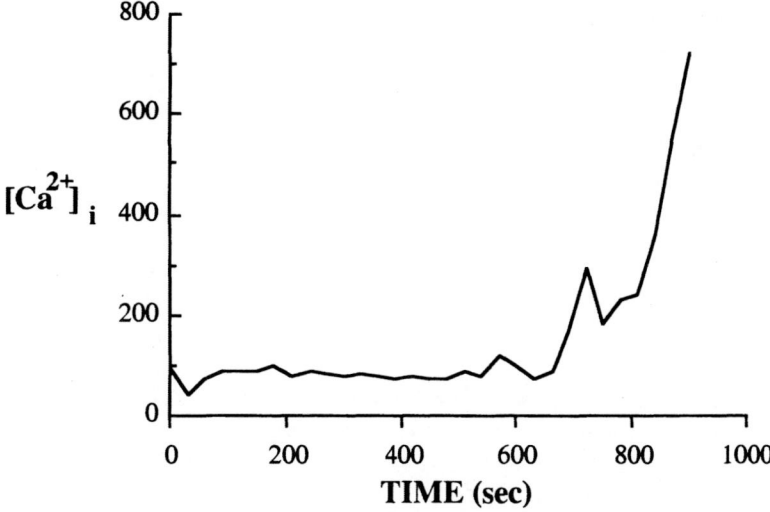

Fig. 6.7. Time-dependent changes in cytosolic free calcium in a single isolated rat cardiac myocyte loaded with Fura-2 and incubated with 1mM tert-butyl hydroperoxide (tBHP). The tBPH was added at time 0. An upward shift in the curve denotes an increase in cytosolic Ca^{2+}. (Data provided by Dr. M.J. Daly, University of Melbourne.)

Oxyradical-Induced Loss of Ca^{2+} Homeostasis

Having mentioned how the various control systems which are responsible for maintaining intracellular Ca^{2+} homeostasis respond to free radical exposure (Table 6.2 and Fig. 6.6) it would be unreasonable to assume that this did not result in a raised cytosolic Ca^{2+}, because Ca^{2+} ions will flood into the cell, along their concentration gradient and across the now permeabilized cell membrane. In addition suppression of the Na$^+$ K$^+$ ATPase enzyme (Fig. 6.6) will cause a temporary gain in Na$^+$, which can then exchange for Ca^{2+} by way of the Na$^+$:Ca^{2+} exchanger, the activity of which is actually enhanced under these conditions (Reeves et al. 1986). Moreover, there is now little chance of the Ca^{2+} which by now is collecting in the cytosol (Fig. 6.6) being transferred to the sarcoplasmic reticulum, because it, too, is now surrounded by "leaky" membranes and its Ca^{2+}-activated uptake pump will be working inefficiently, and at an abnormally slow rate. The end result can only be a raised cytosolic Ca^{2+}, an event which initiates cell death and tissue necrosis. The starting point, however, was either the excessive production of oxyradicals – or the failure of the retrieval systems. That oxyradical production does provoke a raised cytosolic Ca^{2+} is shown by Figure 6.7. Here an isolated cardiac myocyte was exposed to a free radical generating system under conditions which allowed a continuous measurement of cytosolic Ca^{2+} (using Fura-2, a Ca^{2+} sensitive fluorescent dye) to be made. Within ten minutes cytosolic Ca^{2+} had risen alarmingly. The record was terminated because the myocyte simply disintegrated!

Evidence of Excess Oxyradical Production During Myocardial Ischaemia and Post Ischaemic Reperfusion

Two approaches have been used to determine whether oxyradical production is enhanced during myocardial ischaemia and subsequent reperfusion: one indirect, and the other direct.

Indirect evidence of the production of these radicals comes from experiments in which agents such as superoxide dismutase, catalase, allopurinol and dimethyl-thiourea (Table 6.3) have been used as protective agents, with protection being gauged by improved functional and ultrastructural recovery during post-ischaemic reperfusion (Bolli 1990). Although indirect, results (Table 6.3) such as these indicate:

(i)   that oxygen metabolites are generated under these conditions;
(ii) that $.^-O_2$ and $.OH$ may both be involved, and
(iii) because so many systems can participate in the generation of these metabolites (xanthine oxidase, dissociation of the mitochondrial electron transport chain, activated neutrophils, arachidonic acid metabolism and autoxidation of a variety of compounds including the catecholamines (Table 6.4)), effective control of their production, or protection against the havoc they cause, may

Table 6.3. Agents which either limit oxyradical production, or act as scavengers

Agent	Action
A. Inhibition of Oxyradical Production	
1. *Superoxide dismutase* (SOD)	Catalyzes the dismutation of $.O_2^- \rightarrow O_2 + H_2O$
2. *Catalase* (CAT)	Converts $H_2O_2 \rightarrow O_2 + H_2O$
3. *Allopurinol*	inhibits xanthine oxidase, Hydroxanthine + xanthine oxidase $\rightarrow H_2O_2 + O_2 +$ xanthine $\rightarrow$ uric acid $+ H_2O_2 + .O_2^-$
4. *Desferrioxamine* (DFO)	Chelates transition metals; therefore inhibits the Fenton reaction: $O_2^- + M^n \rightarrow O_2 + M^{(n-1)} \; M^{(n-1)} + H_2O_2 \rightarrow M^n + .OH + OH^-$ (M^n is a transition metal, usually Fe or Cu)
B. Free Radical Scavengers	
5. N-2-mercaptoprionylglycine (MPG)	Intracellular oxyradical scavenger
6. Dimethylthiourea	$.OH$ scavenge
7. Mannitol	$.OH$ scavenger
8. Dimethyl sulphoxide	$.OH$ scavenger
9. Captopril*	Oxyradical scavenger

Superoxide dismutase is a large molecule and is therefore restricted to the extracellular space. Usually it is given together with catalase to prevent H_2O_2 accumulating as a potential source of $.OH$ ($H_2O_2 \rightarrow .OH + OH^-$)

* Captopril is an angiotensin converting enzyme inhibitor. For data relating to its scavenging activity see Bagchi et al. (1989), and Koener et al. (1991)

Table 6.4. Sources of oxyradicals

Extracellular	Activated neutrophils
Intracellular	Dissociation of mitochondrial electron transport chain
	Arachidonic acid metabolism
	Auto-oxidation of catecholamines and other compounds
	Sarcoplasmic reticulum

only be obtained by using a combination of scavengers, antioxidants and enzyme inhibitors. Moreover, some of these agents must be capable of penetrating the cell surface (Table 6.3), otherwise the oxyradicals which are produced intracellularly will continue to cause havoc.

Direct evidence of oxyradical production has come from the use of electron spin resonance spectroscopy (Zweier et al. 1987b; Garlick et al. 1987) and measurements of the rate of formation of malondialdehyde (Koller and Bergmann 1989).

Irrespective of which of these techniques is used (direct or indirect) evidence of the accumulation of oxyradicals during prolonged periods of ischaemia, and an exaggerated production upon reperfusion, is now unequivocal (Bolli et al. 1989; Bolli 1990), even in man (Ferrari et al. 1990). The following sequence, therefore may well exist: impaired coronary flow → ischaemia + reperfusion → oxyradical generation → lipid peroxidation → membrane injury → Ca^{2+} overload → necrosis. The duration of the ischaemic episode need not be long – for example, the ischaemia which is artificially induced during balloon angioplasty is often quite sufficient (Ferrari et al. 1990).

The Role of Calcium Antagonists as Protective Agents

Although loss of homeostasis with respect to Ca^{2+} may be one of the end-results of oxyradical generation (Fig. 6.7) and this condition will be exacerbated under conditions of energy depletion, the possibility of using calcium antagonists as protective agents has only recently emerged. This is not altogether surprising, because:

(i)   if oxyradicals render cell membranes freely permeable, then excess Ca^{2+} entry would not be limited to entry through the voltage- and calcium antagonist-sensitive Ca^{2+} channels, and

(ii) the oxyradical-induced failure of the intracellular mechanisms involved in maintaining Ca^{2+} homeostasis involves changes in the activities of key enzymes and organelles – and not simply energy depletion. The energy sparing effects of the calcium antagonists might therefore seem to be of little or no benefit.

However, the calcium antagonists are protective, *presumably because of their ability to protect phospholipid containing membranes against oxidative injury caused by lipid peroxidation.*

Protection Against Oxyradical-Induced Injury: Are the Calcium Antagonists Effective?

Evidence of Protection

There is a growing body of evidence which indicates that oxyradical-induced injury contributes to the damage caused by ischaemia, and post-ischaemic reperfusion (Hammond and Hess 1985; Lucchesi 1990). The precise mechanisms involved in this oxyradical-mediated cellular toxicity are not, as yet, completely established, but lipid peroxidation of cell membranes is a likely candidate. Such an effect is not peculiar to myocardial cell membranes – the endothelial cells of the vasculature are equally sensitive (Demopoulos et al. 1980) and indeed, become hyperpermeable (Yamada et al. 1990).

Evidence has accumulated during the past few years which indicates that some of the calcium antagonists can protect against lipid peroxidation – at least to some extent. Apparently they do this by trapping the oxyradicals and immobilizing them within the lipid bilayers of the membranes. Ondrias and his colleagues (Ondrias et al. 1989), using multilamellar phosphatidylcholine liposomes as a test preparation, found nifedipine to be more potent in this respect than verapamil. Janero and Burghardt (1989) compared the antioxidant effect of a series of dihydropyridine-based calcium antagonists (niludipine, nimodipine, nisoldipine, felodipine, nicardi-pine, nifedipine, and nitrendipine) and found nisoldipine, felodipine and nicardi-

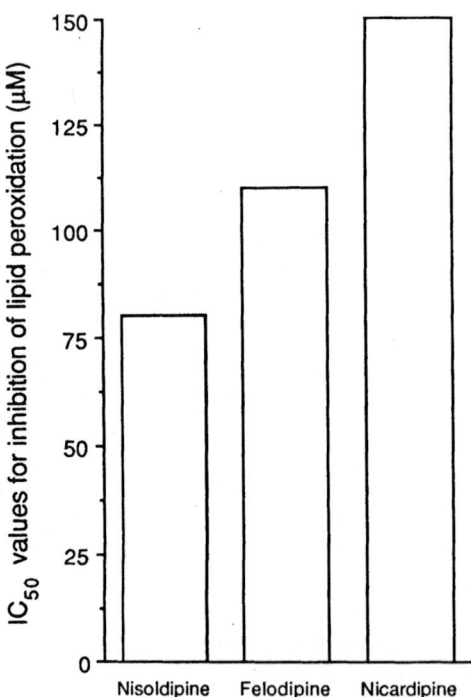

Fig. 6.8. IC_{50} values (concentrations required to reduce the response by 50 percent) for the inhibitory effect of nisoldipine, felodipine and nicardipine on the ability of free radicals generated by hypoxanthine in the presence of xanthine oxidase to cause lipid-peroxidation induced changes in liposomes prepared from rat myocardial membrane phospholipid. (Data from Janero and Burghardt 1989.)

Table 6.5. The protective effect of calcium antagonists against oxyradical-induced lipid peroxidation

Calcium antagonist	Preparation	Reference
Nifedipine > verapamil > diltiazem	Ventricular myocytes	Mak and Weglicki 1990
Diltiazem	Isolated rat hearts	Koller and Bergmann 1989
Nifedipine > verapamil	Phosphatidylcholine liposomes	Ondrias et al. 1989
	Cardiac membranes	Janero and Burghardt 1989

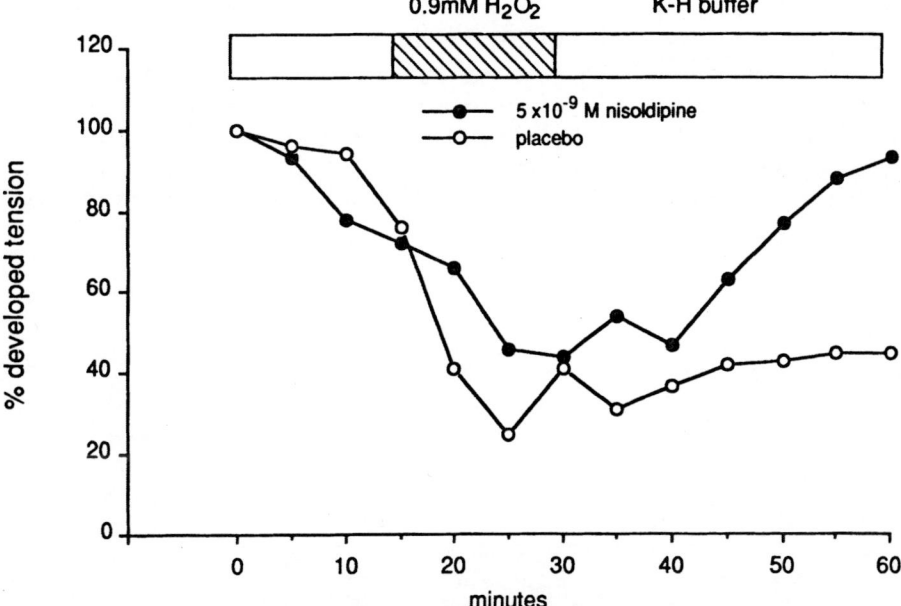

Fig. 6.9. Effect of 5×10^{-9}M nisoldipine on recovery of active tension generation (peak systolic tension) in isolated rat hearts exposed to 0.9mM H_2O_2 for 30 minutes. % developed tension is expressed as percent relative to the peak systolic tension generated immediately before adding the H_2O_2. Nisoldipine was present throughout. Perfusion at 37°C, using Krebs-Henseleit buffer. Note the improved recovery (p < 0.01) in the nisoldipine-treated hearts. (Data from S. Britnell, University of Melbourne.)

pine to be more effective (Fig. 6.8) than niludipine, nimodipine, nicardipine or nifedipine. These compounds lacked any appreciable scavenging activity but, presumably because of their high membrane partition coefficients, prevented the oxyradicals from reaching their target sites within the lipid bilayers of the membrane. *Diltiazem (Koller and Bergmann 1989) has also been shown to protect* against oxyradical-induced lipid peroxidation but relative to nifedipine it's activity in this respect is weak (nifedipine > verapamil > diltiazem, Mak and Weglicki 1990). Other examples of the antioxidant activity of calcium antagonists are listed in Table 6.5. One thing is quite clear – that is, that of all of the available calcium antagonists the dihydropyridines are the most effective – as far as protecting against oxyradical-induced injury is concerned.

An easy way of proving that the calcium antagonists do protect against oxyradical-induced injury is to undertake the type of experiment shown in Figure 6.7. Here, isolated rat hearts were perfused with and without the addition of hydrogen peroxide to the perfusion buffer, and with half of the hearts being treated with 5×10^{-9}M nisoldipine. As this figure (Fig. 6.9) shows treatment with nisoldipine favoured the recovery of function, despite the exposure to H_2O_2.

Evidence of the ability of the calcium antagonists to protect against the consequences of oxyradical production at the cellular level is not restricted to studies on liposomes prepared from cardiac myocyte membrane phospholipids although these have been quite widely used. Other investigators have used isolated endothelial cells, exposing them to hydrogen peroxide to induce peroxidation-evoked injury – as gauged by excessive permeability to albumin (Yamada et al. 1990). Again evidence of a protective effect has been uncovered (Fig. 6.10) and once again dihydropyridine-based calcium antagonists (including the second generation antagonists nilvadipine and nicardipine) (Chapter 2) were found to be effective, albeit at a relatively high dose-level.

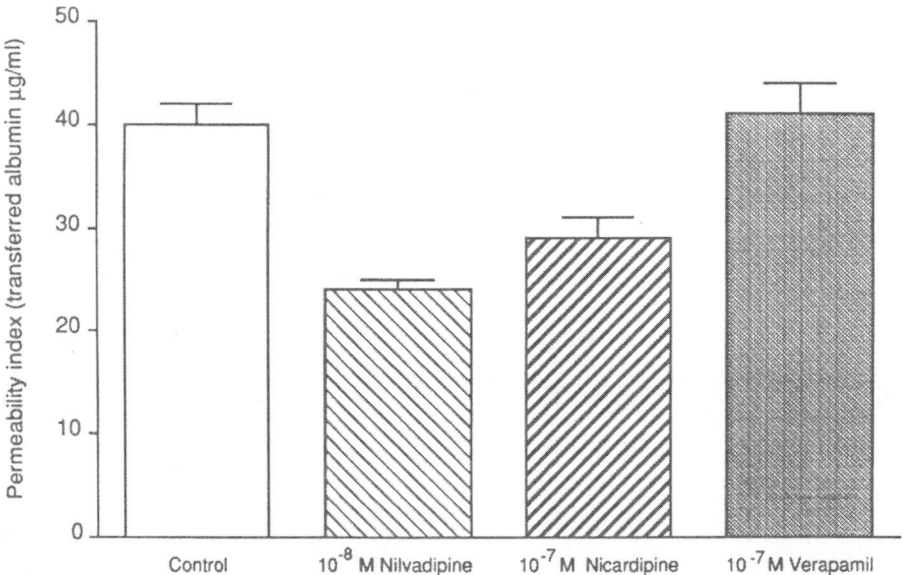

Fig. 6.10. Effect of three calcium antagonists – nilvadipine, nicardipine and verapamil on H_2O_2-induced increase in endothelial membrane permeability measured in terms of albumin transfer. Normally these cells are impermeable to albumin. The permeability shown here is indicative of oxyradical-induced injury. (Data from Yamada et al. 1990.)

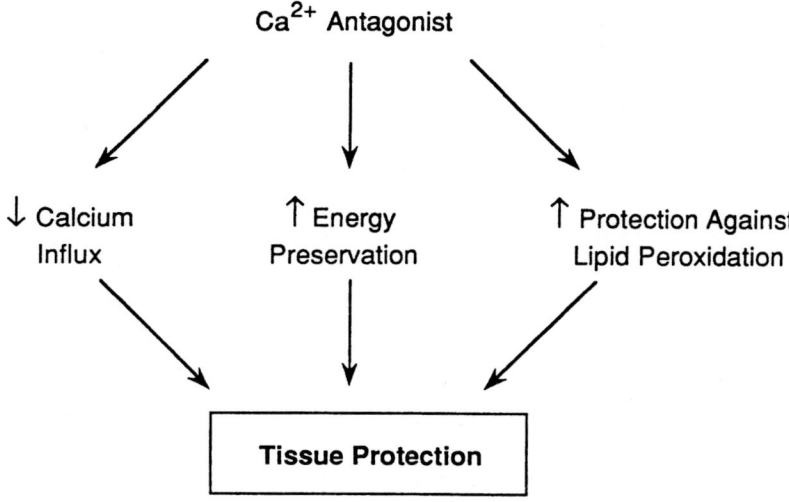

Fig. 6.11. Schematic representation of the way in which calcium antagonists act as tissue protective agents

Mode of Action

Although the dihydropyridine-based calcium antagonists are able to attenuate oxyradical-induced injury, their mode of action in this respect is unclear. The concentrations which are needed are high, far exceeding the concentrations needed to achieve calcium channel blockade – except, perhaps (Fig. 6.9) in the case of nisoldipine. The most likely explanation for their efficacy here revolves around their lipophilicity – a factor which, by allowing them to concentrate in the lipid-containing phase of the plasmolemma, may either stabilize the membrane, or render it less sensitive to oxyradical-induced peroxidation. If this does turn out to be the case, then prophylactic therapy with long-acting calcium antagonists would be desirable if the prevailing conditions were such that oxyradicals might be expected to be generated – viz ischaemia (Fig. 6.11) and possibly atherosclerosis (Chapter 11).

In Summary

1. Oxyradicals are implicated in a wide variety of clinical disorders – ranging from myocardial ischaemia and reperfusion injury to arrhythmias and atherosclerosis.
2. As far as the myocardium is concerned oxyradicals can be generated extracellularly (from neutrophils) and intracellularly (by the sarcoplasmic reticulum, mitochondria, autoxidation of catecholamines etc.).
3. Once formed oxyradicals render lipid containing membranes freely permeable, and disrupt proteins – including enzymes. The end-result is a lethally-injured, Ca^{2+} overloaded cell.

4. Protective mechanisms involve either the prevention of oxyradical formation, the scavenging of the oxyradicals or reducing the likelihood of oxyradicals causing peroxidative-induced damage to membranes and enzymes.
5. Dihydropyridine-based calcium antagonists confer some protection – as indicated by their ability (nisoldipine > felodipine > nicardipine) to attenuate oxyradical-induced lipid peroxidation (Fig. 6.8).
6. This ability of these drugs to protect against oxyradical-induced injury may contribute to their ability to slow atherogenesis (Chapter 11) and to protect against ischaemia-reperfusion induced injury. In either case, however, long-acting antagonists would be required to provide *sustained* protection.

Chapter 7

Endothelin-1 and the Calcium Antagonists

"The way to be a bore is to say everything"
... from Sept Discours en vers sur l'Homme, by VOLTAIRE.

Endothelin-1 is one of a recently discovered family of potent vasoconstrictor polypeptides (Yanagisawa et al. 1988; Yanagisawa and Masaki 1989a; 1989b; Masaki et al. 1990; Luscher 1991). These polypeptides share a common biochemistry in that:

(i)   they contain twenty one aminoacids;
(ii)   they have two intrachain disulphide bridges linking residues 1 and 15, and 3 and 11;
(iii) residues 16-21 provide a hydrophobic tail (Fig. 7.1), and
(iv)   the terminal residue is tryptophan.

Endothelin-1, the first of this family of polypeptides to be isolated, was harvested from the medium bathing cultured porcine endothelial cells and for this reason initially became known as *porcine endothelin*. However, now that the other isoforms – endothelin-2, endothelin-3 and VIC (or mouse β endothelin) – have been identified (Yanagisawa and Masaki 1989a; 1989b) endothelin-1 is the nomenclature which is being used. Why endothelin-1 is of interest centres mainly around its potent constrictor activity – an effect which is causing many investigators to wonder

Structure of Porcine Endothelin

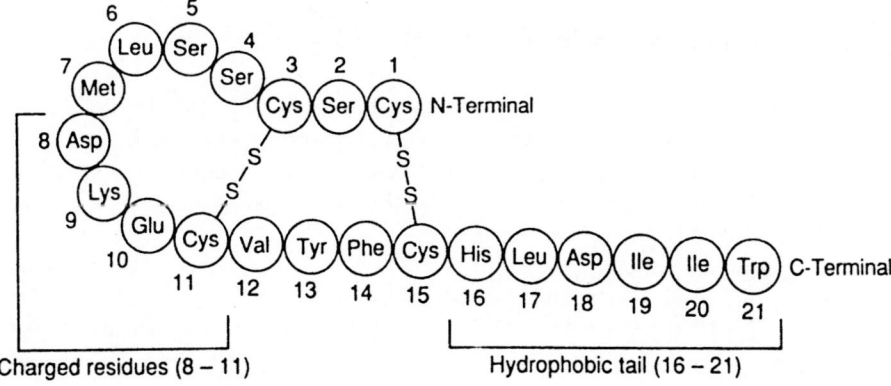

Fig. 7.1. Chemical structure of endothelin-1

whether it may not be involved in the pathophysiology of hypertension (Shepherd 1990), cerebral and coronary vasospasm (Luscher 1991) the phenomenon of "no reflow" as well as disorders of the peripheral circulation, including Raynaud's disease (Masaki et al. 1990; Nayler 1990; Zamora et al. 1990). However, there are many other conditions in which this polypeptide may be implicated, including atherosclerosis (it is a potent mitogen), Buerger's disease and Takayasu's arteritis (Kanno et al. 1990), renal failure (Tomita et al. 1989) and even myocardial infarction (Miyauchi et al. 1989). Irrespective of the pathological condition however, the three prominent activities of endothelin-1 are:

(i)   the potent and sustained vasoconstriction it produces (Yanagisawa et al. 1988);
(ii) its ability to promote smooth muscle cell proliferation (Hirata et al. 1989) – a property which links it to the genesis of atheromatous lesions (Chapter 11), and
(iii) its ability to mobilize intracellular Ca^{2+} (Chapter 10) – a property which may be of significance with respect to the early rise in cytosolic Ca^{2+} which occurs during conditions of inadequate coronary perfusion.

Not wishing to be a bore, and not wanting to regurgitate everything that has already been written about the endothelins, only certain aspects of the chemistry and pathophysiological significance of endothelin-1 will be described here. After all, the main purpose of this chapter is not to describe the pharmacology and biochemistry of endothelin-1 but rather to discuss whether calcium antagonists, including the second-generation antagonists, provide a useful means of attenuating its sustained vasoconstrictor effect. Endothelin-1 is being signalled out for special attention because:

(i)   it is intensely vasoconstrictive;
(ii) vascular endothelial cells produce this isoform selectively – whereas other tissues produce this and other isoforms, and
(iii) the rate of endothelin-1 production is enhanced under certain pathological conditions – including myocardial infarction (Miyauchi et al. 1989), congestive cardiac failure (Margulies et al. 1990), subarachnoid haemorrhage (Chapter 14), and hypertension (Saito et al. 1990).

The Production of Endothelin-1

Endothelin-1 is produced by vascular and other endothelial cells (Nayler 1990) by a process which starts with a mRNA encoded precursor – preproendothelin. The gene encoding for human endothelin-1 mRNA is located on chromosome 6 (Bloch et al. 1989). Not all endothelins are encoded by this gene, however. For example, endothelin-3 is encoded on chromosome 20.

Human preproendothelin, the precursor of "big" endothelin (or proendothelin) contains two hundred and twelve aminoacids, but porcine preproendothelin is slightly smaller, containing only two hundred and three aminoacids. Irrespective of the size of the preproendothelin precursor, however, proteolytic cleavage of the biologically inactive preproendothelin precursor (Cade et al. 1990) yields the intermediate and smaller precursor known variously as "big" endothelin, or

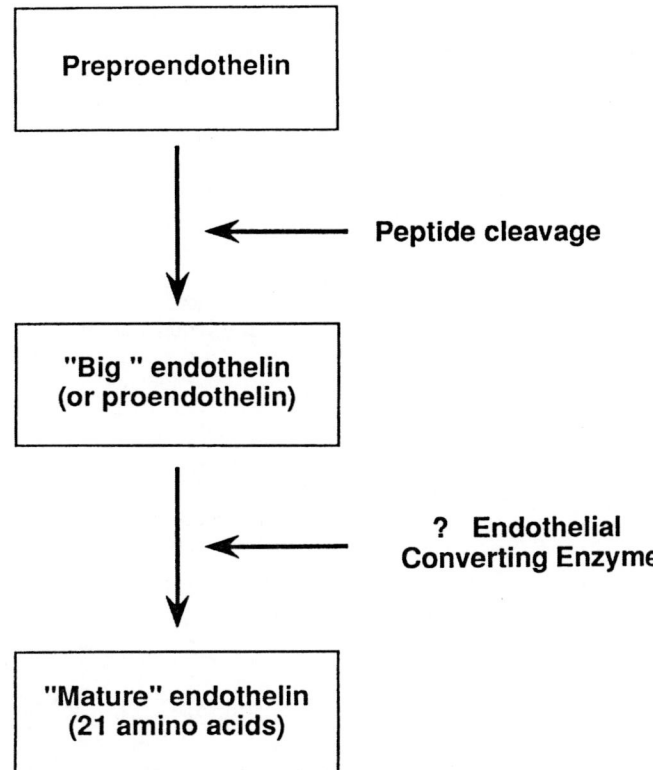

Fig. 7.2. Schematic representation of the steps involved in the production of "mature" (biologically active) endothelin-1

proendothelin (Fig. 7.2). Human "big" endothelin contains thirty eight aminoacids; porcine "big" endothelin contains thirty nine. The liberation of the "mature" biologically active endothelin-1 involves a proteolytic cleavage of a tryptophan-valine link in the "mature" but biologically inactive precursor.

Once the various enzymatic cleavage steps are complete the end-product – in this case endothelin-1 – is not stored in the endothelial cells. Instead it diffuses either into the lumen of the vessel, or abluminally to the adjacent smooth muscle cells. It is for this reason that the relatively low plasma levels which have been detected should not have come as a surprise – in reality it is the interstitial levels which are of greater interest because it is this pool of endothelin-1 which reaches the receptors in the adjacent tissue.

Vascular endothelial cells are assuming an ever increasing role in the mechanisms thought to be responsible for maintaining vascular tone. On the one hand they release endothelin-1, the most potent constrictor agent discovered so far. On the other hand, they release the vasodilator prostanoids, PGI_2 and PGE_2, together with the endothelial-derived relaxing factor – EDRF – or "NO" (Ress et al. 1989; Furchgott and Zawadzki 1980). At any one time, therefore, it is reasonable to assume that the endothelium is an important regulator of vascular smooth muscle tone – with too much endothelin-1, or hypersensitivity to endothelin-1 or too little PGI_2, PGE_2 or EDRF tipping the balance towards constriction – as occurs, for

Table 7.1. Conditions which raise plasma endothelin-1 levels

Condition	Reference
Myocardial infarction	Miyauchi et al. 1989
Renal failure	Tomita et al. 1989
Cardiogenic shock	Cernacek and Stewart 1989
Subarachnoid haemorrhage	Masaoka et al. 1989
Surgery	Saito et al. 1989
Heart failure (experimental)	Margulies et al. 1990
Hypertension	Saito et al. 1990
Renal transplantation	Berbinschi and Ketelslegers 1989
Provoked vasospastic angina	Toyo-Oka et al. 1991
Raynaud's disease	Zamora et al. 1990
Atherosclerosis	Kanno et al. 1990
Buerger's disease	Kanno et al. 1990
Takayasu's arteritis	Kanno et al. 1990

Normal levels are around 1.5 pg/ml (Toyo-Oka et al. 1991)

example in atherosclerotic arteries (Chapter 11), or in coronary or cerebral artery vasospasm (Luscher 1991).

Agents and Conditions Which Stimulate Endothelin-1 Production

Agents which stimulate endothelin-1 production can be subdivided into receptor-operated mechanisms, physical stimuli, and others (Yanagisawa et al. 1988). The receptor operated mechanisms include:
(i)   adrenaline;
(ii) angiotensin II;
(iii) arginine vasopressin;
(iv) thrombin;
(v)   transforming growth factor β;
(vi) interleukin-1.

Physical stimuli include:
(i)   shear stress, and
(ii) ischaemia.

Some of the clinical conditions which provoke raised plasma levels are listed in Table 7.1.

The Endothelin Receptor

The endothelins interact directly with membrane-located binding sites which are quite separate from those occupied by the calcium antagonists (Gu et al. 1989b; Davenport et al. 1989). These binding sites are widely – but not universally –

Table 7.2. Tissue distribution of endothelin-1 binding sites

Heart	Atria and ventricles, atrioventricular nodes, coronary arteries and veins
Kidney	Glomerulus, renal papilla, renal artery, renal veins, mesangial cells
Eye	Retinal capillaries, corneal endothelium, ciliary body, iris
Skin	Fibroblasts
Lung	Bronchi, trachea, alveoli, pulmonary artery
Stomach and gut	Muscosal lining
Adrenal gland	Medulla and cortex
Vasculature	Arteries and veins
Spleen	
Liver	
Placenta	
Vas deferens	
Uterus	

Adapted from Nayler 1990

distributed. For example, they do not occur in adipocytes, connective tissue, cartilage, platelets or red blood cells. In some tissues (Table 7.2) there are regional areas of concentration. In the heart, for example, the density of receptors in the atria exceeds that of the ventricle. In the brain the density in the cerebellum $>$ hypothalamus $>$ striatum. In the kidney the density in the glomeruli $>$ inner medulla $>$ cortex.

The Endothelin-1 Receptor

During the last few months this receptor has been cloned and its aminoacid sequence defined. It:
(i)   contains 427 aminoacid residues;
(ii) has a molecular mass of 48,516 daltons, and
(iii) seven membrane spanning domains with an extracellular N-terminus and a cytoplasmic C terminus (Arai et al. 1990, and Fig. 7.3).

In comparison with the α_1 and α_2 adrenergic receptors, therefore, the endothelin-1 receptor has a relatively small molecular weight. The α_1 and α_2 adrenoceptors also contain seven membrane spanning domains, but they have molecular weights of approximately 80,000 and 60,000–75,000 daltons respectively (Insel 1989).

As far as homology with other receptors is concerned, the endothelin receptor shows significant sequence similarity with G protein-coupled receptors (O'Dowd et al. 1989). As with other large hormone receptors (such as Lutropin and choriogonadotropin) the N-terminus which precedes the first of the transmembrane segments is relatively long (Fig. 7.3) and is probably involved in the binding of endothelin. It also contains two potential glycosylation sites (Sakurai et al. 1990). Potential phosphorylation sites have been identified in the third cytoplasmic loop and in the C-terminal tail (Fig. 7.3) (Sakurai et al. 1990).

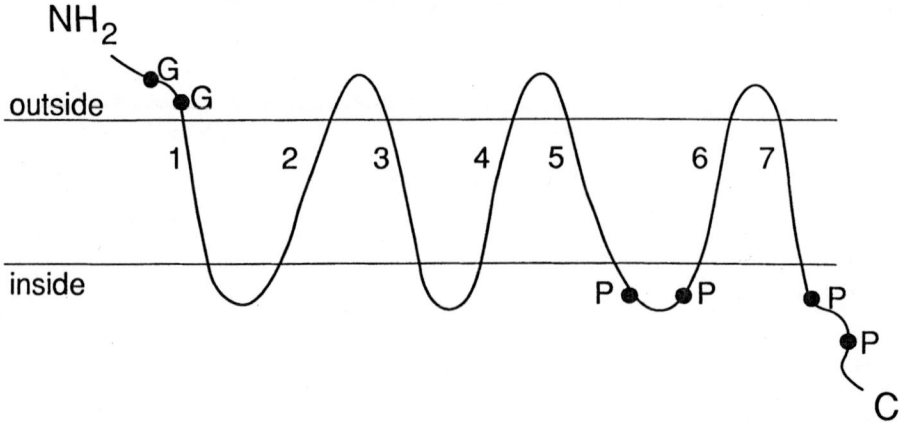

Fig. 7.3. Probable structure of the endothelin-1 receptor. Note that there are seven membrane spanning domains and a long carboxy terminus (C). G = glycosylation sites; P = phosphorylation sites

Receptor Subtypes

Almost as soon as investigators started probing the pharmacology and biochemistry of endothelin-1 (or porcine endothelin as it was then called) it became difficult to do anything other than accept the notion of endothelin isoforms. In fact it took only a few months for Yanagisawa and his colleagues to identify the three isoforms now known as endothelin-1 (ET-1), endothelin-2 (ET-2) and endothelin-3 (ET-3). From a pharmacological point of view it is relatively easy to distinguish between ET-1 and ET-2 on the one hand, and ET-3 on the other, because whereas ET-1 and ET-2 are potent vasoconstrictors, ET-3 is relatively weak. In many other respects, however, the three isoforms are equipotent. For example, it is well known now that the vasoconstrictor response to these endothelin isoforms is usually preceded by a transient vasodilation – due, almost certainly, to the release of EDRF (endothelial derived relaxing factor) and in this respect the three isoforms (ET-1, ET-2 and ET-3) are roughly equipotent (Warner et al. 1989). One way of accounting for these findings is to assume that there are two endothelin receptors:
(i) an ET-1/ET-2 selective subtype, to be known as *the ET_A* receptor, and
(ii) a non-selective endothelin receptor – the ET_B receptor (Sakurai et al. 1990).

Endothelin-1 and the Calcium Antagonists

Stimulation of the endothelin-1 (ET_A) receptor produces a widespread spectrum of responses. Arteries and veins, as well as arterioles and venules, contract – as do the lymphatic, tracheal and bronchiolar smooth muscle (Nayler 1990). At the cellular level cytosolic Ca^{2+} rises (Ohnishi et al. 1989) at the same time as $Na^+:H^+$ exchange activity increases, and phospholipase C, phosphoinositol metabolism, and protein kinase C are activated (Simonson and Dunn 1990). The rise in intracellular Ca^{2+}, coupled with Yanagisawa's original observation concerning the ability of nicardi-pine to attenuate the coronary constrictor effect of endothelin-1 (Yanagisawa et al. 1988) caused some investigators to question whether this polypeptide might not be the missing endogenous Ca^{2+} agonist, directly activating the Ca^{2+} channel? The real situation, it seems, is far more complex because:

(i)   if endothelin-1 does interact with the L-type Ca^{2+} channel then it must be at a site quite distinct from that occupied by the traditional L-type calcium antagonists – because calcium antagonists cannot displace specifically bound endothelin-1 (Nayler 1990), and

(ii)   endothelin-1 induced vasoconstriction is not dependent on the presnce of extracellular Ca^{2+}, and is not *fully* reversible by endothelial-derived relaxing factors released in response to either acetylcholine or bradykinin, or by directly acting nitrovasodilators (Luscher et al. 1990).

Nevertheless the endothelins, including endothelin-1, raise cytosolic Ca^{2+} in a variety of tissues – including vascular smooth muscle cells (Marsden et al. 1989; and Fig. 7.4).

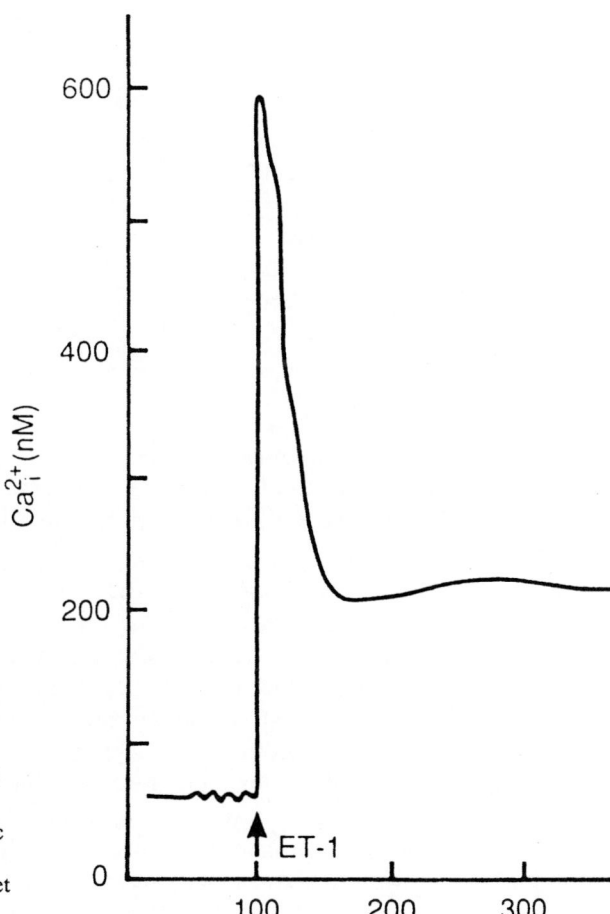

Fig. 7.4. Effect of endothelin-1 on cytosolic Ca^{2+} in vascular smooth muscle cells. Cytosolic Ca^{2+} was measured by using Fura-2. (Data from Marsden et al. 1989.)

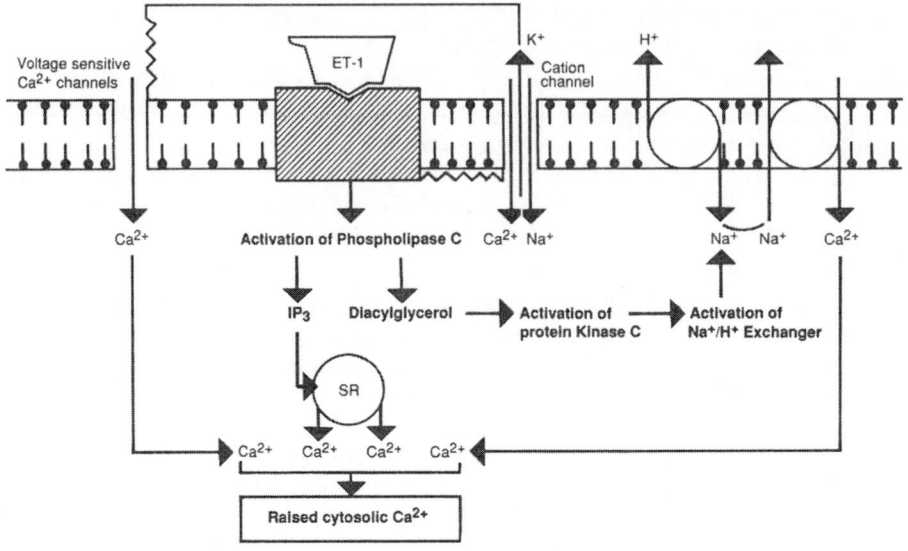

Fig. 7.5. Schematic representation of the mechanisms involved in the endothelin-1 induced increase in cytosolic Ca^{2+}

As far as the contractile effect of endothelin-1 on smooth muscle is concerned the following observations provide the key as to the multifactorial nature of the mechanisms which are involved:
(i)   the response develops slowly, but is sustained;
(ii) it is accompanied by a raised cytosolic Ca^{2+};
(iii) Ca^{2+} uptake is enhanced, as is phosphoinositol metabolism;
(iv) protein kinase C is activated, and the constrictor response is blunted by protein kinase C inhibitors;
(v)   the peptides have no direct effect on the contractile proteins;
(vi) cyclic AMP levels remain unchanged, and
(vii) whereas blockade of the L-type Ca^{2+} channels attenuates the response, blockade of the T- and N-channels, or of the Na^+ channels, is ineffective.

The simplest explanation for these various findings is to assume that the raised cytosolic Ca^{2+} which mediates the constrictor effect of this polypeptide originates from at least two pools – one intracellular, and the other extracellular. The intracellular pool is probably located (Fig. 7.5) within the sarcoplasmic reticulum and is mobilized in response to the enhanced rate of phosphoinositol metabolism. The extracellular Ca^{2+} may enter through several different routes including entry in exchange for Na^+ (Fig. 7.5) and, of course by way of the L-type Ca^{2+} channels. As yet there is no certainty as to how endothelin-1 activates these L-type Ca^{2+} channels. One possibility is that activation occurs because of endothelin-1's ability to partially depolarize the cell membrane, as a secondary consequence of protein kinase C activation (Yang et al. 1990a). Alternatively, activation may be by way of a transduction molecule – such as a membrane-located guanosine triphosphate binding protein.

In general however, as far as this chapter is concerned the main points to grasp are that:

(i)   endothelin-1 causes substantial vasoconstriction in a variety of vascular beds;
(ii)   the response is sustained, and is accompanied by a raised cytosolic Ca^{2+};
(iii) the Ca^{2+} involved in the constrictor response comes from two sources – one intracellular and the other extracellular, and
(iv)   the entry of the extracellular Ca^{2+} component involves entry through a calcium-antagonist sensitive pathway – viz, the L-type Ca^{2+} channel.

The Involvement of Endothelin-1 in the Maintenance of Vascular Tone

Low doses of endothelin-1, when injected intravenously, cause vasodilation – presumably because the polypeptide releases prostacyclin and endothelial-derived relaxing factor from vascular endothelial cells (de Nucci et al. 1988). In the human forearm, for example, an infusion of endothelin-1 at the rate of 0.5ng/min/100ml forearm tissue (Kiowski et al. 1991) produces such a response. Increasing the dose to 2.5 ± 1.5ng/min/100ml forearm tissue, however, causes vasoconstriction (Kiowski et al. 1991) (similar results have been obtained in a wide variety of animal studies). The question is, then, does circulating endothelin-1 play any role at all in the local control of blood pressure? Many investigators have answered this question in a negative manner, simply because the measured circulating levels of endothelin-1 are usually around 1pg/ml – and therefore below the threshold needed to activate a constrictor response. There are at least two reasons why this negative argument should be put aside:

(i)   plasma levels almost certainly provide a misleading idea of the interstitial levels of endothelin-1 – remembering that the polypeptide is released from the endothelium and diffuses abluminally – and not solely into the lumen of the associated blood vessel, and
(ii)   threshold concentrations of the polypeptide *potentiate* the constrictor response to other vasoactive agents, including serotonin and noradrenaline (Yang et al. 1990b).

It seems probable, therefore, that there are several ways in which endothelin-1 may contribute to the local regulation of vascular tone:

(i)   it may provoke relaxation, by stimulating prostacyclin and EDRF release;
(ii)   it may enhance the constrictor response to other agents, including noradrenaline and serotonin, and
(iii) in sufficiently high concentrations, the polypeptide may directly activate a constrictor response.

Some of the agents which promote endothelin-1 release have already been listed in Table 7.2. There are others including the oxidation of low density lipoproteins (Boulanger et al. 1990).

Endothelin-1 and the Coronary Circulation:
The Role of the Calcium Antagonists

The coronary constrictor effect of endothelin-1 is well documented. It is dose-dependent, develops slowly, and is insensitive to α adrenergic, serotonergic, or histaminergic blockade and to angiotensin converting enzyme inhibitors. It does not require an intact endothelium, is accompanied by an increased rate of Ca^{2+} uptake (Pang et al. 1989) and requires extracellular Ca^{2+} (Yanagisawa et al. 1988). More importantly the response is antagonized by calcium antagonists – including second generation antagonists (Fig. 7.6).

There are two ways in which endothelin-1 could be involved in the genesis of coronary artery spasm – or sustained constriction:
(i)   by way of its own *direct* constrictor effect, and
(ii) by exacerbating the constrictor effect of other locally-released vasoactive agents – including noradrenaline and serotonin.

Irrespective of which mechanism is involved, however, it now seems probable that endothelin-1 may well be involved in the genesis of myocardial ischaemia (Chapter 10), and possibly vasospastic angina (Luscher 1991).

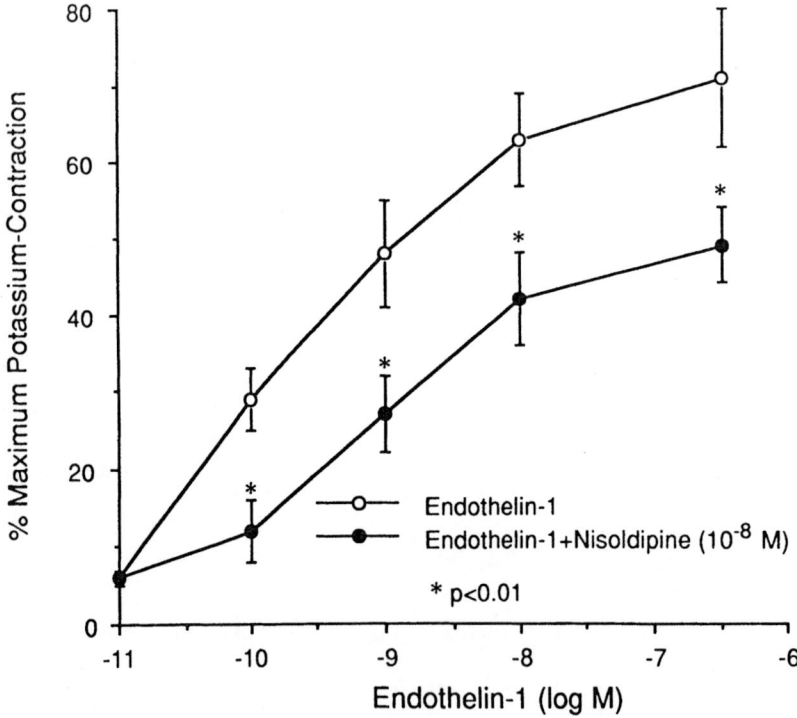

Fig. 7.6 Effect of 10^{-8}M nisoldipine on the constrictor effect of endothelin-1 on dog coronary artery. The constrictor response is expressed in terms of the maximum constriction obtained during K^+-evoked contractions

Endothelin and Hypertension

Just as endothelin-1 may be involved in the aetiology of coronary vasospasm and myocardial ischaemia, it may equally well be involved in the genesis of hypertension. There are two reasons for reaching this conclusion:
(i) when injected into the left brachial artery, endothelin-1 causes a sustained pressor response (Clarke et al. 1989), and
(ii) plasma endothelin-1 levels are abnormally high in patients with essential hypertension (Shichiri et al. 1990).

The relevance of these observations to this chapter is that the calcium antagonists (verapamil, nifedipine and nicardipine) block this vasoconstrictor effect, and in so doing unmask a weak vasodilator response to endothelin-1 (Kiowski et al. 1991). This is not a non-specific response, because non-specific vasodilators fail to block the constrictor response.

Endothelin-1 and Atherosclerosis

There are many reasons for arguing that endothelin-1 is probably involved in the genesis of atherosclerosis. These reasons include:
(i)   its potency as a mitogenic agent (Hirata et al. 1989);
(ii) because of its intrinsic constrictor activity and its ability to promote the release of other vasoconstrictors – including vasopressin, noradrenaline and angiotensin, it is likely to increase vessel wall injury caused by shear stress;
(iii) endothelin-1 potentiates the mitogenic activity of other mitogenic agents – including transforming growth factor, and
(iv) many of the substances which are released in response to tissue injury – including thrombin and platelet derived growth factor, stimulate the production of endothelin-1 (Nayler 1990).

Although it is well established now that endothelin-1 is a mitogen, that smooth muscle cell proliferation plays an important role in the atherogenic processes (Chapter 11) and that the calcium antagonists slow the growth of new atherogenic lesions, whether calcium antagonists suppress the mitogenic effect of endothelin-1 has not yet been established.

In Summary

1. Endothelin-1 has a dual effect on the vasculature, low doses causing a dilator and high doses a constrictor response.
2. The dilator response can be accounted for in terms of the release of endothelial *derived relaxing factors* – including prostacyclins and EDRF.

3. The constrictor effect involves:
   (i)   a *direct* effect, and
   (ii) sensitization of the vasculature to the constrictor effect of other agents, including serotonin and noradrenaline.
4. The direct constrictor effect of endothelin-1 involves activation of an endothelin-1 specific receptor (ET_A), resulting in activation of the phosphoinoside system with the consequent release of Ca^{2+} from the sarcoplasmic reticulum, and Ca^{2+} influx through a Ca^{2+} antagonist sensitive pathway – presumably the L-type Ca^{2+} channel.
5. Pathological conditions which are characterized by increased vascular resistance – vasospastic angina, and hypertension – may involve either increased rates of endothelin-1 production, slowed rates of clearance, or a hypersensitive response.
6. The calcium antagonists, including second generation antagonists, attenuate the constrictor effect of this peptide.
7. Since the release of endothelin-1 is triggered by a number of factors – including thrombin, adrenaline, angiotensin II, ischaemia, shear stress, and lipid peroxidation – long-acting vascular selective calcium antagonists may be the preferred form of control.

Chapter 8

Calcium Antagonists and the Stunned Heart

> *"I can discover facts, Watson, but I cannot change them."*
> Sir A. CONAN DOYLE in "The Bridge".

The heart is essentially an aerobic organ, with comparatively little capacity for anaerobic metabolism. It should come as no great surprise, therefore, to find that a sudden, sustained and severe reduction in coronary blood flow can be hazardous, or even lethal. The myocardium, however, does not respond in an "all-or-none" manner. Instead, depending on the duration and severity of the ischaemic episode (viz, the total ischaemic load), the heart either becomes "stunned" (Heyndrickx et al. 1975), *hibernates* (Rahimtoola 1985; 1989), or *infarcts* (Jennings and Reimer 1981). This chapter (Chapter 8) is concerned with the first of these conditions – that of "stunning" – but before considering whether the calcium antagonists can alleviate this condition it may be useful to distinguish between these three sequelae of ischaemia.

Stunning, Hibernation or Infarction?

It is quite easy to distinguish between stunning and hibernation on the one hand, and infarction on the other, because *stunning* and *hibernation* are fully reversible, non-lethal conditions, whereas infarction is lethal, and irreversible. The conditions of stunning and hibernation however, although both non-lethal, are subtly different from one another.

The Stunned Heart

When applied to the mammalian heart the term "stunning" might be envisaged as being a way of describing its delicate morphology and intricate physiology. Instead it is used to describe the contractile dysfunction which occurs when coronary flow is restored after a relatively short period (10 – 15 minutes) of ischaemia (Braunwald and Kloner 1982). *Stunning*, therefore, is a *post-ischaemic* condition characterized by the depressed functioning of potentially jeopardized myocardium which has been salvaged by reperfusion before the ischaemic event has had time to cause irreversible damage. This state of contractile dysfunction can persist for hours, or even days, but ultimately (Fig. 8.1) the myocardium recovers (Heyndrickx et al. 1975; Braunwald and Kloner 1982; Kloner et al. 1989; Bolli 1990).

The Hibernating Heart

This is an entirely different phenomenon and is the main subject of the next chapter (Chapter 9). When applied to the heart, the term "hibernation" describes a state of sustained mechanical dysfunction which occurs when coronary flow is impaired, but not to such an extent as to cause lethal injury. The hibernating heart, therefore, is a chronically underperfused heart. In marked contrast to the "stunned" heart, however, the *hibernating heart rapidly recovers its normal contractile state once coronary flow is restored* (Rahimtoola 1985).

The Infarcted Heart

This condition is all too familiar to cardiologists – and pathologists. It describes the *irreversibly* injured heart, in which cell death and tissue necrosis is the inevitable outcome. Hence,

(i)   *"stunning"* refers to the prolonged but reversible mechanical dysfunction encountered during reperfusion after a short period of ischaemia;

(ii) *"hibernation"* refers to the loss of contractility caused by a sustained reduction in coronary blood flow which, although severe, does not jeopardize the myocardium, and

(iii) *"infarction"* refers to the irreversible loss of structure and function caused by prolonged periods of ischaemia – irrespective of whether reperfusion is attempted or even accomplished.

The Clinical Relevance of Myocardial Stunning

During the past few years interest in the pathophysiology of myocardial stunning has intensified – in part because it's clinical relevance has been recognized (Table 8.1) and it therefore is no longer thought of as being just a laboratory artifact, or curiosity (Patel et al. 1988). Maybe there are subtle differences between laboratory models of "stunning" and the "stunning" which occurs clinically. One such difference could be that in most laboratory models of this phenomenon the hearts are healthy prior to the induction of the ischaemia-reperfusion incident, whereas in clinical practice pre-existing episodes of ischaemia may have already injured the myocardium. Nevertheless, if delayed recovery despite the restoration of coronary perfusion is used to define myocardial stunning it is not difficult to find evidence of it's natural occurrence. For instance, the administration of thrombolytic agents during evolving myocardial infarction (Anderson et al. 1983; Christian et al. 1990), coronary bypass surgery (Ballantyne et al. 1987; Breisblatt et al. 1990), coronary vasospasm (Mathias et al. 1987), exercise-induced angina (Camici et al. 1986), unstable angina (Nixon et al. 1982) and even acute accidentally-induced myocardial infarction – such as that which is occasionally caused by a wasp sting (Jones and Joy 1988) or by cocaine (Ascher et al. 1988) – can result in myocardial stunning.

Table 8.1. Conditions which result in or contribute to myocardial "stunning", in man

Condition	Reference
Thrombolytic therapy during involving acute myocardial infarction	Anderson et al. 1983 Reduto et al. 1981 Stack et al. 1983 Patel and Kloner 1987 Christian et al. 1990
Exercise-induced ischaemia	Camici et al. 1986
Coronary bypass surgery	Breisblatt et al. 1990 Ballantyne et al. 1987
Unstable angina	Nixon et al. 1982
Coronary vasospasm	Mathias et al. 1987
Cardiomyopathies	Sagie et al. 1988 Yasutomi et al. 1989 Pasternac 1989 Fine et al. 1989
Wasp sting	Jones and Joy 1988
Cocaine-induced infarction	Ascher et al. 1988
Accidentally-induced ischaemia caused by investigational procedures	Lette et al. 1989

Animal Models of Myocardial Stunning

There are almost as many animal models of myocardial stunning as there are clinical conditions which give rise to it. As Table 8.2 shows, the animal models include reperfusion following short periods of global or regional ischaemia in either isolated or *in situ* hearts and exercise-induced ischaemia (Heyndrickx et al. 1975) with and without left ventricular hypertrophy (Hittinger et al. 1990), and without pre-existing coronary artery stenosis (Thaulow et al. 1989). The common and essential characteristics of each of these models is successful reperfusion after a short period of ischaemia which, if not terminated, would have progressed to infarction. In many of the studies – including those of Reimer et al. (1986) and Nayler et al. (1988) – repetitive episodes of ischaemia and reperfusion have been employed, with the interesting finding that successive episodes of stunning do not have a cumulative effect – as if the heart learns to protect itself!

Even the limited list of experimental models given in Table 8.2 allows certain conclusions to be reached concerning the conditions under which stunning occurs.

(i)   It is *not* species specific.
(ii) It occurs in isolated crystalloid-perfused hearts, and therefore cannot depend entirely upon:
   (a)   formed elements of the blood, including platelets and neutrophils;
   (b)   innervation, including sympathetic innervation, or
   (c)   the peripheral circulation.
(iii) It occurs in anaesthetized and conscious animals.

Table 8.2. Experimental models of myocardial stunning

Model	Reference
1. Isolated Hearts (global ischaemia)	
Ferret	Kusuoka et al. 1990
Rabbit	Krause 1990
	Ambrosio et al. 1987
Rat	Nayler et al. 1988
	Limbruno et al. 1989
	Henry et al. 1990
2. In Situ Hearts	
A. Anaesthetized animals (acute regional ischaemia)	
(i) Dogs	Swain et al. 1984
	Reimer et al. 1986
	Greenfield and Swain 1987
	Bolli et al. 1989
	Przyklenk et al. 1989
(ii) Pigs	Buchwald et al. 1989
B. Conscious animals (exercise-induced ischaemia)	
(i) Dogs	Heyndrickx et al. 1975
	Thaulow et al. 1989
	Hittinger et al. 1990

(iv) It can be induced in previously normal, and therefore presumably, healthy hearts – indicating that pre-existing injury is not a prerequisite.

The Electrical, Mechanical, Morphological and Biochemical Properties of the Pre-Stunned and Stunned Myocardium

A. The Pre-Stunned Myocardium

The term "pre-stunned" is used here to denote the condition of the myocardium as it exists after a relatively short period of ischaemia, but prior to reperfusion and the associated expression of the "stunned state". The changes which occur after only a few minutes of ischaemia, and before reperfusion is attempted include:

(i) a decline in peak developed tension followed by mechanical quiescence (Fig. 8.1);

(ii) a substantial fall in the tissue reserves of adenosine triphosphate (ATP) and creatine phosphate (CP) (Fig. 8.2), and a reduction in the total adenylate charge (Jennings et al. 1985; 1990);

(iii) a concommitant rise in the inorganic phosphate (P_i), hydrogen ion (H^+) and magnesium (Mg^{2+}_i) concentration (Fig. 8.3), and

(iv) a reduction in tissue glycogen (Jennings et al. 1985).

STOP PERFUSION

REPERFUSION

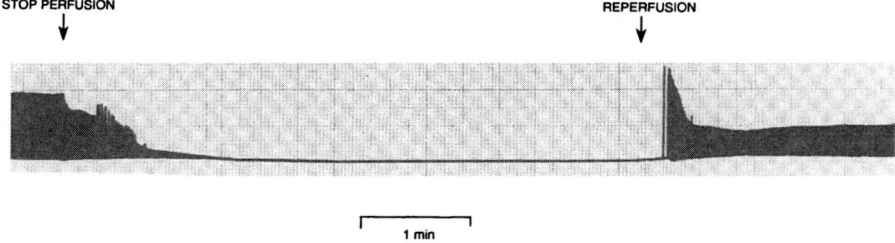

1 min

Fig. 8.1. Mechanical activity recorded from an isolated rat heart before, during and after ten minutes of normothermic ischaemia. Note the partial recovery of contractile function upon reperfusion. Complete recovery requires hours

(v) Electrical activity usually persists, but with some ST segment depression, a small fall in the transmembrane resting potential and a decrease in the amplitude of the action potential (Levine et al. 1987). These changes, however, are relatively trivial, and rapidly disappear upon reperfusion.

(vi) Returning to the intracellular environment,

(a) the metabolic capacity of the mitochondria is maintained, provided that sufficient substrate is available;

(b) the sarcolemmal enzymes (the Na^+-K^+ and the Ca^{2+}-activated ATPases), and the ion exchangers (the Na^+:Ca^{2+} exchanger and the Na^+:H^+ exchanger) remain functional;

(c) the sarcoplasmic reticulum (SR, Chapter 4) shows an apparent decrease in its Ca^{2+} accumulating activity (Limbruno et al. 1989; Feher et al. 1989), with decreases in the rate of Ca^{2+} uptake of up to thirty five percent after only ten minutes of ischaemia. Use of agents such as ruthenium red and ryanodine to block the SR Ca^{2+} release channels has shown, however, that this apparent decrease in the rate of Ca^{2+} uptake is really an *increased rate of Ca^{2+} efflux* through the SR Ca^{2+} release channels (Feher et al. 1989). The structure and functioning of these channels was described in Chapter 4. As far as the stunned myocardium is concerned, it is only important to realize that after only a few minutes of ischaemia the SR channels, which normally permit a controlled efflux of Ca^{2+} from the lumen of the SR into the cytosol, begin to leak Ca^{2+}. At the same time,

(d) there is a small, but significant and persistent rise in cytosoli Ca^{2+} (Ca^{2+}_i) (Table 8.3) which is readily detectable by NMR spectroscopy at a time when total tissue Ca^{2+} is unchanged (Jennings et al. 1985). Since the total tissue Ca^{2+} is unchanged, the additional Ca^{2+} ions which accumulate in the cytosol prior to reperfusion (Fig. 8.4) must have come from an intracellular pool. There are several possible sources, including the sarcoplasmic reticulum, the mitochondria and H^+-induced displacement of previously bound Ca^{2+} (Langer and Nudd 1983; Blanchard and Solaro 1984; Allen and Orchard 1984, and Fig. 8.5). Of these three sources the sarcoplasmic reticulum seems to be the largest contributor (Feher et al. 1989).

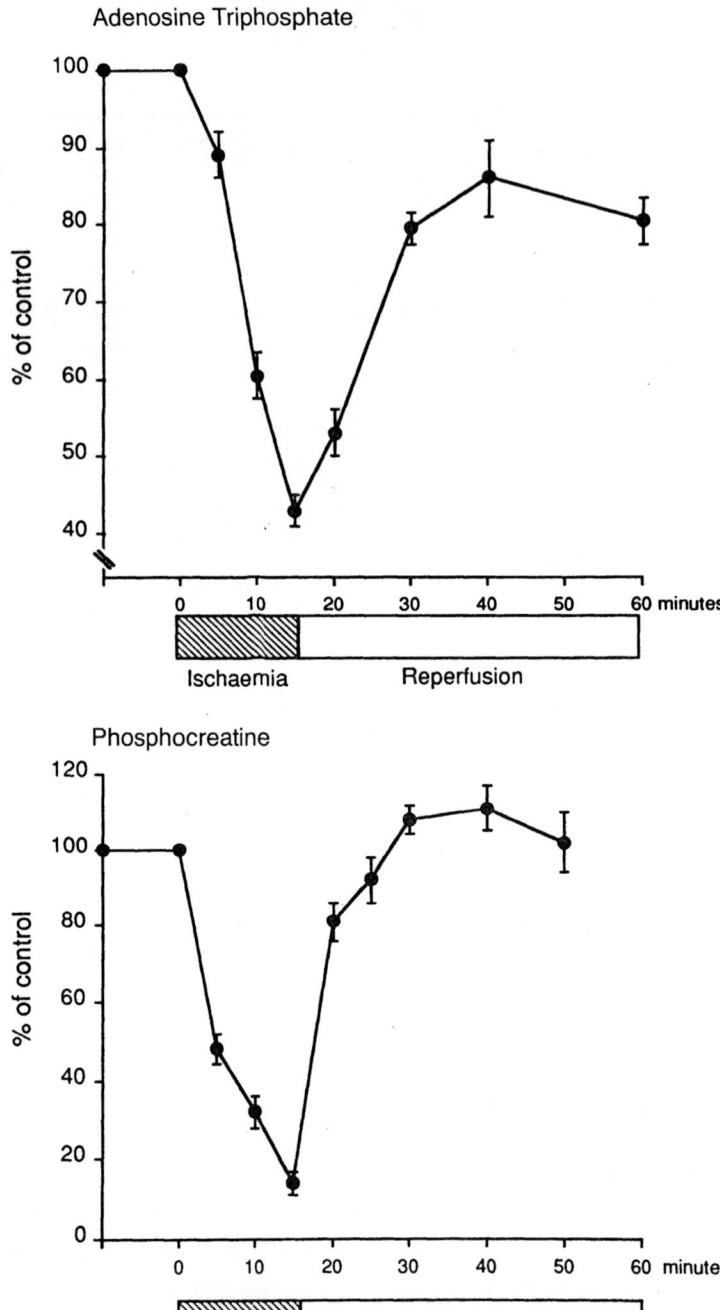

Fig. 8.2. Effect of fifteen minutes global ischaemia followed by reperfusion on the tissue levels of adenosine triphosphate (ATP) and creatine phosphate (CP) in isolated, crystalloid-perfused rat hearts. Each result is mean ± SEM of 6 experiments. Note the precipitous decline in ATP and CP during the ischaemic episode, and their recovery upon reperfusion. % Control refers to percentage relative to values obtained during aerobic perfusion

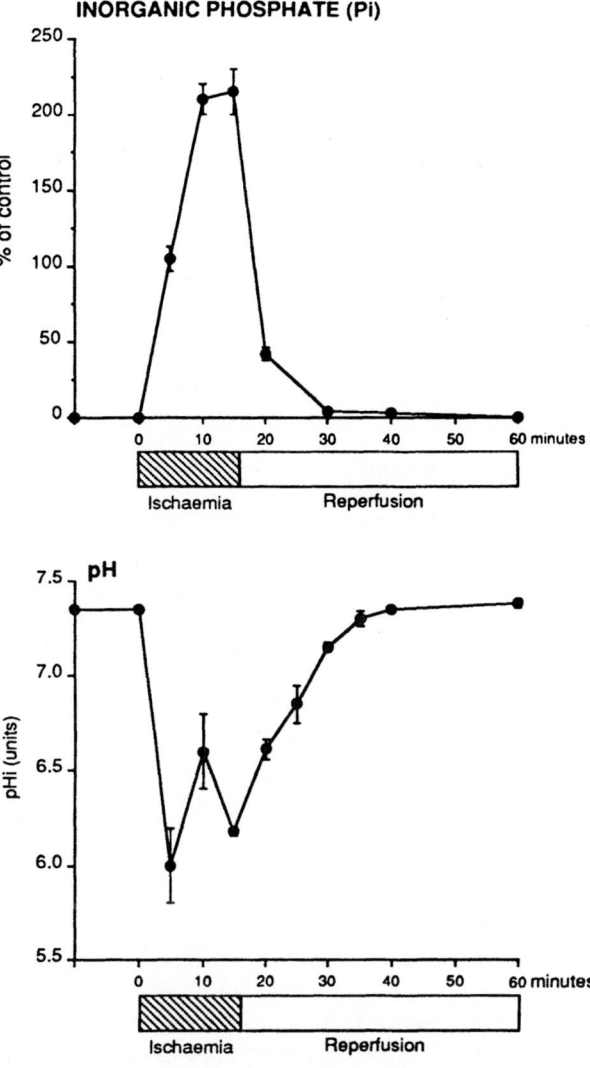

Fig. 8.3

(iv) As far as the ultrastructure of the myocardium is concerned the changes are minimal (Jennings et al. 1990). Perhaps the most obvious is the disappearance of the glycogen granules – but this would be expected with the switch from aerobic to anaerobic metabolism. Other changes include mild margination of the nuclear chromatin, marked relaxation of the myofibrils and some mitochondrial swelling (Jennings et al. 1985). Compared with the changes which occur after longer periods of ischaemia, however, these changes are minimal and would not be expected to impede recovery. In any case they are reversible.

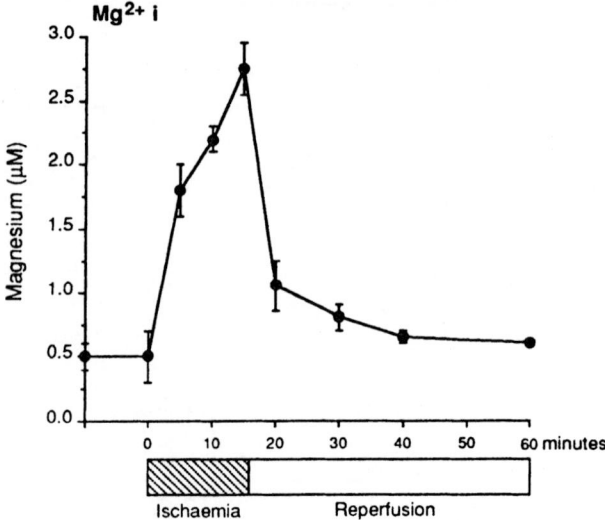

Fig. 8.3. Effect of 15 minutes global ischaemia on inorganic phosphate (P_i), intracellular pH (pH_i) and intracellular Mg^{2+} (Mg^{2+}_i) in isolated rat hearts. Global ischaemia was at 37°C. P_i, pH_i and Mg^{2+}_i were measured by NMR spectroscopy. Each value is mean ± SEM of 6 experiments

Table 8.3. Evidence of an early ischaemia-induced increase in cytosolic Ca^{2+} (Ca^{2+}_i)

Model	Minutes of ischaemia	% Increase	Reference
Rat heart	9–15	5 fold	Steenbergen et al. 1987
Ferret heart	10–15	4 fold	Marban et al. 1987
Rabbit heart	3	3 fold	Lee et al. 1988
Rat heart	9–15	4 fold	Watts et al. 1990

These, then, are the conditions which prevail after 10–15 minutes of ischaemia, immediately prior to the restoration of coronary perfusion and the consequent „stunning" of the heart. Peak developed tension has decreased – or the affected area may even become mechanically quiescent – but electrical activity persists. The adenosine triphosphate reserves have fallen, but are not necessarily exhausted, and the cytosolic levels of P_i, Mg^{2+}, H^+ and Ca^{2+} have risen. The glycogen granules will have disappeared, but otherwise the ultrastructure of the myocardium remains relatively normal – apart from some margination of the nuclear chromation and relaxation of the myofibrils (Table 8.5). Of all of these changes the rise in cytosolic Ca^{2+} (Ca^{2+}_i) is probably the most significant. Such a rise is not unique to the "pre-stunned" heart, however; a similar rise occurs during periods of hypoxic perfusion (Koretsune and Marban 1990b) – although the mechanisms which are responsible for the increase may differ.

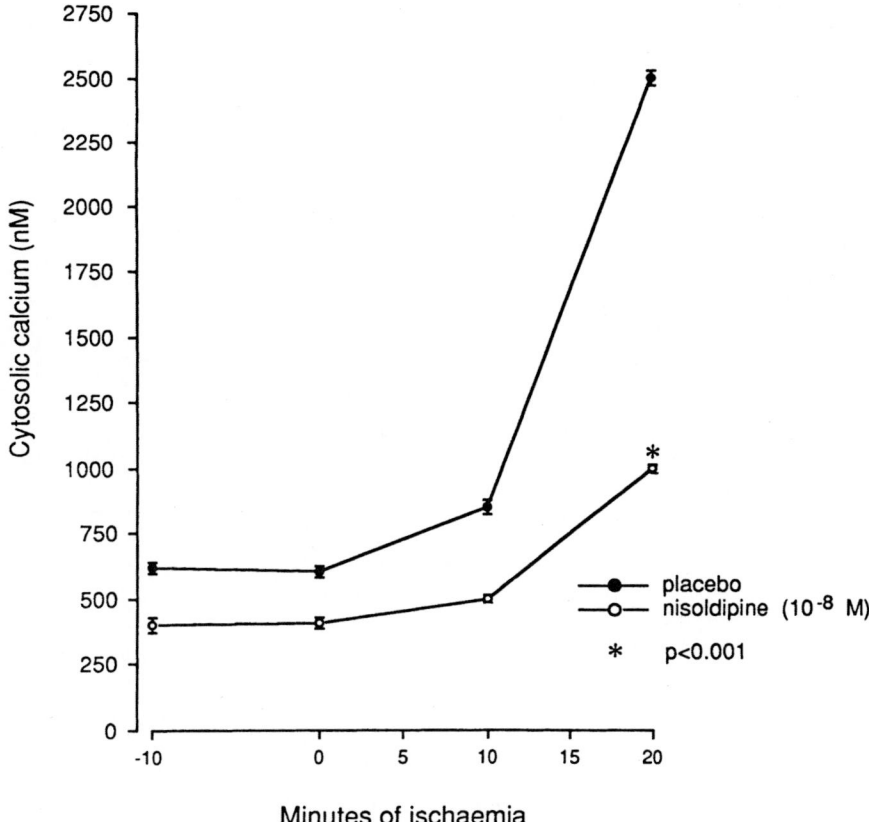

Fig. 8.4. Effect of twenty minutes global ischaemia, with and without 10^{-8}M nisoldipine, on cytosolic Ca^{2+} (Ca^{2+}_i) in isolated rat hearts. Cytosolic Ca^{2+} was measured by NMR spectroscopy, using F-BAPTA. The NMR spectra were averaged over a 7.5 minute collection period. Perfusion until 0 minutes was under aerobic conditions. The cytosolic levels of Ca^{2+} (Ca^{2+}_i) are the average of the systolic and diastolic levels

B. The Post-ischaemic "Stunned" Myocardium

When reperfused after a relatively short period of ischaemia the hearts become "stunned". At this time there is:

(i)   a rapid restoration of contractile activity (Fig. 8.1). During the first one or two minutes the active tension generating activity of the myofibrils often approaches that of the pre-ischaemic period but then declines to around sixty or seventy percent of the pre-ischaemic level. At the same time as systolic shortening is decreasing, the actual onset of shortening is delayed. As already noted this state of contractile dysfunction can persist for hours, or even days but ultimately the tension generating activity of the myofibrils returns to the pre-ischaemic level. Sometimes recovery seems to be particularly delayed in the endocardium. At the same time,

Table 8.4. Procedures which enhance the contractile performance of the "stunned" heart

Intervention	Reference
Additional Ca^{2+}	Ito et al. 1987
	Kusuoka et al. 1987
Paired pacing	Becker et al. 1986
Adrenaline	Przyklenk and Kloner 1987b
Beta-adrenergic stimulation	Bolli et al. 1985
Dopamine	Arnold et al. 1985
Pyruvate	Mentzer et al. 1989
Isoprenaline	Ambrosio et al. 1987

Table 8.5. Effect of 10–15 minutes ischaemia, and of reperfusion on the metabolic and functional status of the myocardium

Parameter	Ischaemia (relative to aerobic control)	Post-ischaemic (reperfused) (relative to aerobic control)
ATP	↓↓↓↓	↓
CP	↓↓↓↓	↑
P_i	↑	=
$Mg^{2+}{}_i$	↑	=
$H^+{}_i$	↑	=
$Ca^{2+}{}_i$	↑	=
S.R.	↓	↓
T_{max}	O	↓
Cardiac Efficiency	↓↓	↓
Coronary Flow	O	=

Where ↓ denotes a decline, ↑ an increase, = no change, O denotes not detectable, and $_i$ denotes cytosolic (or intracellular)
P_i = inorganic phosphate; $Mg^{2+}{}_i$, $H^+{}_i$ and $Ca^{2+}{}_i$ = intracellular free magnesium, hydrogen and calcium ion concentrations. SR = sarcoplasmic reticulum. T_{max} is time to develop peak tension, ATP (adenosine triphosphate), CP (creatine phosphate)

(ii) the tissue reserves of ATP are partially restored, and more often than not there is a complete restoration – sometimes with an overshoot – of the CP reserves (Fig. 8.2), and

(iii) intracellular P_i, Mg^{2+}, H^+ (Fig. 8.3) and Ca^{2+} (Marban et al. 1987) return to their pre-ischaemic levels – well ahead of the recovery of contractile function.

As far as the sarcoplasmic reticulum is concerned, although reperfusion ultimately results in the restoration of its normal function, complete recovery is always delayed. This applies to its Ca^{2+} accumulating activity and the activity of the associated Ca^{2+}-activated ATPase (Limbruno et al. 1989; Krause et al. 1989). As for the relatively trivial changes in ultrastructure which occurred during the ischaemic episode (glycogen depletion, mild margination of the nuclear chromatin and the swelling of an occasional mitochondrion), these rapidly disappear (Jennings et al. 1985), leaving an apparently normal ultrastructure at a time when the contractile function remains depressed.

Any thought of accounting for the persistent mechanical dysfunction of these hearts in terms of either suppressed oxidative metabolism or an inability of the mitochondria to generate energy-rich phosphate compounds can be discarded (Ambrosio et al. 1987; Headrick et al. 1990). Certainly basal oxygen consumption may be modestly depressed, unchanged, or even enhanced (Krukenkamp et al. 1986; Liedtke et al. 1988; Stahl et al. 1988) but the ratio of the mean rate of oxygen consumption to the work output of the heart is inappropriately high (Laster et al. 1989) – as if with "stunning" the heart has become mechanically inefficient. However, even when the active tension generating activity of the myocardium is depressed it retains it's capacity to respond to inotropic interventions – such as (Table 8.4) the addition of extra Ca^{2+} (Ito et al. 1987; Kusuoka et al. 1987), paired pacing (Becker et al. 1986) and the introduction of a variety of inotropic drugs – including dopamine and adrenaline (Table 8.4). Because of this ability to respond to such a variety of inotropic interventions it is impossible to avoid the conclusion that despite their depressed contractile state these "stunned" hearts, like their hibernating counterparts (Chapter 9), retain a contractile and metabolic reserve.

There are two other possibilities concerning the aetiology of stunning which should be mentioned at this stage – has the coronary vasculature remained patent, and has the excitatory process survived? These questions are easily answered because:

(i) transmural coronary flow is well preserved upon reperfusion (Jeremy et al. 1989); in addition, there is no evidence of a large "no reflow" area (Nayler et al. 1990a), and

(ii) although the conduction velocity of the excitatory stimulus is slowed, the transmembrane resting potential reduced, and the overall amplitude of the action potential diminished during the ischaemic episode (Levine et al. 1987) these changes rapidly disappear upon reperfusion. It is hard to see, therefore, how they could be responsible for the suppressed contractile state of the myocardium which persists during the first few hours (or days) of reperfusion.

In general therefore, the stunned heart retains significant contractile (Table 4.5) and metabolic reserves and coronary flow, its ultrastructure appears to be relatively normal as does the ionic composition of its cytosol, and its electrophysiology. Why then is it stunned?

Possible Mechanisms of Myocardial Stunning

From a purely theoretical point of view mechanisms which might be responsible for, or at least be involved in, the "stunning" process include:
(i)   abnormal energy production;
(ii)   impaired energy utilization;
(iii)   subtle changes in ultrastructure not readily identified at electronmicroscopy;
(iv)   impaired myocardial perfusion;
(v)   abnormal Ca^{2+} flux;
(vi)   oxyradical-mediated contractile dysfunction;
(vii)   abnormal functioning of the sarcoplasmic reticulum, and
(viii) a decreased sensitivity of the myofilaments to Ca^{2+}.

Probably there is no single cause – but some of these proposed mechanisms can discarded.

Is Abnormal Energy Production Involved?

The answer seems to be no! There are several reasons for reaching this conclusion. *Firstly*, although the ATP levels of the stunned myocardium are lower than normal, and they may recover slowly, with a time course which sometimes resembles the time course for the recovery of contractile function (Ellis et al. 1983), this parallelism does not always occur (Glower et al. 1987). *Secondly*, the CP content of these hearts is either normal, or supranormal (Kloner et al. 1983 and Fig. 8.2), indicating that the phosphorylating activity of the mitochondria is well preserved. *Thirdly*, these hearts can respond to a variety of inotropic stimuli (Table 8.4) *without* depleting their ATP and CP stores (Arnold et al. 1985). *Finally*, manipulations that foster ATP synthesis do not hasten the recovery of these hearts (Hoffmeister et al. 1985).

Is Energy Utilization Impaired?

This is an improbable explanation, at least as far as the myofibrils are concerned, because the reversal of post-ischaemic dysfunction by a wide range of inotropic interventions implies that the ability of the myofibrils to use ATP for contraction (via the myofibrillar ATPase enzyme) is not only retained, but survives with considerable functional reserve. Nevertheless it must be admitted that the myocardium in the affected zone has become mechanically inefficient (Stahl et al. 1988).

Is the Altered Ultrastructure Responsible?

Again, the answer must be in the negative, because the changes which do occur appear to be minimal and rapidly reverse upon reperfusion (Jennings et al. 1985). With repeated episodes of ischaemia there may be some slight damage to the extracellular collagen matrix (Zhao et al. 1987) but it is difficult to see how this could explain the loss of contractility, because the rate of collagen resynthesis is far slower than the recovery of myocardial function. In any case, the loss of collagen is modest (Charney et al. 1989).

Is Perfusion Adequate During Reperfusion?

In the past investigators have argued that occlusion of the coronary microvascular, possibly mediated by microthrombi or leucocytes, contributes to myocardial stunning (Engler and Covell 1987). This hypothesis seemed to be supported by the fact that when the coronary flow of these hearts is increased to supranormal levels by infusion of papaverine or dipyridamole, their contractility is returned towards normal (Stahl et al. 1986). However, inadequate coronary perfusion does not seem to play a critical role – to the contrary, the stunned hearts retain their coronary flow reserve (Jeremy et al. 1989), and there is no evidence of a no-reflow condition (Nayler et al. 1990a). Even if the coronary flow was regionally inadequate, the defect could not be explained simply in terms of microthrombitic or leucocyte plugging of blood vessels, because crystalloid-perfused hearts are also subject to stunning. Probably the benefit which is derived from increased coronary perfusion is due to the "garden hose" effect – an effect which involves physical stretching of the sarcomeres.

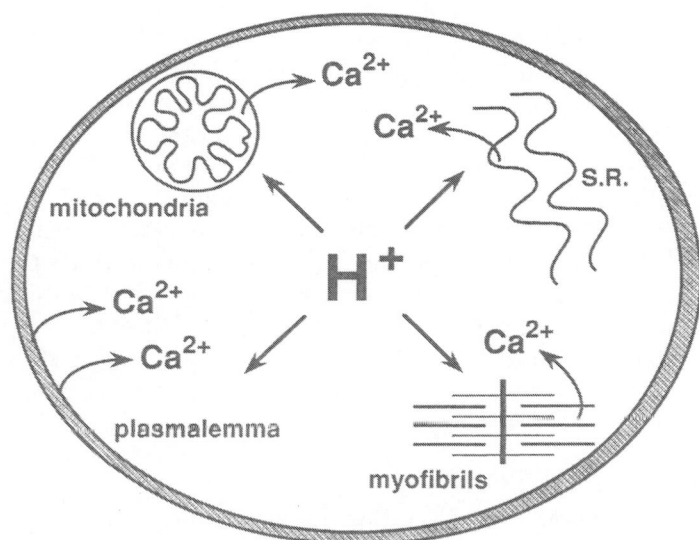

Fig. 8.5. Schematic representation of the intracellular sources from which Ca^{2+} can be displaced by H^+. Since cytosolic H^+ increases during ischaemia (Fig. 8.3) these sources could contribute to the pool of Ca^{2+} which accumulates in the cytosol (Fig. 8.4)

Is There an Abnormal Ca^{2+} Influx?

Since "stunned" hearts exhibit sustained, but reversible contractile dysfunction it might have been argued that they are receiving insufficient Ca^{2+} for excitation contraction coupling. This may happen, but the cytosolic levels of Ca^{2+} (Ca^{2+}_i) actually *increase* during the ischaemic episode (Table 8.3), presumably, in part, because of the slowed Ca^{2+} accumulating activity of the sarcoplasmic reticulum (Krause and Hess 1985) and its tendency to leak Ca^{2+}. Other possible causes of the raised Ca^{2+}_i include entry in exchange for Na^+, entry across a leaky sarcolemma, and H^+-induced displacement of previously bound Ca^{2+} (Fig. 8.5). Whatever its cause, cytosolic Ca^{2+} rises both during the early stages of the ischaemic episode (Table 8.3 and Fig. 8.4) as well as during the first few minutes of reperfusion (Marban 1991). Accordingly there seems to be a paradox, because these stunned hearts are exhibiting a depressed contractile state despite the presence of adequate Ca^{2+}, an almost normal ultrastructure, considerable metabolic reserve, comparatively minor changes in electrophysiology and under conditions in which microthrombitic or leucocyte plugging of the vasculature cannot occur.

Do the Myofibrils Become Relatively Insensitive to Ca^{2+}?

This seems to be a real possibility, because exposing myocytes to a raised Ca^{2+} is known to desensitize them to Ca^{2+}, and to produce a condition comparable with that of stunning (Kitakaze et al. 1987; Kusuoka et al. 1990). The desensitization cannot be due to a continued effect of the accumulated P_i or H^+, because although both P_i and H^+ decrease the maximal Ca^{2+}-activated force and myofilament Ca^{2+} sensitivity in chemically skinned muscle preparations (Kentish 1986; Fabiato and Fabiato 1978) and intact hearts (Kusuoka et al. 1986), intracellular H^+ and P_i rapidly return to normal during post-ischaemic reperfusion (Fig. 8.3), at a time when tension development remains depressed. The raised cytosolic Ca^{2+} also disappears soon after reperfusion (Marban et al. 1987; 1990; Marban 1991) but by this time the myofibrils presumably have become relatively desensitized to Ca^{2+}, leaving the hearts "stunned". The precise cause of this Ca^{2+}-desensitization of the myofibrils is unknown – but since recovery is slow it can be presumed to involve structural damage caused by the activation of Ca^{2+}-dependent proteases (or phospholipids). Since the damage is not evident at electronmicroscopy it presumably involves a delicate but small component of the contractile machinery.

Oxyradical-Mediated Dysfunction: Is this Relevant?

Oxy- and hydroxy-radicals also seem to contribute to the stunning process (Bolli et al. 1988; Bolli 1990). There are at least four reasons for reaching this conclusion. Thus, these radicals:

Table 8.6. Oxyradicals and the subcellular functioning of the myocardium

Organelle	Effect of oxyradicals	Reference
Myofibrils		
Tension generation	↓	Shattock et al. 1982
		Burton et al. 1984
		Jackson et al. 1986
		Blaustein et al. 1986
		Przyklenk et al. 1990
Sarcoplasmic Reticulum (SR)		
Ca^{2+} uptake/retrieval of cytosolic Ca^{2+}	↓	Rowe et al. 1983
Ca^{2+} ATPase activity	↓	Thompson and Hess 1986
Sarcolemma		
Ca^{2+} ATPase (extrudes Ca^{2+} across the sarcolemma) into the extracellular space	↓	Kaneko et al. 1989
$Na^+ K^+$ ATPase (prevents Na^+ accumulation)	↓	Kramer et al. 1984
		Xie et al. 1990
$Na^+:Ca^{2+}$ exchanger	↓	Reeves et al. 1986

The altered activity of the SR would tend to slow the retrieval of Ca^{2+} from the cytosol. At the sarcolemma depressed Ca^{2+} ATPase activity would slow the etrusion of Ca^{2+} across the sarcolemma, giving further support for a raised cytosolic Ca^{2+}. This will be further exaggerated by the decline in $Na^+ K^+$ ATPase activity, the resultant accumulation of Na^+ being available for exchange with Ca^{2+} by way of the $Na^+:Ca^{2+}$ exchanger. The end result is raised cytosolic Ca^{2+}.

Table 8.7. Oxyradical scavengers and inhibitors of oxyradical production which improve functional recovery of "stunned" hearts

Agent	Reference
Agents which act as free radical scavengers	
Superoxide/dismutase and catalase	Gross et al. 1986
	Buchwald et al. 1989
	Jeroudi et al. 1990
	Myers et al. 1985
N-2-mercaptopioprionylglycine	Myers et al. 1986
Dimethylthiourea	Bolli et al. 1987
Agents which prevent free radical generation	
Allopurinol	Headrick et al. 1990
Oxypurinol	Puett et al. 1987
Deferoxamine	Farber et al. 1987

(i)   are produced in limited amounts during conditions of inadequate perfusion. More importantly the restoration of full perfusion is accompanied by a burst of oxy- and hydroxy-radical production (Bolli 1990). Also,
(ii) they have a direct depressant effect on the tension generating activity of myofibrils (Table 8.6).

In addition,
(iii) they interfere with many of the systems which either directly, or indirectly, regulate cytosolic Ca^{2+} (Table 8.6), with the nett effect of raising cytosolic Ca^{2+}, and
(iv) inhibitors of oxyradical production and the addition of free radical scavengers attenuate, or even prevent, the post-ischaemic dysfunction which is so characteristic of the stunned heart. Some of the agents which have been used are listed in Table 8.7.

The Sarcoplasmic Reticulum: Is it Involved?

As with the possible involvement of the oxyradicals it is difficult not to conclude that the sarcoplasmic reticulum participates in the stunning process. This is because:
(i)   the activity of the Ca^{2+}-stimulated, Mg^{2+}-dependent ATPase enzyme which is responsible for pumping Ca^{2+} ions back from the cytosol into the lumen of the sarcoplasmic reticulum (SR) is depressed under these conditions (Limbruno et al. 1989), and
(ii) Ca^{2+} efflux through the SR Ca^{2+} release channels is augmented (Krause et al. 1989) – i.e., the SR Ca^{2+} release channels leak Ca^{2+} into the cytosol.

Myocardial Stunning: A Multifactorial Event

Having considered the major events which *theoretically* might be involved in the aetiology of myocardial stunning it is now possible to discard some of them – or at least to assign them to a secondary role. Defective excitation, inadequate energy (as ATP) to support contraction, severe ultrastructural damage, injury to or plugging of the microvasculature, inhibition of tension generation by H^+, P_i, and Mg^{2+} ions that accumulated during the ischaemic episode, and inadequate Ca^{2+} for excitation-contraction coupling are all theoretically possible causes which, for one reason or another (Table 8.8), can now be put aside or assigned a secondary role. This leaves three possible primary causes.
(i) Ca^{2+} overloading-induced decrease in the Ca^{2+} sensitivity of the myofibrils (Kitakaze et al. 1987);
(ii) Free-radical mediated damage (Bolli 1990).
(iii) Impaired functioning of the sarcoplasmic reticulum (Rowe et al. 1983; Thompson et al. 1986).

Table 8.8. Possible causes of myocardial "stunning"

Possible, and Probable Causes

1. Decreased myofibrillar Ca^{2+} sensitivity.
2. Oxyradical mediated damage.
3. Sarcoplasmic reticulum malfunction.

Unlikely, but possible causes

1. Ultrastructural damage – but this is unlikely, and in any case the changes are rapidly reversed.
2. Defective excitation – but the changes in the action potential are minimal and disappear upon reperfusion.
3. Inadequate Ca^{2+} – for excitation-contraction coupling – but *cytosolic Ca^{2+}* is high during the early stages of reperfusion.
4. Inadequate reperfusion, possibly due to neutrophil plugging, vasospasm or vessel injury – but this does not necessarily occur.
5. Inhibitory effect of the P_i, H^+ or Mg^{2+} which accumulates intracellularly, on excitation-contraction coupling – but these ions are rapidly washed out upon reperfusion.
6. Impaired myofibrillar energy usage – but the hearts have adequate functional reserve as shown by their ability to respond to inotropic interventions.
7. Inadequate energy production – but the hearts respond to inotropically active drugs and interventions, *without* further depleting their endogenous stores of ATP and CP.
8. Damage to the collagen matrix – but this requires repetitive episodes of transient ischaemia.
9. Impairment of sympathetically-mediated, neural response – this cannot be essential, because even denervated hearts become "stunned" upon reperfusion after a short period of ischaemia.

These three potential causes of stunning are not listed in any particular order of importance, because they are not mutually exclusive. Instead it is likely that they each contribute to the process which culminates in the temporary loss of contractile function. Cytosolic Ca^{2+} overloading, for example, augments oxyradical production (McCord 1985) which in turn causes lipid peroxidation and membrane damage, which, if the sarcoplasmic reticulum is involved, will cause a further rise in cytosolic Ca^{2+} (Fig. 8.6). A similar argument can be made with respect to the sarcolemma, because here, too, oxyradical-induced lipid peroxidation promotes an increase in Ca^{2+} permeability (Kutryk et al. 1991), and with the Ca^{2+} gradient favouring Ca^{2+} influx, Ca^{2+} from the extracellular space would move into the cytosolic pool.

As yet there is no certain explanation as to why a sustained increase in cytosolic Ca^{2+} should desensitize the myofibrils to Ca^{2+}. One possible explanation is that the transient cellular Ca^{2+} overload may activate Ca^{2+}-sensitive proteases, thereby facilitating the proteolysis of one or more components of the contractile proteins (Marban 1991). An equally viable hypothesis is that it is the SR membrane which is attacked – either by oxyradicals or by the Ca^{2+}-activated proteases – including calpain II (Rardon et al. 1990) – or phospholipases.

If a transient Ca^{2+} overload provides the key to myocardial stunning, then agents which attenuate the ischaemia induced rise in cytosolic Ca^{2+} – either directly, or indirectly – should be protective, as should agents which limit oxyradical induced injury.

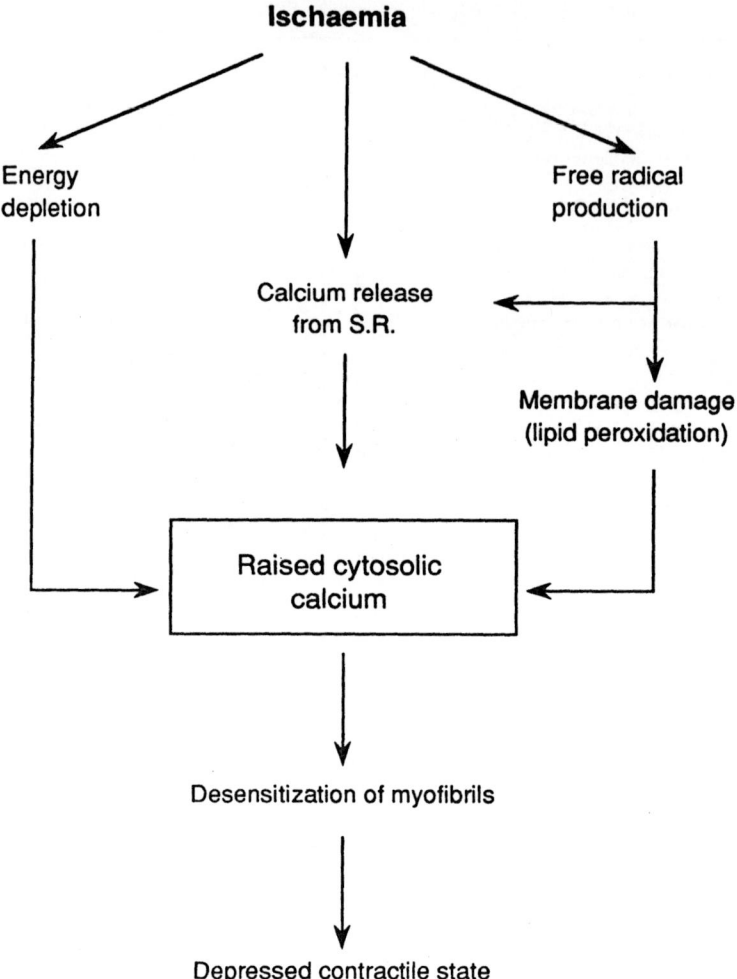

Fig. 8.6. Schematic representation of the possible involvement of oxygen-derived free radicals, calcium release from the sarcoplasmic reticulum and a raised cytosolic Ca^{2+} in the aetiology of the stunned myocardium

Calcium Antagonists and the Stunned Myocardium

If Ca^{2+} ions are involved in the stunning process the next question to be answered centres around the possibility of using calcium antagonists to provide protection. In the last few years this possibility has been quite vigorously investigated, and if restoration of contractile function is used as a measure of protection then the prototype calcium antagonists – nifedipine (Lamping and Gross 1985; Przyklenk and Kloner 1987a; Przyklenk et al. 1989), verapamil (Przyklenk and Kloner 1988) and diltiazem (Watts et al. 1990) are all protective, even, it seems, when treatment is delayed until the time of reperfusion (Przyklenk and Kloner 1988; Przyklenk et al.

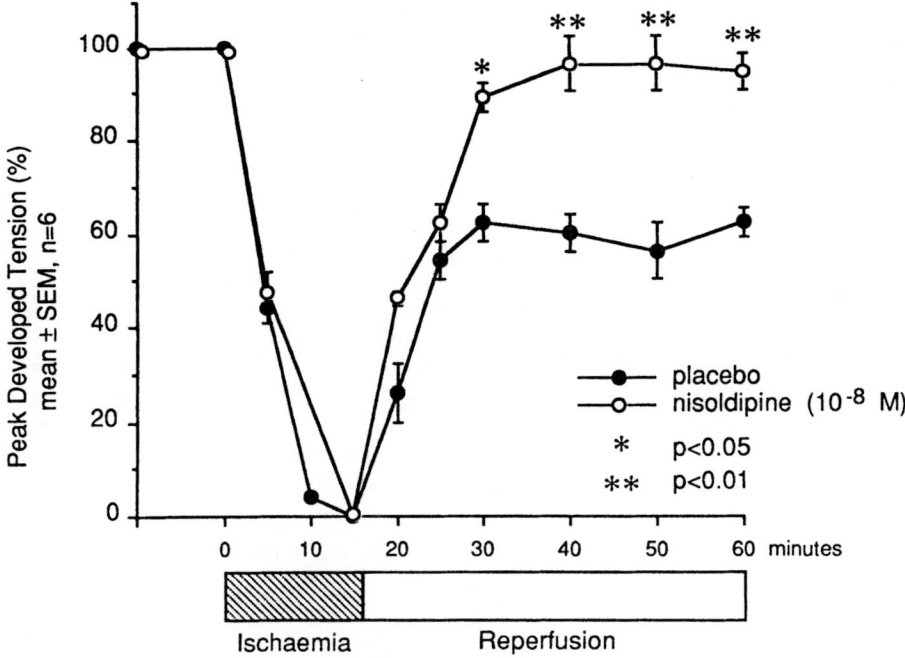

Fig. 8.7. Effect of 10^{-8}M nisoldipine on recovery of contractile function in isolated rat hearts that were "stunned" by fifteen minutes of global ischaemia, at 37°C. Note that nisoldipine – added here before the hearts were made ischaemic, improved functional recovery

1989). The second generation calcium antagonists – for example, nisoldipine – (Fig. 8.7) are equally effective.

There are at least five mechanisms which might be involved in this protective effect of the calcium antagonists:

(i) by acting as "energy sparing drugs" they will attenuate the ischaemia-induced rise in cytosolic Ca^{2+} simply by preserving the ATP needed to pump Ca^{2+} out of the cytosol into either the SR or across the sarcolemma into the extracellular space. Nisoldipine, for example (Fig. 8.4) has such an effect;

(ii) by virtue of their inhibitory effect on slow Ca^{2+}-channel mediated Ca^{2+} influx, they will attenuate that component of the ischaemia-induced cytosolic Ca^{2+} overload which might originate from this source;

(iii) in blood perfused hearts they may attenuate vascular plugging due to thrombi, as well as dilating the coronary vasculature. Such an effect would reduce the area "at risk" of being "stunned", and

(iv) some of them, and more particularly the second generation calcium antagonists can act as antioxidant agents (Chapter 6) and therefore might be expected to protect lipid-containing membranes against oxyradical-induced damage (Janero and Burchardt 1989) – damage which includes enhanced Ca^{2+} permeability (Kutryk et al. 1991).

In Summary

1. When applied to the heart, the term "stunning" refers to the slowly reversible contractile dysfunction exhibited by hearts which are reperfused after a relatively short period of ischaemia.
2. This state of temporary contractile dysfunction is not accompanied by ultrastructural damage, severe electrophysiological disturbances or persistent energy depletion.
3. The "stunned" hearts respond to inotropic stimuli and therefore have contractile (and metabolic) reserve.
4. A sustained increase in cytosolic Ca^{2+} is the likely cause of the contractile dysfunction, since this desensitizes the myofibrils to Ca^{2+}. Factors responsible for the raised cytosolic Ca^{2+} include oxyradical-induced changes in membrane permeability, energy depletion and a "leaky" SR.
5. Agents which protect against "stunning" include oxyradical scavengers and calcium antagonists – the latter acting to reduce cytosolic Ca^{2+}, thereby minimizing the Ca^{2+}-induced desensitization of the myofibrils.
6. This ability of the calcium antagonists to protect against "stunning" probably involves an "energy-sparing" effect associated with their effect on the peripheral vasculature, a direct inhibitory effect on Ca^{2+} influx, dilation of the coronary vasculature and, in some instances, their ability to protect against oxyradical induced injury. Some of these protective measures would apply to the prophylactic use of these agents, whilst others would be more important upon reperfusion.

Chapter 9

Calcium Antagonists and the Hibernating Myocardium

"I won't think of it now ... I'll think of it tomorrow."
Scarlett O'Hara, in "Gone With The Wind", by MARGARET MITCHELL

As mentioned in Chapter 8, there are at least three potential outcomes of myocardial ischaemia – viz:

(i)   *infarction* – a condition caused by prolonged ischaemic episodes which culminates in *irreversible* loss of contractile activity, cell death, and tissue necrosis (Jennings et al. 1990);

(ii) *stunning* – a post-ischaemic condition characterized by prolonged, but *reversible* contractile dysfunction (Kloner et al. 1989; Marban 1991), and

(iii) *hibernation* (Rahimtoola 1985; 1989) (Fig. 9.1).

This chapter is concerned with the last of these conditions – hibernation.

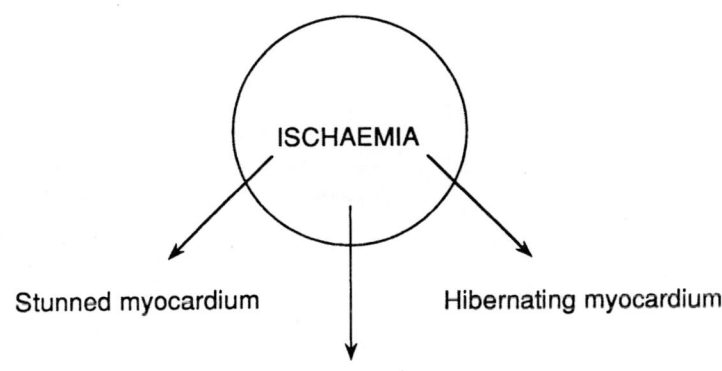

Fig. 9.1. Schematic representation of three possible sequelae of ischaemia

The Hibernating Myocardium

The term "hibernation", as applied to the mammalian heart, means a *persistent state of contractile dysfunction caused by chronic coronary hypoperfusion* (Rahimtoola 1989). Atherosclerotic-induced narrowing of a major coronary artery is probably one of the commonest causes but there are others – including residual low-grade stenosis after thrombolytic therapy (Marshall et al. 1990) and unsatisfactory angioplasty.

Although the aetiologies of "hibernation" and "stunning" differ hibernating and stunned hearts share some common features. For example, in neither condition is there any evidence of tissue injury or sustained electrophysiological disturbances (Table 9.1) and in each case the depressed contractile state is reversible (Kloner et al. 1989). However, the two conditions should not be confused with one another as whilst *myocardial stunning is a post-ischaemic event associated with the restoration of coronary perfusion after a short period of ischaemia (Fig. 9.2 and Table 9.1), the hibernating heart is in a state of chronic, but mild hypoperfusion.* Thus, the hibernating heart is an ischaemic heart in which the severity of the reduction in coronary blood flow falls short of that needed to cause either sustained dysfunction upon reperfusion, or lethal injury (Rahimtoola 1989; Braunwald and Rutherford 1986). Perhaps the best way of describing how the myocytes respond to this situation is to assume that they down-regulate their contractile activity – as if attempting to balance energy usage and energy supply.

In general, therefore, hibernation is a chronic ischaemic event which is terminated by reperfusion (Fig. 9.2) whereas stunning is an acute event provoked by post-ischaemic reperfusion (Chapter 8).

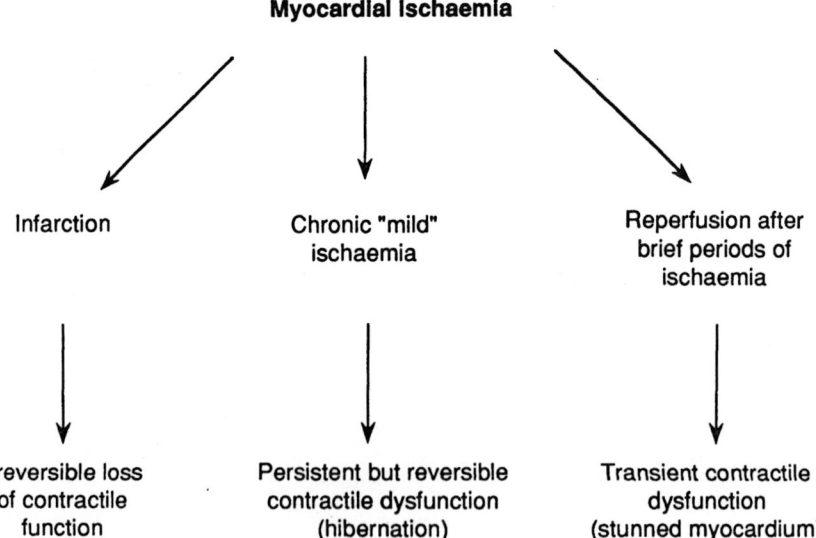

Fig. 9.2. Schematic representation of the differences between the aetiology of myocardial infarction, hibernation, and stunning

Table 9.1. Comparison between stunned and hibernating hearts

	Stunned	Hibernating
Occurrence	Post-ischaemic	Ischaemic
Myocyte Injury	Absent	Absent
Sustained electrophysiological disturbances	Absent	Absent
Coronary Flow	Restored	Reduced
Duration of contractile dysfunction	Hours, or days	Prolonged (months or years)
Reversibility	Delayed	Immediate

Is Myocardial Hibernation an Adaptive Process?

Although teleological arguments are considered to be unfashionable, they can be useful. From a teleological point of view the ability of the myocytes to down regulate their contractile state in response to hypoperfusion can be regarded as an adaptive process likely to favour survival. Quite obviously the longer energy usage and energy production are matched, or balanced, the greater the delay in the onset of lethal injury. Rahimtoola (1989) who, incidentally, was the first to use the term "hibernation" to describe this hypoperfusion syndrome, has often argued that the response should be considered as one of "self-preservation (little blood, little work)", and he is probably right! One thing is certain, the condition is readily and rapidly reversible. All that is needed is the restoration of normal coronary perfusion – as accomplished, for example, by revascularization at coronary bypass surgery (Chatterjee et al. 1973; Brundage et al. 1984) or by laser – or balloon-assisted-angioplasty (Litvack et al. 1988).

The Identification of the Hibernating Myocardium

The two essential characteristics of the hibernating myocardium – chronic underperfusion and sustained contractile dysfunction – are not only readily reversible: they are also easy to identify. This is fortunate because although the hibernating tissue may be responsible for a low cardiac output and even cardiac failure, the situation, once recognized, can be reversed. The contractile dysfunction – or more accurately, the regional wall abnormality it causes – can be monitored in several different ways (Table 9.2). For example, ventricular angiography, radionuclide ventriculography and two dimensional echocardiography can be used. The other component of the syndrome – the chronic perfusion defect – is even easier to detect (Table 9.2). Commonly used techniques include:
(i)   positron emission tomographic imaging – using [13]nitrogen-ammonia, or rubidium-82, for example, as markers;
(ii) monitoring the reversal of the regional wall abnormality (or asynergy) *following either* the administration of nitroglycerine to reduce myocardial

Table 9.2. Techniques used to detect hibernating myocardium

Technique	Basis of response
1. Nitroglycerine or isosorbide dinitrate administration	Reduced myocardial O_2 consumption
2. Adrenaline administration or postextrasystolic potentiation	Proof of contractile and metabolic reserve
3. Positron emission tomography	Persistence of metabolism despite perfusion defect
4. 2D echocardiographic ventriculogram, or radionuclide ventriculogram	Abnormal wall motion Delayed ventricular emptying

oxygen consumption (McAnulty et al. 1975; Bodenheimer et al. 1976; 1978; Banka et al. 1976) or coronary revascularization, to improve coronary perfusion (Chatterjee et al. 1972; Breisblatt et al. 1986; 1990), and
(iii) either the administration of a positive inotropic agent (Klausner et al. 1976; Massie et al. 1978; Nesto et al. 1982) or the induction of post-extrasystolic potentiation (Morton et al. 1978), to prove the existence of contractile and metabolic reserve, and the absence of lethal injury. Alternatively
(iv) the detection of delayed ventricular emptying monitored by radionuclide ventriculography can be used (Fernandes et al. 1991).

If the hibernating myocardium is hypokinetic and the immediate cause of that hypokineticity a sustained hypoperfusion, three questions follow as a matter of course:
(i) Under what clinical conditions, if any, does this situation occur?
(ii) What is the basis of the depressed contractile state?
(iii) What remedial measures can be taken, and in particular are the second generation calcium antagonists – or their prototypes – likely to be beneficial?

The Hibernating Myocardium: It's Clinical Occurrence

There are at least four conditions in which myocardial hibernation can be assumed to occur in patients with coronary heart disease. Susceptible patients include patients with either unstable or chronic stable angina, post-myocardial infarction or silent ischaemia.

(i) *Unstable Angina*
Patients with unstable angina often exhibit reduced wall motion at rest, painless and minor ST-T changes in their electrocardiograms (Chierchia et al. 1983) and unsatisfactory coronary perfusion. It can be assumed, therefore, that some segments of the myocardium are hibernating.

Table 9.3. Conditions which may promote myocardial hibernation

Condition	Reference
Unstable angina	Chierchia et al. 1983
Post myocardial infarction	Schuster et al. 1981
Chronic stable angina	Rankin et al. 1985
Left ventricular dysfunction of unknown aetiology	Akins et al. 1980
Silent ischaemia	Kannel 1989
Cardiac ischaemia in the neonate	Downing and Chen 1990

(ii) *Chronic Stable Angina*

Since coronary bypass surgery almost immediately improves and stabilizes left ventricular wall motion in approximately one third of patients with chronic stable angina (Rankin et al. 1985) this provides another group of patients with segments of hibernating myocardium – or at least the segments were hibernating prior to bypass surgery and the consequent restoration of perfusion (Table 9.3).

(iii) *Post Myocardial Infarction*

Acute myocardial infarction is usually a multivessel disease and whilst the area of infarction is well defined, areas adjacent to the infarct often exhibit wall motion abnormalities (Schuster et al. 1981). Again, it is likely that these adjacent zones contain hibernating tissue.

(iv) *Silent Ischaemia*

This is another subgroup of patients who show signs of abnormal left ventricular wall motion and compromised coronary blood flow. Developing atherogenic lesions are the most common cause. However, because these patients remain asymptomatic until the late stages of the occlusive event and their ECG's fail to reveal the tell-tale signs of ischaemia, the "hibernating" state of the affected myocardium often remains unrecognized.

These examples of conditions under which segments of the myocardium almost certainly *"hibernate"* are mentioned here only to establish that, as with the stunned hearts (Chapter 8), the hibernating myocardium is a clinically identifiable syndrome and not just a laboratory curiosity. The list is by no means exhaustive. Ischaemic neonatal hearts, for example, are probably hibernating (Downing and Chen 1990).

The Possible Causes of the Depressed Contractile State

By definition, the "hibernating" heart suffers from only one major defect – that of chronic underperfusion. The end-result is hypokinesis of the ventricular wall, not infarction – unless the underlying perfusion defect intensifies. When considered at the cellular level, possible causes of the hypokinetic state include:

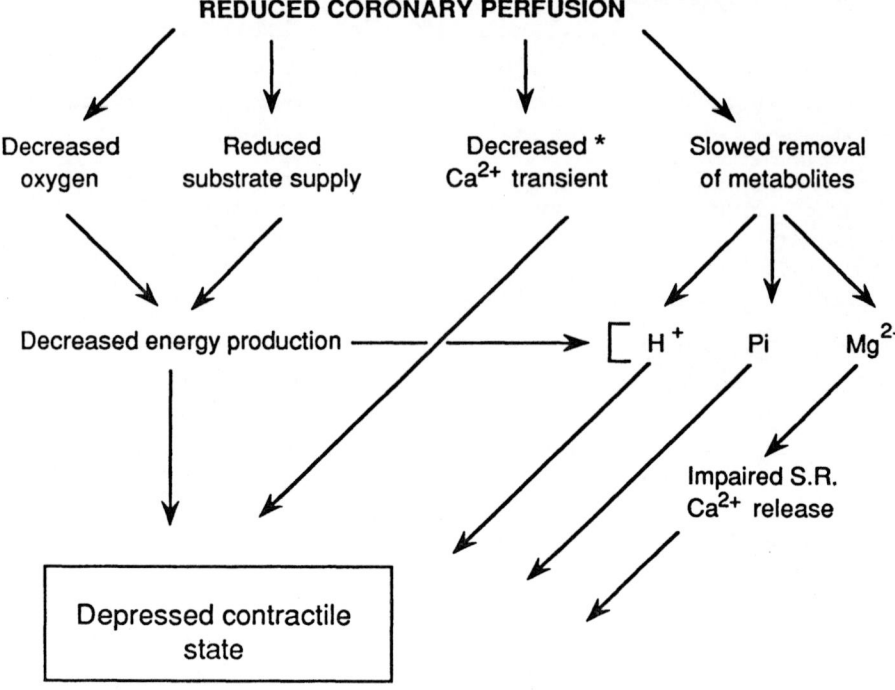

Fig. 9.3. Schematic representation of the possible consequences of a chronic reduction in coronary blood flow. * denotes the response which is largely responsible for the state of contractile dysfunction known as "hibernation"

(i)   the metabolic consequences of the hypoperfusion;
(ii) the physical consequences of the accompanying reduction in coronary perfusion pressure – as in the "garden hose" effect (Arnold et al. 1968);
(iii) an altered intracellular ionic homeostasis, and
(iv) an excitation-contraction coupling defect.

Metabolic Consequences of Hypoperfusion

The metabolic consequences of persistent hypoperfusion can be subdivided into two main categories (Fig. 9.3) – impaired energy production due to substrate and oxygen insufficiency, and a slowed removal of metabolites. Theoretically either, or both, of these sequelae could contribute to the hypokineticity of the hibernating myocardium. However, although insufficient energy production to meet the requirements for contraction would seem to be the most logical reason for the poor contractile function, such an explanation is untenable. Difficulties with an explanation of this sort centre around:

(i)   the rapid reversibility of the hypokinetic state – as for example, after nitroglycerine administration (Helfant et al. 1974), after revascularization

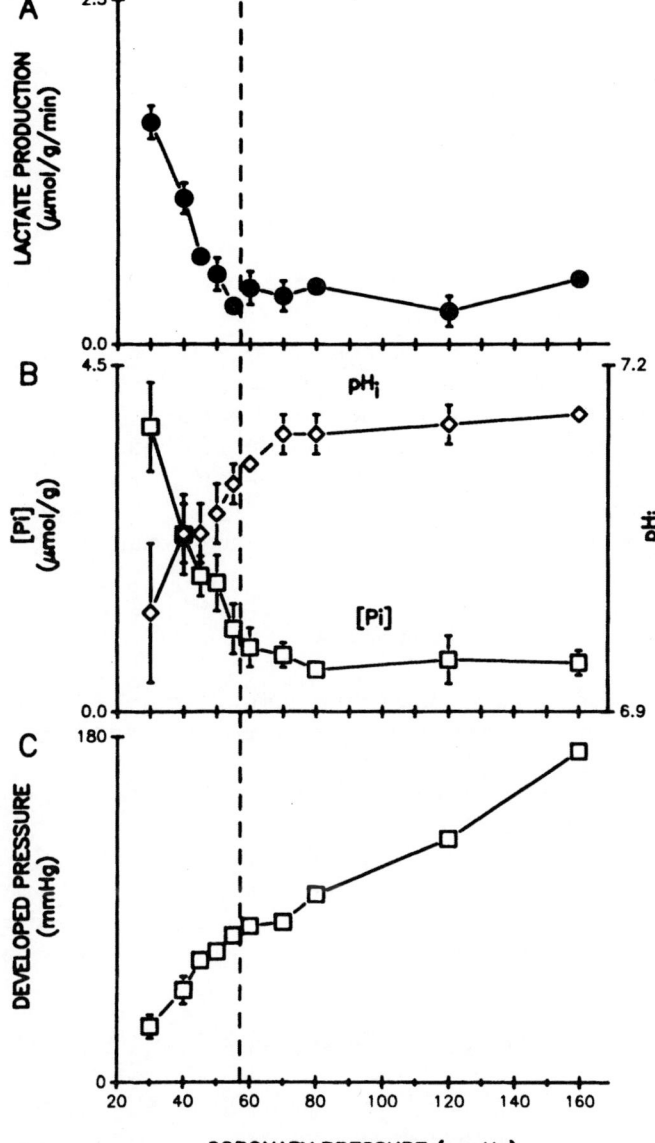

Fig. 9.4. Effect of perfusion pressure on lactate production (panel A), inorganic phosphate (P$_i$) and intracellular pH (pH$_i$) (panel B), and developed pressure (panel C) during twitch contractions in ferret hearts perfused with 2mM Ca^{2+}. Note that a reduction in perfusion pressure (from 80 to 60mm Hg) does cause a small rise in cytosolic P$_i$ and a fall in pH$_i$. (Reproduced from Marban 1991, with permission.)

(Chatterjee et al. 1972; 1973) and following the introduction of positive inotropic interventions (Dyke et al. 1974; Horn et al. 1974). This rapid reversibility must mean that although hypokinetic, the hibernating heart retains considerable metabolic and functional reserve, which for some reason, it does not use – unless "prodded". In addition,

(ii) NMR spectroscopy (Marban 1991) has failed to reveal any evidence of either significant metabolic failure or ischaemia-induced changes in metabolism which could account for the dysfunction. The rate of lactate production does not change significantly, nor are there marked changes in cytosolic P_i or H^+, although there is a tendency for each of these parameters to increase as perfusion pressure falls (Fig. 9.4). Moreover, as far as can be gauged from NMR spectroscopy, the tissue reserves of adenosine triphosphate (Fig. 9.5) are well maintained, even after a positive inotropic agent or manoeuvre has been introduced.

Physical Consequences of Hypoperfusion

According to the "garden hose" effect, distention of the intracardiac coronary arteries stretches the myocytes adjacent to the vessels, causing an increase in contractile force by way of the Frank-Starling mechanism. It is difficult to account for the contractile dysfunction of the hibernating heart in this way, because although increasing the coronary perfusion pressure leads to an increase in the contractile state of these hearts, this increase occurs without any accompanying change in sarcomere length (Kitakaze and Marban 1989).

Altered Intracellular Homeostasis

Although the changes in cytosolic inorganic phosphate (P_i) and hydrogen ion (H^+) concentration which occur under these conditions are small (Fig. 9.4), they could theoretically contribute to the hypokinetic state. H^+ ions, for example, displace Ca^{2+} from their binding sites on the contractile proteins, and P_i desensitizes the myofibrils to Ca^{2+} (Kentish 1986). Such effects are rapidly reversible, and certainly contribute to the contractile dysfunction exhibited by hypoxic hearts (Koretsune and Marban 1990a; 1990b). Theoretically, therefore they could contribute to the contractile dysfunction of hibernating hearts – and any effect they might have would rapidly disappear when normal coronary perfusion was re-introduced.

Impaired Excitation-Contraction Coupling

At the present time this seems to be the most likely cause of the depressed functional state. Using 5,5'F_2-BAPTA and NMR spectroscopy to monitor changes in cytosolic Ca^{2+} on a beat to beat basis Marban (Marban 1991) has recently shown that a reduction in coronary perfusion pressure actually reduces the Ca^{2+}-transient – that is, *it reduces the amount of Ca^{2+}* made available to the contractile proteins on a beat to beat basis for use in active tension development. Such an effect is evident in the records reproduced as Fig. 9.5. This decrease in the amount of Ca^{2+} which becomes available for use in excitation-contraction coupling contrasts sharply with the conditions described in the last chapter for myocardial stunning, where despite the concommitant decline in the contractile state of the myocardium cytosolic Ca^{2+} actually rises!

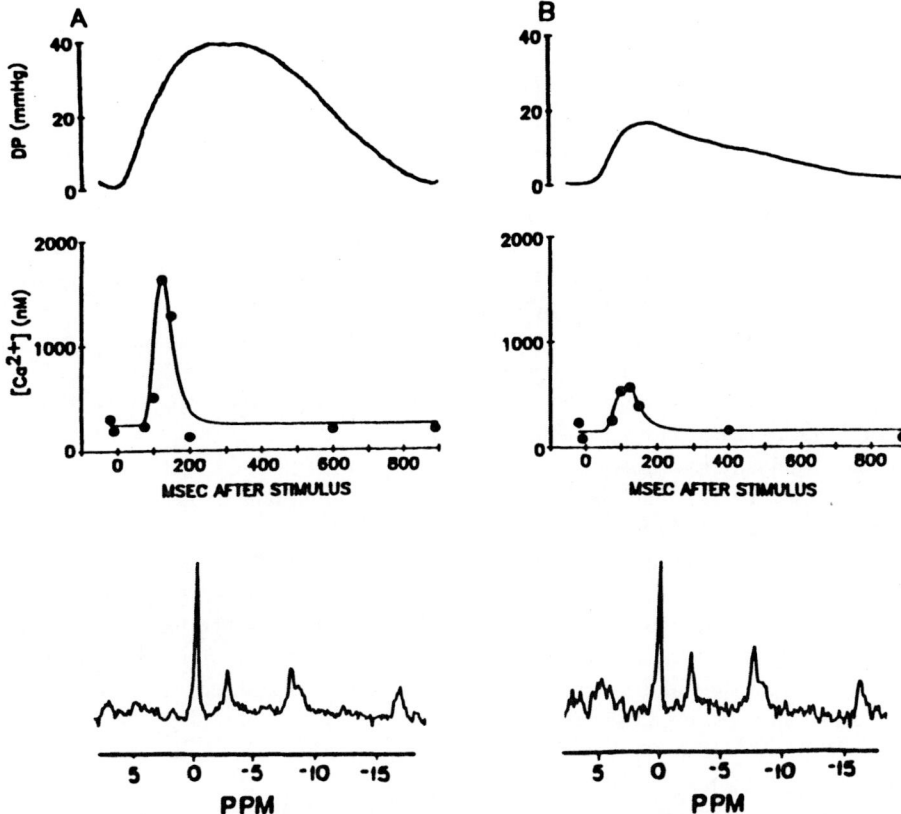

Fig. 9.5. Measurement of $[Ca^{2+}]_i$ (cytosolic Ca^{2+}) in a perfused heart with $5,5^1F_2$-BAPTA at two perfusion pressures. Panel A: contractile pressure, Ca^{2+} transient and phosphorous-31 spectrum during control perfusion (perfusion pressure 80mm Hg), and (B) during hibernation induced by lowering the perfusion pressure to 60mm Hg. Note the decrease in force and systolic intracellular Ca^{2+} with little change in energy metabolism as gauged by the ^{31}P spectrum. This fall in $[Ca^{2+}]_i$ is probably responsible for the hypokinetic state of the myocardium (reproduced from Marban 1991, with permission)

As yet, there is no unequivocal explanation as to why hypoperfusion causes a decline in the amount of Ca^{2+} which becomes available for use in excitation-contraction coupling. Theoretically it could result from either:

(i)   reduced inward Ca^{2+} current, or

(ii) a failure of the Ca^{2+}-induced Ca^{2+}-release process of the sarcoplasmic reticulum (Chapter 4). In this latter case,

    (a) the magnitude of the "trigger" Ca^{2+} may be reduced;

    (b) the intraluminal Ca^{2+} stores of the reticulum may be depleted, or "locked" in and therefore unavailable for release, or

    (c) the Ca^{2+} release channels associated with the junction "feet" processes may be functioning imperfectly. As to this latter possibility Mg^{2+} ions may be the culprit because cytosolic Mg^{2+} increases during episodes of ischaemia and, as discussed in Chapter 4, these ions close the Ca^{2+}-release channels of the sarcoplasmic reticulum (Williams and Ashley 1989).

Probably there is no single cause of the hibernation-induced decline in contractility but one thing is certain – the decline in the magnitude of the "trigger" Ca^{2+} is a major contributor to the response, and whatever its cause, it is easily overcome.

In general, although the precise cause of this hypoperfusion-induced state of contractile dysfunction is unknown, some potential causes can be *rejected*, just as others can be accepted. Rejected potential causes include:

(i)   energy depletion, NMR spectroscopy having failed to provide any evidence of this (Marban 1991). However the associated but small rise in P_i may be involved, either by decreasing the phosphorylation potential or by a direct inhibitory effect on myofibrillar activity;

(ii)   electrophysiological disturbances, since these are minimal;

(iii) ultrastructural changes, because the changes are minimal and largely restricted to glycogen depletion;

(iv)   failure of mitochondrial oxidative phosphorylation, and

(v)   free radical accumulation. Although this contributes to myocardial "stunning" and many other conditions, it is unlikely to be involved in myocardial hibernation, because, by definition, the restoration of normal coronary perfusion results in the prompt recovery of function – and recovery from free-radical induced injury is never prompt!

On balance, it seems probable that the most likely cause of this "hibernation" process involves the restricted supply of "activator" Ca^{2+}. There is no need to postulate a decrease in the Ca^{2+} sensitivity of the myofilaments – as there is in the stunned hearts. However, knowing that the Ca^{2+} which is available for excitation-contraction coupling is reduced on a beat to beat basis is only half of the story – what is required now is a description of the mechanisms which are involved. As yet, these mechanisms are unknown. The possible involvement of a small rise in cytosolic Mg^{2+} should not be disregarded, however, because, as discussed in an earlier chapter, these ions are remarkably efficient at prolonging the closing of the SR Ca^{2+} release channels.

Effective Remedial Measures

Since the hibernating myocardium has considerable contractile and metabolic reserve (Table 9.2, and Marban 1991) but suffers from a restricted supply of activator Ca^{2+}, it is logical to suggest that positive inotropic drugs or interventions (as in paired pacing) should be used to overcome the contractile defect. After all, if the primary defect is a reduced availability of activator Ca^{2+}, then any agent which either increases the amount of Ca^{2+} that enters by way of the voltage-sensitive Ca^{2+}-selective channels or via the $Na^+:Ca^{2+}$ exchanger, or which enhances Ca^{2+} release from the sarcoplasmic reticulum, should be of benefit – as indeed such agents are

(Klausner et al. 1976; Massie et al. 1978; Rahimtoola 1985). Conversely, agents which decrease Ca^{2+} entry through the Ca^{2+} selective channels are probably contraindicated, since they would further reduce the amount of Ca^{2+} available for excitation-contraction coupling. For this reason calcium antagonists which have a direct negative inotropic effect on the heart – and this includes all of the first generation calcium antagonists – would have to be excluded, *unless* their effect on either afterload, venous return or end-diastolic volume was such that it outweighed their direct negative inotropy. Obviously vascular selective second generation calcium antagonists would be more appropriate.

From a purely theoretical point of view there are at least two reasons why some of the vascular selective *second generation* calcium antagonists may improve the functional state of the hibernating myocardium. These reasons are as follows:

(i) because of their vascular selectivity peripheral vascular resistance will fall without any accompanying negative inotropy. Instead of declining, the inotropic state of the myocardium will be enhanced, because of the change in end-diastolic volume associated with the altered venous return and the Frank-Starling mechanism, and

(ii) those second generation antagonists which lack negative inotropy and which, as well as being vascular selective, are particularly selective for the coronary vasculature, will enhance coronary flow, thereby directly attenuating the underlying perfusion defect. The second generation calcium antagonist

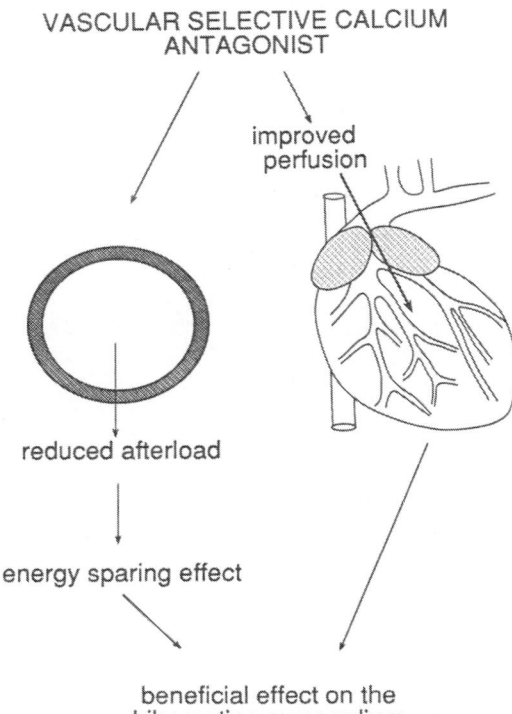

VASCULAR SELECTIVE CALCIUM ANTAGONIST

improved perfusion

reduced afterload

energy sparing effect

beneficial effect on the hibernating myocardium

Fig. 9.6. Schematic representation of the way in which vascular selective calcium antagonists might benefit the hibernating heart

nisoldipine would seem to act in this way (de Cock et al. 1990; Koolen et al. 1990), probably because it lacks any appreciable negative inotropy, enhances coronary flow and reduces peripheral vascular resistance.

In Summary

1. Myocardial "hibernation" describes a reversible state of contractile dysfunction caused by chronic hypoperfusion and does not involve tissue injury or marked electrophysiological disturbances.
2. At the cellular level the predominant cause of the contractile dysfunction appears to involve, or centre around, a decreased availability of Ca^{2+} for excitation-contraction coupling ("activator Ca^{2+}").
3. Despite being in a state of contractile dysfunction, hibernating hearts possess contractile and metabolic reserve and therefore respond to inotropic stimuli, including paired pacing.
4. Second generation calcium antagonists which are vascular selective appear to be beneficial (Fig. 9.6) particularly if they selectively dilate the coronary vasculature.

Chapter 10

Second Generation Calcium Antagonists and the Ischaemic Myocardium

> *"I put the words down and push them around a bit."*
> EVELYN WAUGH

As outlined in the last two chapters, ischaemia-induced injury which progresses to infarction is the third and by far the least desirable consequence of inadequate coronary perfusion. The other two sequelae ("stunning" and "hibernation") are reversible conditions which occur without marked electrophysiological abnormalities or ultrastructural damage. By contrast prolonged episodes of ischaemia precipitate a cascade of events which results in irreversible loss of structure and function, irrespective of whether coronary blood flow is satisfactorily restored. Recognized causes of this latter condition include:
(i)   sustained coronary spasm (Luscher 1991);
(ii)   aggregates of thrombi (Davies 1990);
(iii) disruption and fracturing of atherogenic plaques (Fuster et al. 1990);
(iv)   arterial narrowing – usually due to the formation of atherosclerotic lesions;
(v)   a sudden and catastrophic reduction in perfusion pressure, and
(vi)   a disproportionately large cardiac work load relative to the available coronary blood flow – as, for example in a hypertrophied heart with calcified arteries or in the presence of an abnormally high peripheral vascular resistance.

The question which interests us here is will the second generation calcium antagonists provide protection under these conditions, just as they do for the "stunned" and "hibernating" hearts? The rationale behind this questions includes the following:
(i)   many of these second generation antagonists are vascular selective and therefore might be used to "unload" the heart and hence to act as energy sparing agents without aggravating any existing left ventricular dysfunction;
(ii)   at least one of them – nisoldipine – is relatively selective for the coronary vasculature (Kazda et al. 1980) and therefore might be used to restore flow to the affected area, as well as unloading the heart;
(iii) some have long half-lives (e.g. amlodipine and the slow release formulations of the prototypes), and therefore can be used to provide effective calcium channel antagonist activity on a twenty four hour basis without the need for repetitive dosing;
(iv)   another member of the group – felodipine – tends to normalize the impaired baroreceptor control found in patients with compromised left ventricular function (Kassis and Amtorp 1987);

(v) some of them protect against lipid-peroxidation induced injury to myocytes and vascular cell membrane (e.g. nisoldipine, Chapter 6), and

(vi) at least one of the second generation drugs (anipamil) has relatively little effect on AV conduction, relative to its prototype, verapamil, and therefore can be used to unload the circulation and to protect the myocardium without the risk of causing prolonged bradycardia.

Ischaemic syndromes (excluding "stunning" and "hibernation") include effort- and rest-induced angina pectoris, vasospastic (or Prinzmetal's) angina, silent ischaemia and finally, infarction. Only the last of these conditions – infarction – is relative to this chapter. The others (angina pectoris, vasospastic angina, and silent ischaemia) are discussed in Chapter 15).

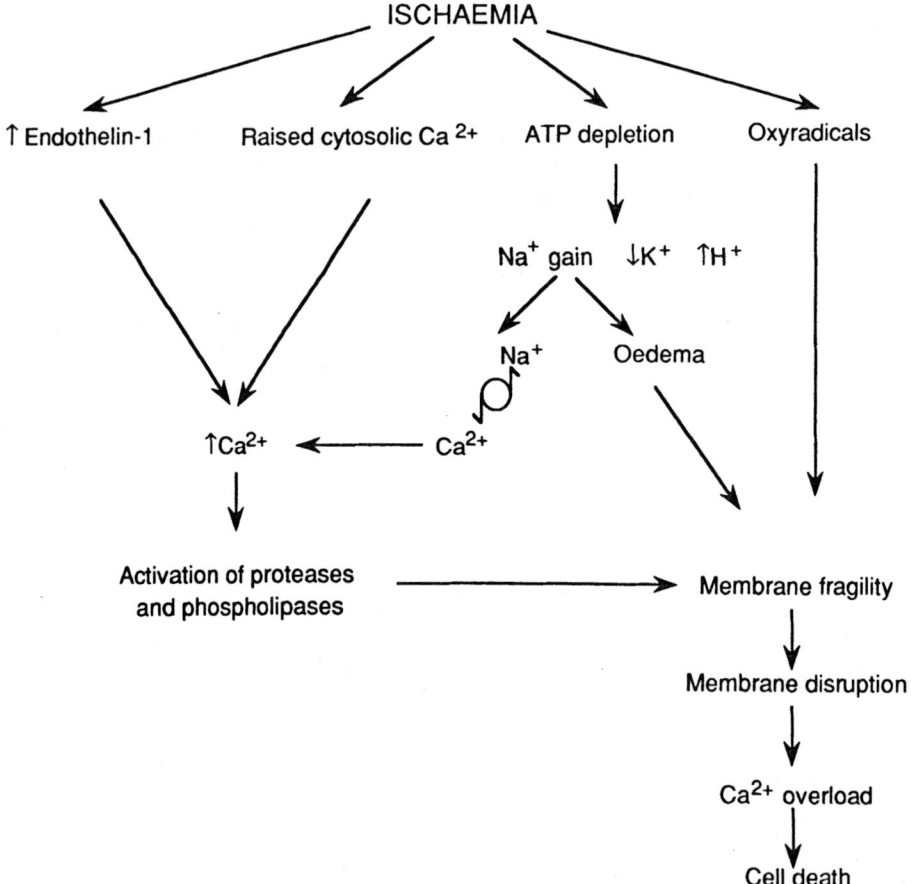

Fig. 10.1. Schematic representation of the consequences of a prolonged ischaemic episode

Myocardial Infarction

Early Biochemical Changes

The biochemical consequences of a prolonged and severe reduction in coronary perfusion are now fairly well established (Fig. 10.1). They include the depletion of the high energy phosphate reserves and their precursors (Jennings et al. 1990), acidification – largely due to the accumulation of lactate and phosphate ions – loss of ionic homeostasis with respect to Ca^{2+}, Na^+ and K^+, and malfunctioning of the SR Ca^{2+} release channels such that they leak Ca^{2+} into cytosolic (Chapter 4). Other changes include:

(i)   externalization of α and β adrenergic and endothelin-1 receptors;
(ii) disruption of the cytoskeleton (Ganote and Vander Heide 1987; Jennings et al. 1990);
(iii) the generation of free radicals (Weisfeldt 1987; Lucchesi 1990);
(iv) the release of endogenously stored catecholamines (Schomig 1990), and
(v)   an increase in cytosolic Ca^{2+} (Fig. 10.2) at a time when total tissue Ca^{2+} is either unaltered, or may even have fallen.

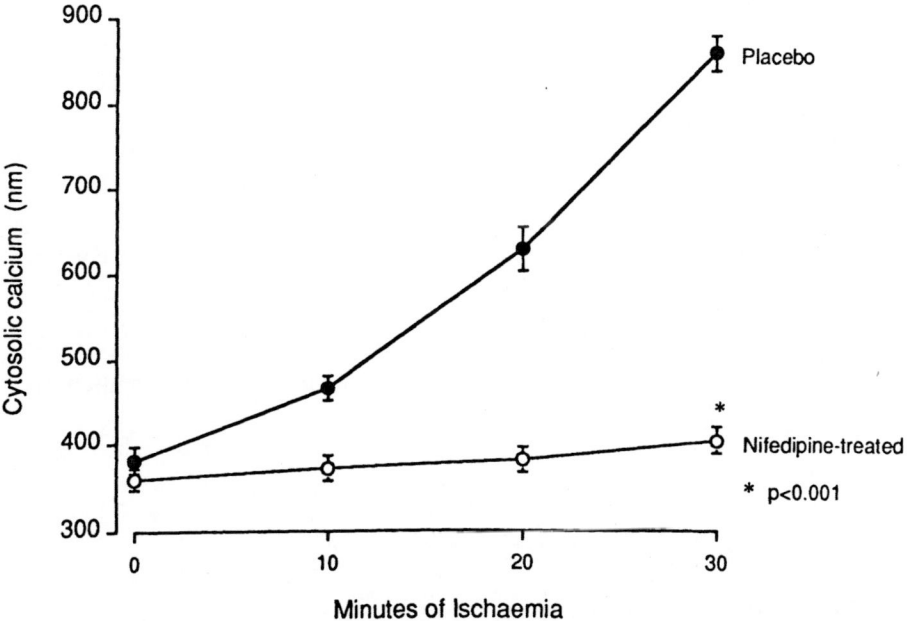

Fig. 10.2. Effect of ischaemia on cytosolic Ca^{2+} (measured by NMR spectroscopy using 5-5′ FBAPTA as a Ca^{2+} indicator) in isolated rat hearts. The measurements relate to the signal averaged measurements made over a 5–7 minute time interval. Each result is mean ± SEM of 5–6 measurements. Nifedipine was added 15 minutes prior to making the hearts globally ischaemic, to provide a final concentration of $10^{-7}M$

Early Ultrastructural Changes

The events which have been listed so far occur relatively early during the ischaemic episode, at a time when recovery is still possible. These changes are accompanied by evidence of progressive morphological damage – including swelling of the mitochondria, distortion of the sarcolemma, disappearance of the glycogen granules, swelling of the sarcoplasmic reticulum and the disruption of an occasional Z band. Even at this stage, however, the sarcolemma remains intact, although increasingly fragile.

Late Biochemical and Ultrastructural Changes

As the duration of the ischaemic episode progresses cytosolic Ca^{2+} (Fig. 10.2) continues to rise and oedema develops, until finally the plasmalemma loses its integrity to such an extent that cytosolic enzymes – which are relatively large macromolecules begin appearing in the extracellular fluid. By this time the Ca^{2+}-dependent endogenous proteases and phospholipases are activated, the myofibrils show signs of lysis and many of the mitochondria are vacuolated and contain deposits of calcium apatite. Reperfusion at this stage causes a burst of oxyradical production (Weisfeldt 1987), massive Ca^{2+} overloading, and explosive swelling of the myocytes. The affected myocytes soon die and necrose.

The Significance of the Early Rise in Cytosolic Ca^{2+}

The rise in cytosolic Ca^{2+} which occurs relatively early during ischaemia, long before there is any overall increase in total tissue Ca^{2+} and whilst the sarcolemma is still intact is probably a crucial event here. Various investigators have used a variety of intracellular Ca^{2+}-sensitive indicators to document this rise, including the 5.5′ difluoro derivative of 1,2-bis (O-aminophenoxy) ethane – N, N, N^1 – 1-tetraacetic acid (5F-BAPTA) (Steenbergen et al. 1987; Koretsune and Marban 1980b). Presumably much of this Ca^{2+} originates from the sarcoplasmic reticulum and cannot be retrieved because of the limited availability of adenosine triphosphate as substrate for the relevant Ca^{2+}-activated ATPase enzymes. Irrespective of its origin, the significance of this early rise in cytosolic Ca^{2+} involves:
(i)   its ability to activate the lysosomal proteases and phospholipases;
(ii) its stimulant effect on oxyradical production, and
(iii) its involvement in the increase in end-diastolic resting tension which occurs at this time (Apstein et al. 1988).

If the magnitude of this early rise in cytosolic Ca^{2+} is a key event in determining whether reperfusion is accompanied by the recovery of a normal ultrastructure and function (systolic and diastolic) then it is logical to expect that the attenuation of this rise in cytosolic Ca^{2+} will favour recovery. Pretreatment with either diltiazem,

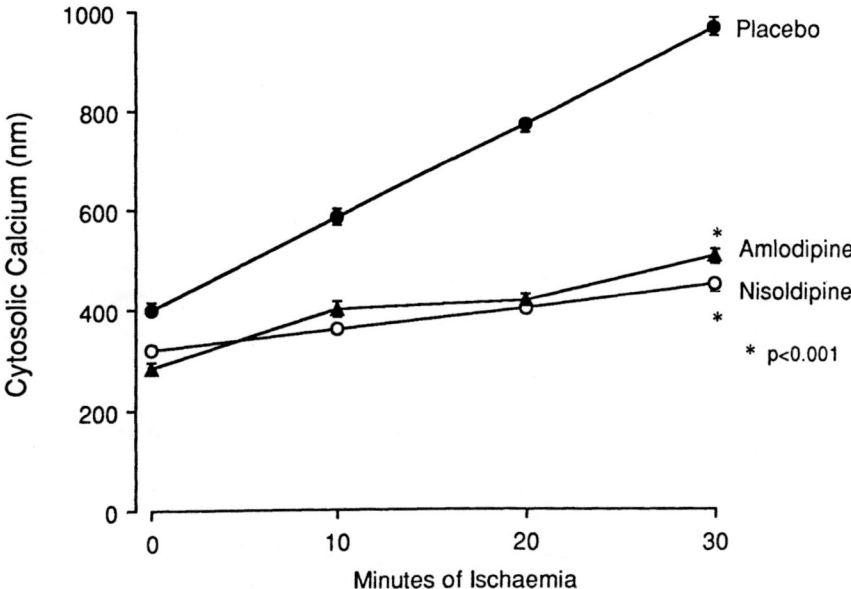

Fig. 10.3. Effect of pretreatment with nisoldipine (10^{-7}M) (added directly to the perfusion buffer) and amlodipine (0.25mg·kg^{-1} given intravenously, 3 hours before starting the experiment) on the ischaemia-induced rise in cytosolic Ca^{2+} in isolated Langendorrf-perfused rat hearts. Cytosolic Ca^{2+} was measured as described in Figure 10.2

verapamil (Watts et al. 1990) or nifedipine (Fig. 10.2) does have such an effect – so does nisoldipine and amlodipine (Fig. 10.3).

The Possible Contribution of Endothelin-1 to Ischaemia-Reperfusion Injury

In Chapter 7 of this book some information was provided relating to the intense vasoconstrictor effect of the polypeptide, endothelin-1. This polypeptide is extremely relevant to current discussions relating to the aetiology of irreversible ischaemia-induced injury to the myocardium because:

(i)   not only is this polypeptide a potent vasoconstrictor, it also mobilizes intracellular Ca^{2+};

(ii) cardiac myocytes, as well as the coronary vasculature, contain endothelin-1 specific binding sites;

(iii) the plasma levels of endothelin-1 increase quite dramatically during ischaemia, due to an enhanced rate of production at the mRNA level (Miyauchi et al. 1989);

(iv) latent endothelin-1 receptors are externalized and become functional during ischaemia and post-ischaemic reperfusion (Nayler et al. 1990b; Liu et al. 1990), and

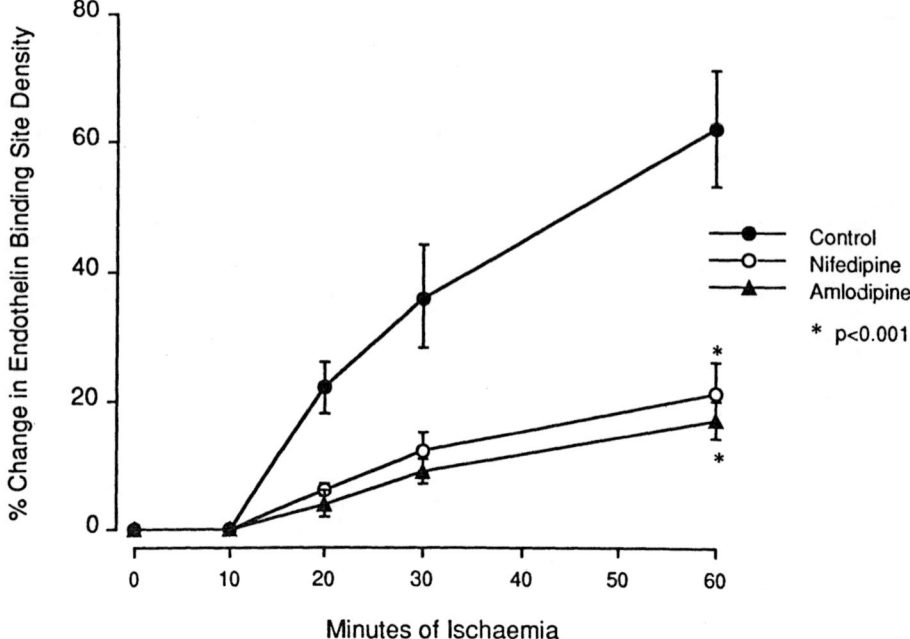

Fig. 10.4. Effect of 10^{-6}M nifedipine, added to the isolated hearts 15 minutes before making them ischaemic, and 0.25mg/kg amlodipine given intravenously three hours before isolating the hearts and making them globally ischaemic, on the ischaemia-induced increase in endothelin-1 binding site density

(v) calcium antagonist drugs – including first and second generation drugs, attenuate this ischaemia-reperfusion induced externalization of these receptors (Nayler et al. 1990b, and Fig. 10.4).

These observations relating to the possible involvement of endothelin-1 in the events which are triggered by an ischaemic episode and which may trigger or contribute to the early rise in cytosolic Ca^{2+} which occurs during ischaemic conditions are relevant to this discussion – because if left to progress unhindered, the sequel can only be a raised end diastolic resting tension followed by cell death and tissue necrosis (Nayler 1990). Precisely why the calcium antagonists attenuate the ischaemia-induced internalization of the endothelin-1 receptors is unknown – possibly it is a secondary consequence of their ability to prevent excessive Ca^{2+} influx by way of the L-type Ca^{2+} channels at a time when the energy reserves have fallen to such an extent as to allow the Ca^{2+} to remain in the cytosol.

Hence, the second generation calcium antagonists share with their prototypes, the ability to attenuate the early rise in cytosolic Ca^{2+} which occurs under conditions of severe ischaemia (Figs. 10.3 and 10.4), and which precedes any rise in total tissue Ca^{2+} or loss of membrane integrity. This, together with their ability to act as energy-sparing agents (by reducing the work load on the heart), to dilate the coronary vasculature (Chapter 15) and to prevent the externalization of the endothelin-1

receptors provides a logical rationale for their use as protective agents. In this context some of the second generation antagonists will possibly be less complicated to use than their prototypes because:
(i)   they possess relatively little negative inotropy, and
(ii) their prolonged duration of action will ensure protection on a twenty four hour basis.

Clinical Evidence of a Protective Role
for the Second Generation Antagonists

It is too early, as yet, to decide whether the second generation antagonists do reduce infarct size and decrease the risk of re-infarction. Preliminary evidence, however, suggests that they will be of benefit. Some of this evidence comes from the study of de Cock et al. (1990), who monitored systolic and diastolic function in patients receiving nisoldipine following myocardial infarction. They concluded that "nisoldipine reduced exercise-induced ischemia and improved exercise capacity and diastolic left ventricular function in post-infarction patients with reduced left ventricular function". Tzivoni et al. (1991) reached a similar conclusion in a small but double-blind, placebo-controlled trial using repeated exercising to provoke an ischaemic episode.

In Summary

1. Prolonged episodes of ischaemia result in a progressive rise in cytosolic Ca^{2+}, in addition to the gradual depletion of the high energy phosphate reserves.
2. This rise in cytosolic Ca^{2+} involves the redistribution of internally stored Ca^{2+}, possibly due to:
   (i)   leakage of Ca^{2+} from the SR (Chapter 4);
   (ii) a failure of the Ca^{2+} retrieval mechanisms, and
   (iii) endothelin-1 mediated mobilization of intracellular Ca^{2+}.
3. The early rise in cytosolic Ca^{2+} precedes any increase in total tissue Ca^{2+} and may be responsible for triggering the cascade of events which results in cell death and tissue necrosis.
4. The second generation calcium antagonists resemble their prototypes in attenuating this early rise in cytosolic Ca^{2+}, possibly because they:
   (i)   act as energy sparing agents, and
   (ii) attenuate the ischaemia-induced externalization of the endothclin-1 receptors at a time when the plasma levels of endothelin-1 are rising.
5. Clinical trials are needed now to establish whether these second generation calcium antagonists which are relatively selective for the vasculature can be administered early during an ischaemic episode without running the risk of exacerbating existing ventricular dysfunction.

Chapter 11

The Molecular Mechanisms Involved in the Anti-Atherogenic Effect of the Calcium Antagonists

> *"A fool is a man who never tried an experiment in his life."*
> Sir FRANCIS DARWIN, 1877.

Atherosclerosis is neither a new nor a particularly pleasant disease. The ancient Greek physicians were familiar with it, as were the Egyptians, but they could neither treat nor control it. Even today it remains the leading cause of death in many countries (Castelli 1984; American Heart Association Report 1990), but this surely must change, now that so many risk factors have been identified (Luria et al. 1991; Zemel et al. 1990) and the molecular mechanisms involved in the early stages of lesion formation unravelled (Ross 1986; Henry 1990a; 1990b). Effective treatment regimes are beginning to appear, some involving dietary control (Thompson 1991), others making use of lipid-lowering agents (Brown et al. 1990; Rossouw et al. 1990). When tackling the problem of atherosclerosis, however, it should be remembered that atherosclerosis is a multifactorial disease which involves not just lipid accumulation but also the localized accumulation of collagen, elastin and calcium, together with monocyte infiltration, endothelial injury, and smooth muscle cell proliferation and migration (Nayler 1988; Weinstein and Heider 1988; 1989; Henry 1990a; 1990b). Many of these events are calcium-dependent (Henry 1990a) and principally for this reason laboratory and clinical trials have been undertaken to determine whether calcium antagonists interrupt the cascade of events which culminate in lesion formation (Fig. 11.1). Until recently the only results which were available came from laboratory studies in which fat-fed animals were used, but now several carefully designed clinical trials have been completed (Table 11.1). They show, unequivocally, that calcium antagonists slow the growth of spontaneously developing atherosclerotic lesions in human coronary arteries (Table 11.1). These trials include the INTACT study (Lichtlen et al. 1990) in which nifedipine was used, and the Montreal study (Waters et al. 1990) which used nicardipine. These, and the other trials listed in Table 11.1 are important because:

(i) they re-inforce the data already obtained from studies on fat-fed animals (Table 11.2);

(ii) the results relate specifically to spontaneous lesion formation in *coronary* arteries;

(iii) they provide the basis for an alternative form of treatment (as apposed to the use of lipid-lowering agents – or diet), and

(iv) since clinically relevant doses were used they remove the concern which used to be expressed concerning the relatively high doses used in some of the earlier animal studies.

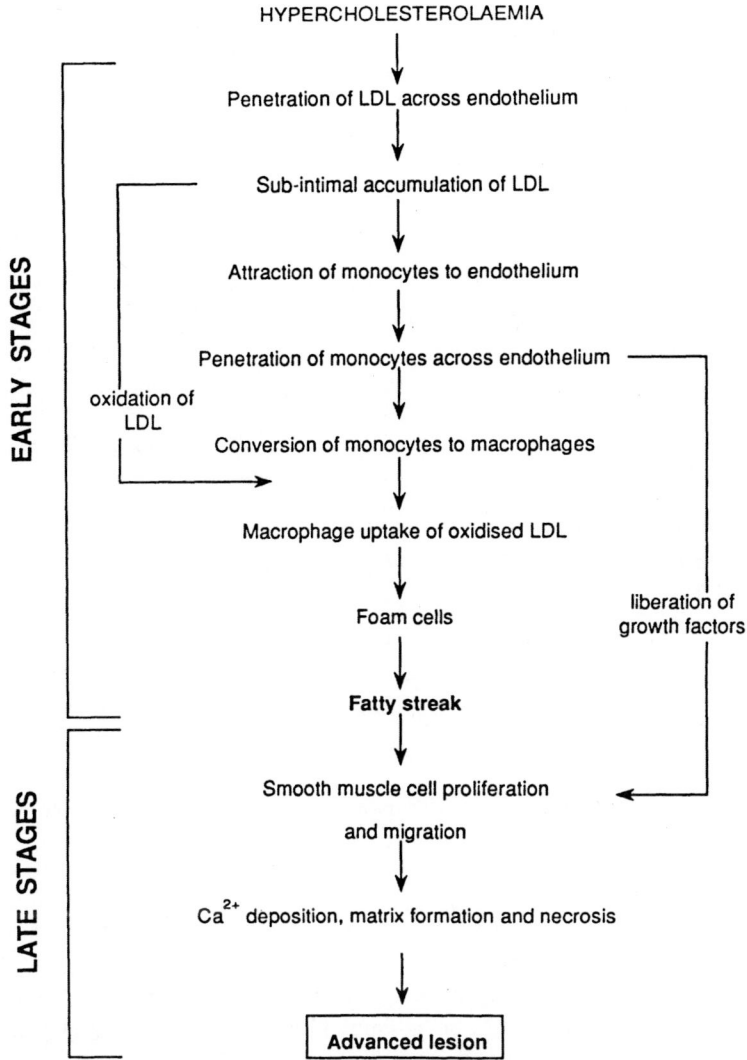

Fig. 11.1. Schematic representation of the cascade of events which culminates in the formation of an advanced atherosclerotic lesion

However, it is no longer sufficient to know that the calcium antagonists are antiatherogenic; it is also important to establish the reason. Is it because they affect one or more of the risk factors – hypertension, for example – or do they alter plasma lipids? Neither of these possibilities seems to be important in this context. For example, in the cholesterol-fed rabbit model of atherosclerosis the antiatherogenic effect occurs without any accompanying change in blood pressure (Henry and Bentley 1981). The same applies to the human studies (Lichtlen et al. 1990; Waters et al. 1990), where the decline in blood pressure in the drug-treated patients is matched

Table 11.1. The inhibitory effect of calcium antagonists on the progression of atherosclerotic lesions in humans

Calcium antagonist	Patient no	Vessel	Treatment period	Result	Reference
A. 1st Generation Calcium Antagonists					
Nifedipine (INTACT study)* (80 mg/day)	425	Coronary	3 years	Positive	Lichtlen et al. 1990
Nifedipine (60 mg/day)	72	Coronary	1 year	Positive	Gottlieb et al. 1989
Nifedipine (80 mg/day)	39	Coronary	2 years	Positive	Loaldi et al. 1989
Verapamil (124–480 mg/day)	26	Coronary	5–34 months	Positive	Kober et al. 1989
B. 2nd Generation Calcium Antagonists					
Nicardipine (80 mg/day)	383	Coronary	2 years	Positive	Waters et al. 1990
Trials in Progress					
A. 1st Generation Calcium Antagonists					
Verapamil (FIPS trial) (124–480 mg/day)	147	Coronary	5 years		Kober et al. 1989
Isradipine (Midas trial) (5–10 mg/day)		Carotid	3 years		Borhani et al. 1990

* denotes the trial is being extended. Positive result denotes slowed plaque formation

by an almost equal decline in the placebo-treated groups. Nor can the antiathero-genic effect of these drugs be explained in terms of a plasma cholesterol lowering effect – because the levels in both the animal and human trials were largely unchanged (Henry and Bentley 1981; Lichtlen et al. 1990; Waters et al. 1990). Admittedly the human trials covered a time scale of only two (Waters et al. 1990) or three (Lichtlen et al. 1990) years – which is a relatively short time when gauged against the time required for lesion formation – but other studies have failed to reveal any evidence of a cholesterol lowering effect even when the duration of treatment has extended beyond five years (Midtbø 1990) – although in these latter studies a *small* increase in plasma high density lipoprotein (HDL) cholesterol was observed.

In general, therefore, it now seems to be established that the calcium antagonists slow the growth of atherogenic lesions without altering two of the main risk factors – plasma cholesterol and hypertension. Their efficacy in this regard can no longer be assumed to apply only to artificially-induced atherosclerosis in fat-fed laboratory

Table 11.2. First and second generation calcium antagonists which slow atherogenesis in animal models

Compound	Model	Reference
A. 1st Generation Calcium Antagonists		
Nifedipine	Cholesterol-fed rabbit	Henry and Bentley 1981
		Willis et al. 1985
		Nayler and Panagiotopoulos 1986
Verapamil	Cholesterol fed rabbit	Blumein et a. 1984
		Rouleau et al. 1983
		Sievers et al. 1987
		Parmley 1990
Diltiazem	Cholesterol-fed rabbit	Ginsburg et al. 1983
		Habib et al. 1986a
B. 2nd Generation Calcium Antagonists		
Nicardipine	Cholesterol-fed rabbit	Willis et al. 1985
Isradipine	Cholesterol-fed rabbit	Habib et al. 1986b
Nisoldipine	Cholesterol-fed rabbit	Fronek 1988 and Fig. 11.4
Amlodipine	Cholesterol-fed rabbit	Nayler 1991
Darodipine	Cholesterol-fed rabbit	Weinstein and Heider 1988
Anipamil	Cholesterol-fed rabbit	Catapano et al. 1988
Nilvadipine	Rabbit cuffed carotid	Nomoto et al. 1987

animals because, as was shown in Table 11.1, they are equally effective in combating naturally occurring atherosclerosis in man. The question to be answered therefore, is not whether these drugs are effective – but why? To do this we first need to consider the events which contribute to plaque formation – not with respect to the risk factors but rather in terms of the molecular mechanisms involved in the growth of these lesions.

Lesion Formation: Sequence of Events

One way of describing an end-stage atherogenic plaque is to think of it as an acellular fibrotic "rubbish basket" for lethally injured cells which are laden with cholesterol, calcium and other debris. There are several reasons why these advanced plaques can be life-threatening. They may protrude into the lumen of the affected blood vessel, thereby restricting blood flow – as in the hibernating heart (Chapter 8). They provide a surface which attracts thrombi, and they are prone to rupture – and hence to precipitate acute occlusive events, which, if left unattended, promote infarction.

Calcium deposition and cell necrosis are relatively *late* events in the sequence of events which mediate lesion formation (Fig. 11.1). *Early* events include:
(i)   hypercholesterolaemia;
(ii) the focal accumulation of low density lipoproteins (LDL) in the subintimal space of an apparently normal artery;

(iii) the adhesion of monocytes (and lymphocytes) to endothelial cells, some of which may be injured – possibly because of:
   (a) excessive shear stress associated with either hypertension or acute vasospasm,
   (b) oxyradical-induced lipid peroxidation (Chapter 6) or
   (c) perhaps just because of the presence of abnormally high plasma cholesterol levels (Kutryk et al. 1991). In addition,
(iv) monocytes and lymphocytes infiltrate into the subendothelial intimal space;
(v) a variety of growth factors are liberated – including the platelet-derived growth factor, and endothelin-1 (Kanno et al. 1990);
(vi) monocytes convert into activated macrophages which then proceed to accumulate lipoproteins from the intimal space, thereby becoming foam cells. They also release growth factors, and
(vii) the released growth factors act on smooth muscle cells causing them to proliferate and migrate from the media to the intima. This is when the lesion starts to become bulky.

Relatively *late* events include (Fig. 11.1):
(i)   continued smooth muscle cell proliferation and migration;
(ii) excess deposition of ground substance and collagen, and
(iii) calcium deposition (as calcium apatite) and cell necrosis.

Factors Concerned with the *Initiation* of Plaque Formation

It is the endothelial cells and their response to the presence of relatively high levels of circulating low density lipoproteins (LDL) which initiate the cascade of events shown in Figure 11.1 (Steinberg et al. 1989; Schwenke and Carew 1989a). The initiating or priming event seems to involve a focal subintimal accumulation of the low density lipoproteins (Fig. 11.2) – an event which precedes any detectable change in the morphology of the overlying endothelial cells and occurs at a time when the selective permeability of the endothelial cell membranes is fully preserved (Schwenke and Carew 1989a; 1989b). Precisely why this happens is unknown, but there is a possibility that it involves the oxidation of membrane-located lipids. The next step involves the circulating monocytes. Instead of continuing to circulate these organelles start to adhere to the luminal surface of the endothelium overlying the focal LDL accumulations – as if there is a cause and effect relationship – possibly involving the local generation of chemotactic factors (Witztum 1990).

The monocytes which are attracted to the endothelium and which start migrating into the subintimal space (Fig. 11.2) presumably enter by way of the gap junctions which separate neighbouring endothelial cells, since by this stage the endothelium is still confluent – but not for much longer, because the monocytes, which by now have congregated in the subintimal space below the endothelium, become lipid-"scavengers", and rapidly "load-up" with cholesteryl ester. This is when the monocytes become "foam" cells. Unfortunately, as they accumulate more and more cholesterol these cells increase in volume, with the inevitable end-result of stretching

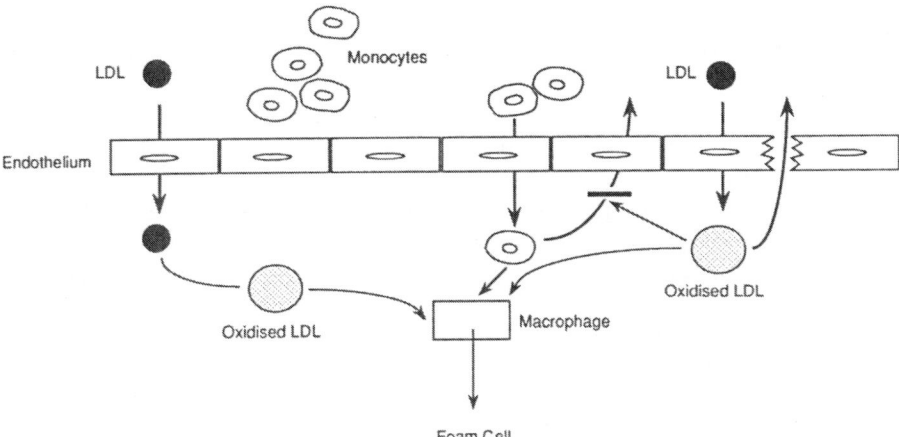

Fig. 11.2. Schematic representation of the role of oxidized low density lipoproteins (LDL) in the atherogenic process. (Adapted from Quinn et al. 1987.)

the endothelial layer until the already fragile endothelial cells simply fracture, or fall apart. The end result is that the macrophages, now laden with cholesteryl ester, become exposed to the circulating platelets. The sequence of events to date, therefore, is as follows: lipid infiltration → monocyte adherence to the endothelium → monocytic invasion of the subintimal space → conversion of monocytes to macrophages → cholesteryl ester loading of the macrophages → foam cells → endothelial disruption.

Even this description of the cascade is incomplete because it ignores some pivotal questions including:

(i)   why do the gap junctions between neighbouring endothelial cells suddenly admit LDL?

(ii)   what attracts the monocytes to the endothelium above the focal accumulations of LDL?

(iii) why, after invading the subintimal space, do the monocytes convert to macrophages?, and

(iv)   why do these organelles become such avid accumulators of the low density lipoproteins?

Comparatively little is known about the mechanisms involved in the initial entry of the LDL, or the factors which facilitate the conversion of monocytes into macrophages, once they become resident in the subintimal space. This is surprising, because these are critical events in the cascade that culminates in plaque formation. By contrast, the mechanisms involved in the rapid uptake of the low density lipoproteins by the macrophages have been more clearly delineated.

The Mechanism Involved in the Macrophage Accumulation of Low Density Lipoproteins (LDL)

Classical LDL receptor pathways cannot play a major role in this process because:

(i)   LDL receptors down-regulate when exposed to LDL;

(ii) humans with homozygous familial hypercholesterolaemia (HFH) develop severe atherosclerosis (accompanied by the conversion of monocytes to foam cells), and yet they lack LDL receptors, and

(iii) simply exposing monocytes to LDL's does not convert them into foam cells.

Obviously some other mechanism which does not require functioning LDL receptors must be involved. The discovery that the macrophages avidly accumulate LDL's *once these complexes have been modified in some way* may have provided the clue as to why the macrophages suddenly start accumulating LDL because the macrophages probably recognize the modified LDL particles as being foreign, and promptly accumulate them. This may be why LDL peroxidation is so important here (Steinberg et al. 1989), because it converts the LDL into a form which is recognized as being foreign and therefore attractive to the macrophages. Peroxidation of the LDL's involves the peroxidation of their polyunsaturated fatty acids and depends upon the presence of heavy metals – such as copper or iron. Obviously, therefore, it will be chelator-sensitive. Maybe this is why chelators such as ethylenediamine tetraacetic acid have antiatherosclerotic properties (Wartman et al. 1967).

Oxidatively-modified LDL contributes to the atherosclerotic process in other highly significant ways. For example:

(i)   it is a potent chemoattractant for monocytes, and accordingly may be responsible for attracting these organelles into the subintimal space. Secondly,

(ii) it actually inhibits the egress of macrophages (Quinn et al. 1987) so that once oxidized LDL has coaxed the monocytes into the subintimal space and the monocytes become macrophages, the oxidized LDL makes sure that the macrophages remain trapped there (Fig. 11.2). In addition the peroxidation products of LDL are highly reactive, and therefore probably promote tissue injury – including injury to the overlying endothelium.

Obviously oxidized LDL is rapidly becoming the villain of this epic. However, the hypothesis that oxidatively modified LDL plays a crucial role in the aetiology of atherosclerosis can only be accepted *if* it can be proved that oxidized LDL is a normal constituent of atherosclerotic arteries. Witztum and his colleagues (Witztum 1990) have recently established the validity of this claim. Their evidence includes the following:

(i)   LDL eluted from atherosclerotic arteries resembles oxidized LDL in terms of its electrophoretic mobility, cholesterol content and high lysophosphatidylcholine content;

(ii) immunological probes for oxidized LDL react positively with LDL isolated from atherosclerotic lesions;

(iii) immunological reagents stain positively for oxidation-specific LDL derivatives in atherosclerotic but not in non-atherosclerotic sections of aorta, and antioxidant agents, including probucol, slow atherosclerotic lesion formation. At the same time, and without lowering plasma cholesterol, probucol inhibits the uptake and degradation of LDL (Carew et al. 1987; Kita et al. 1987).

The avid accumulation of lipids by macrophages, and their accumulation in the subintimal space only takes us part of the way into the development of an atherosclerotic lesion. In fact, it only takes us to the "fatty streak" phase. Nevertheless, these "fatty streak" lesions are known to develop early in human atherosclerosis – they are present, for example, in the coronary arteries of relatively young children long before there is any symptomatic evidence of atherosclerosis (Stary 1987; 1989).

The Progression of the Fatty Streak to the Adult Plaque

The progression of the early "fatty streak" stage of an atherosclerotic lesion to the adult calcified and rigid plaque involves the migration of smooth muscle cells into the arterial intima. Here these cells proliferate – and some of them undergo phenotypic changes, becoming more like macrophages than smooth muscle cells. There are two reasons why arterial smooth muscle cells are an important component of the developing lesion:
(i)   they contribute enormously to its bulk, and
(ii) they secrete the connective tissue matrix which holds the lesion together.

Proliferation of the smooth muscle cells involves their stimulation by a variety of growth factors – including angiotensin II (Daemen et al. 1991), interleukin-1 (IL-1), transforming growth factor beta (TGFβ), and tumour necrosis factor alpha (TNFα) (Nathan 1987). Obviously, the macrophages are not the only source of growth factors. Others include the endothelium – endothelin-1 (Chapter 7) being a potent smooth muscle cell mitogen (Hirata et al. 1989). However, of all the mitogens that are present, platelet derived growth factor (PDGF) is probably the most important as far as the intimal proliferation of smooth muscle cells is concerned – and its production is not limited to macrophages. As its name implies it is also produced by platelets. The endothelium and smooth muscle cells are other sources.

    In summary, the events which are involved in the formation of an atherosclerotic lesion are extraordinarily complex. The initiating factor appears to be lipid infiltration followed closely by the adhesion of monocytes to the endothelium. The monocytes then migrate and locate in the subendothelial layer where they assume the role of macrophages. With time these early lesions increase in size and begin to include smooth muscle cells from the arterial wall. Ultimately the mass of the lesion is such that it disrupts the delicate endothelium, thrombi form, and the smooth muscle cells begin to die, necrose and calcify. It is a sobering thought to realize that it is only when the lesion has reached this advanced stage that it is angiographically detectable – or causes perfusion defects.

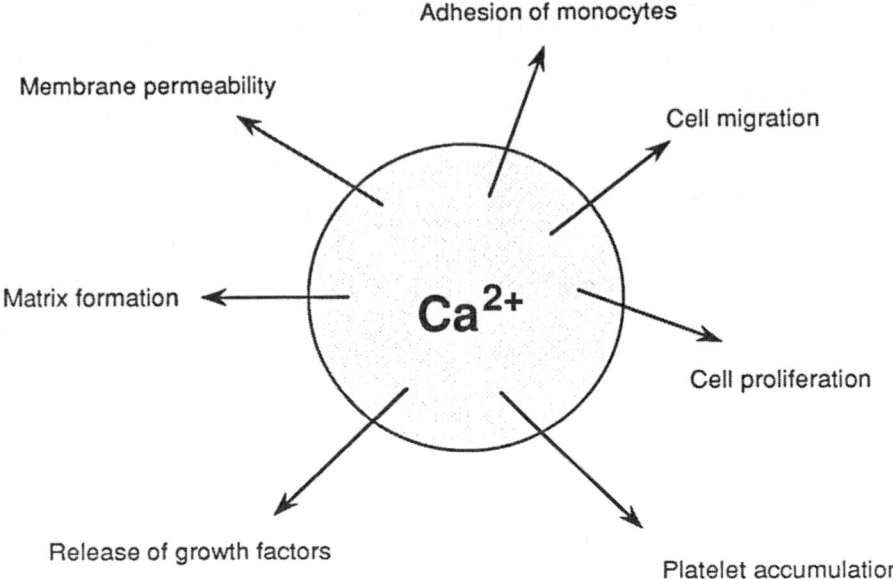

Fig. 11.3. Calcium-dependent processes involved in the formation of an atherogenic plaque

Calcium-Dependent Processes Which Contribute to the Formation of Atherosclerotic Lesions

As a prelude to discussing how calcium antagonists interrupt the sequence of events which starts with monocyte and leucocytes being attracted to the endothelium and terminates in the formation of an atherosclerotic lesion, it may be useful to summarize those processes in the intervening cascade (Fig. 11.1) which are Ca^{2+} dependent.

Calcium seems to be inextricably linked to the events which culminate in lesion formation (Fig. 11.3). For example, myocyte infiltration as well as smooth muscle cell proliferation and migration are Ca^{2+}-dependent processes (Ross 1986). Hypercholesterolaemia increases membrane Ca^{2+} permeability (Strickberger et al. 1988). At the late stage of lesion formation Ca^{2+}-deposition – usually as calcium apatite – in the newly formed lesions contributes to it's stability, rigidity and increasing bulk (Fleckenstein et al. 1990). Even the release of the various growth factors – including the platelet-derived growth factor – is Ca^{2+} dependent, and of course hypertension, one of the major risk factors for atherosclerosis – is Ca^{2+}-dependent. However, just because Ca^{2+} is involved in the events which terminate in formation of an advanced atherosclerotic lesion does not necessarily mean that the calcium antagonists must be protective – but of course they are (Tables 11.1 and 11.2).

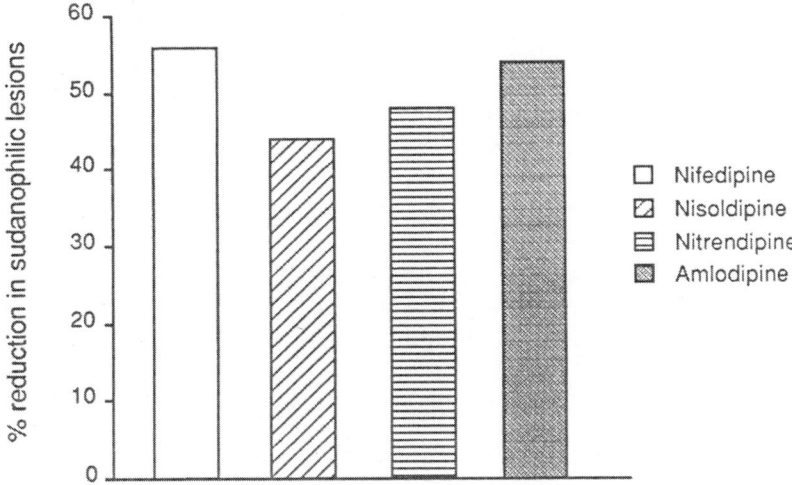

Fig. 11.4. Effect of nifedipine (5mg/kg/day), nisoldipine (5mg/kg/day), nitrendipine (5mg/kg/day) and amlodipine (5mg/kg/day) on the rate of lesion formation in the thoracic aorta in rabbits maintained on a high cholesterol diet (2% cholesterol plus 1% peanut oil) for up to eight weeks. The lesions were detected by Sudan III stain

Human Studies Showing an Antiatherosclerotic Effect of Calcium Antagonist Therapy

As already mentioned, Table 11.1 shows that four clinical studies have reported positive findings relating to the proposed antiatherosclerotic activity of the calcium antagonists. Of these trials two were large scale, purpose-designed trials, a third (Kober et al. 1989) depended upon retrospective analysis and the fourth (Gottlieb et al. 1989) concerned graft survival after coronary bypass surgery. The results are remarkably uniform in showing suppression of lesion formation and slowed growth of developing lesions. The two largest trials (425 patients treated over three years in the INTACT trial (Lichtlen et al. 1990) and 383 patients in the Montreal trial with a treatment period of two years (Waters et al. 1990)) showed that the positive outcome could not be accounted for in terms of either a lowered plasma cholesterol or a significant drop in blood pressure. The same applies to the other two trials (Table 11.1). Moreover these trials, when considered together, show that the beneficial effect is not limited to first generation antagonists, because Waters and his colleagues used nicardipine – a second generation antagonist (Chapter 2) (Waters et al. 1990).

Hence, the clinical trials which have been undertaken so far to investigate whether calcium antagonists slow the progression of naturally occurring atherosclerosis in man have yielded positive results for both first and second generation calcium antagonists.

Laboratory Studies Relating to the Antiatherosclerotic Effect of First and Second Generation Calcium Antagonists

Long before the clinical trials which were referred to in the preceding section had even been completed, laboratory investigations had shown that calcium antagonists slow experimentally-induced atherosclerosis in animals. Several different species were used (Table 11.2), and either cholesterol-loading or artificially-induced arterial intimal thickening employed to provoke lesion formation. The vast majority of studies have been positive (Henry 1990a; 1990b and Table 11.2) and the few which have been negative can readily be accounted for in terms of inadequate dosage, inadequate placebo controls, short duration of treatment or familial biochemical abnormalities (Henry 1990a).

The Molecular Mechanisms Involved in the Antiatherogenic Effect of the Calcium Antagonists

Specific, Ca^{2+}-associated mechanisms – including (Fig. 11.3) cell proliferation, cell migration, secretion of extracellular matrix proteins, the adhesions of monocytes to the endothelium and the release of growth promoting factors – contribute to the sequence of events (Fig. 11.1) which ultimately results in the formation of an atherosclerotic lesion. Just because Ca^{2+} is involved, however, does not necessarily mean that calcium antagonists will impede this sequence because after all, the primary site of action of these drugs is at the L-type Ca^{2+} channel (Chapter 2), and there are many other sources of Ca^{2+}, apart from that which enters by way of these channels. However, even to assume that the calcium antagonists slow the progression of atherosclerosis simply by reducing Ca^{2+} entry through the L-channels is an idea which must be relegated to the "dark ages" because, as Table

Table 11.3. Inhibitory effect of calcium antagonists on events involved in the formation of atherosclerotic lesions

Event	Calcium antagonist	Response	Reference
1. Adhesion of leucocytes	Nitrendipine	Inhibitory	Neuser and Rosen 1990
2. Smooth muscle cell proliferation and migration	Nifedipine	Inhibitory	Nilsson et al. 1985
	Nisoldipine	Inhibitory	Neuser and Rosen 1990
	Nitrendipine	Inhibitory	Neuser and Rosen 1990
3. Cholesteryl ester deposition	Verapamil	Inhibitory	Orekhov et al. 1986 Orekhov 1990
4. Platelet aggregation*	Nifedipine	Inhibitory	Ware et al. 1986
	Verapamil	Inhibitory	Ware et al. 1986
	Diltiazem	Inhibitory	Ware et al. 1986

* Platelet aggregation precedes release of the platelet derived growth factor

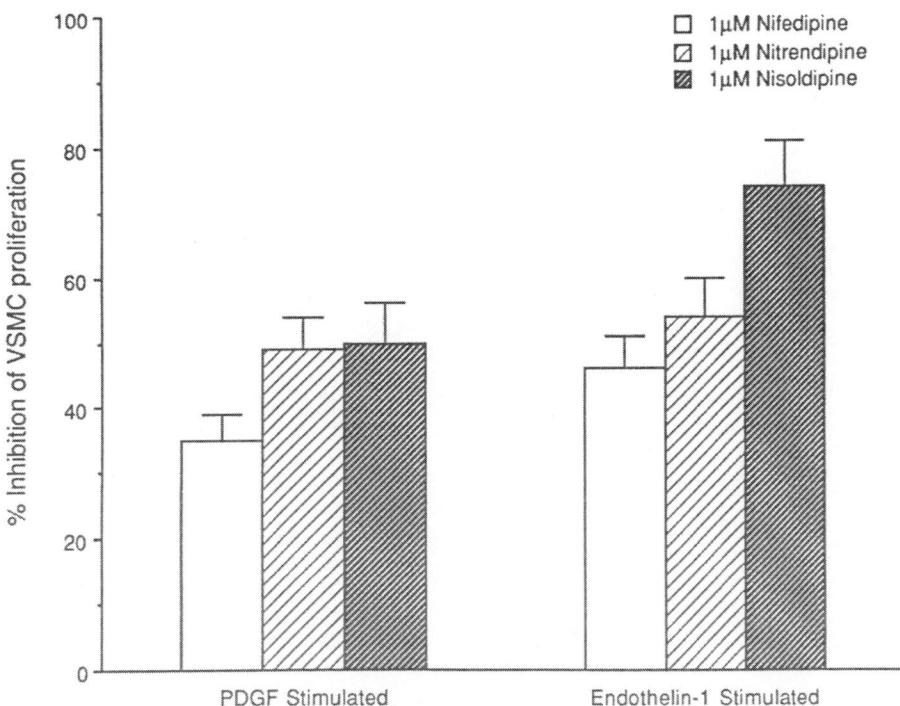

Fig. 11.5. Effect of nifedipine, nitrendipine and nisoldipine on the proliferation of vascular smooth muscle cells. Quiescent cells were stimulated with 1ng/ml platelet-derived growth factor (PDGF), 10^{-7}M endothelin-1, or 10^{-7}M angiotensin II, as indicated. (Data from Neuser and Rosen 1990.)

11.3 shows, these drugs interfere directly with many of the events which are involved in the formation of these lesions. For example, they inhibit the migration of vascular smooth muscle cells (Nakao et al. 1983) and slow their proliferation (Nilsson et al. 1985; and Fig. 11.5). They also inhibit the adhesion of polymorphonuclear leukocytes to endothelial cells (Fig. 11.6), inhibit platelet aggregation (Ware et al. 1986), inhibit intracellular cholesteryl ester deposition (Daugherty et al. 1987) and inhibit collagen synthesis (Orekhov et al. 1986). They have even been shown to inhibit the uptake of LDL cholesterol into cells cultured from the "fatty streak" stage of a developing lesion (Orekhov 1990) – and once again, and as Table 11.4 shows, second generation antagonists – as well as the prototype drugs – are effective. Yet another possibility which should be considered is that the ability of these drugs to protect against lipid peroxidation-induced injury (Chapter 6) is of some consequence here – particularly with respect to preserving the integrity of the endothelium. Some of these effects of the calcium antagonists obviously depend upon the drugs being distributed intracellularly. Because of their lipophilicity this is not a problem – to the contrary, many of the calcium antagonists do accumulate intracellularly and bind to a variety of low affinity but high capacity receptors (Lullmann and Mohr 1987; Zernig 1990).

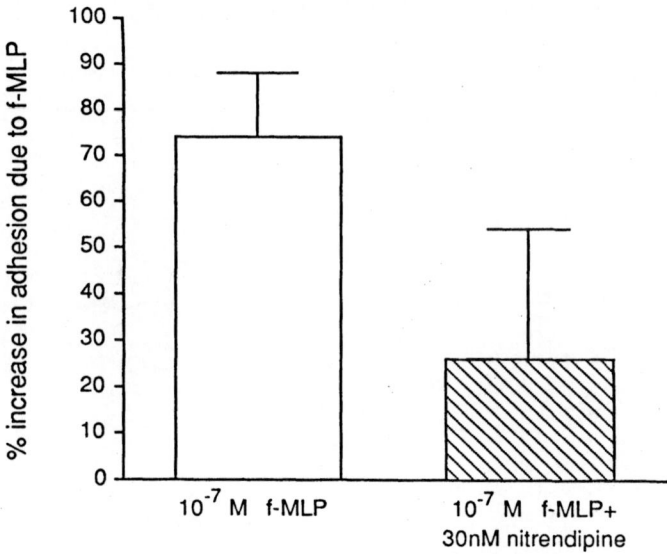

Fig. 11.6. Inhibitory effect of nitrendipine (0.3 and 30nM) on the N-formyl-L-methionyl-L-leucyl-L-phenylalamine (F-MLP)-induced adhesion of polymorphonuclear leucocytes to cultured porcine endothelial cells. (Results from Neuser and Rosen 1990.) F-MLP is used simply to promote cell adhesion

Table 11.4. Inhibitory effect of calcium antagonists on the uptake of cholesterol into atherosclerotic cells cultured from "fatty streaks"

Calcium antagonist	% Decrease in cholesterol uptake
1st Generation Antagonists	
Verapamil	100 ± 6
Nifedipine	100 ± 5
Diltiazem	91 ± 6
2nd Generation Antagonists	
Nicardipine	88 ± 9
Darodipine	83 ± 9
Isradipine	74 ± 9

Data from Orekhov (1990), (unfortunately the concentrations used in these experiments were not given)

In general, therefore, there is no longer any need to suggest that the antiatherogenic effect of the calcium antagonists is due simply to their ability to lower blood pressure. Instead, their mode of action involves interference with the basic events involved in lesion formation. Probably their efficacy in this regard partly reflects their ability to restrict Ca^{2+} entry, an effect which would result in less Ca^{2+} being available to foster cell growth and proliferation, collagen synthesis etc. In addition, other more direct mechanisms may also be involved (Table 11.3). One thing that is certain is that the second generation calcium antagonists are as effective as their prototypes (Fig. 11.5, and Habib et al. 1986b).

Although the development of atherosclerosis is usually regarded as being triggered by a variety of risk factors – including hypertension, raised plasma LDL and the habit of smoking – there are other conditions which can promote lesion formation. These include cardiac bypass surgery, angioplasty and organ transplantation.

Effect of Calcium Antagonists on Restenosis after PTCA

Restenosis after successful coronary angioplasty is a recurrent problem, and since growth factor-dependent stimulation and migration of smooth muscle cells into the intima of the vessel wall plays an important role it has some analogy with atheromatous lesion formation. Theoretically, therefore, calcium antagonists would be expected to delay such an event. Initial trials investigating this possibility were disappointing, but recently favourable results have emerged. For example, using a relatively high dose of verapamil (240mg, twice daily) Hoberg and Kubler (1991) found a significant delay in the rate of stenosis over a treatment period of six months. Maybe this is one area where the longer acting second generation drugs will be needed – to ensure *sustained* protection against the mechanisms involved in lesion formation.

Effect of Calcium Antagonists on Coronary Graft Patency

Allied to the problem of atherosclerosis and restenosis after PTCA, is the restenosis seen after coronary artery bypass surgery (Verheul et al. 1991), and which is due to the development of intimal lesions rather than altered vessel reactivity (Ku et al. 1991). Here again the calcium antagonists have been shown to be protective both acutely (Seitelberger et al. 1991) and long-term (Gottlieb et al. 1989) – with the long-term benefit being expressed as an improved patency over a twelve month period.

Graft patency after cardiac transplantation is another area in which accelerated atherosclerosis presents difficulties – although its precise cause is as yet unidentified. Again, there is emerging evidence of a protective role for calcium antagonists (Fowler et al. 1991).

In general, therefore, structural lesions which impair coronary perfusion and which exhibit accelerated rates of smooth muscle cell proliferation and migration include not only spontaneous atherosclerosis but also restenosis after PTCA, after coronary bypass surgery and after cardiac transplantation. In each case the calcium antagonists have been shown to have a favourable effect, but so far, the vascular selective, long-acting second generation antagonists have not been used for this purpose to any great extent, which is surprising!

Endothelial Dysfunction Early in the Atherogenic Process

Plaque formation is undoubtedly the terminal event in the atherosclerotic saga – and the one which is most readily detected and most familiar to pathologists. One of the earliest events – apart from the raised plasma cholesterol level and lipid infiltration – is an altered vascular reactivity which is expressed as *impaired relaxation* (Zeiher et al. 1991; Merkel et al. 1990). This occurs in humans (Nabel et al. 1990; Bossaller et al. 1987) as well as in laboratory animals (rabbits, monkeys and pigs), is not peculiar to the coronary blood vessels (Yamamoto et al. 1987; Jayakody et al. 1985), and is triggered by hyperlipidaemia.

This altered vessel reactivity has the following characteristics:
(i)   it is triggered by raised plasma cholesterol;
(ii) it embodies augmented constrictor responses to agents such as serotonin, histamine, ergonovine and endothelin-1 (Shimokawa et al. 1983; Kawachi et al. 1984; Lopez et al. 1990), and
(iii) endothelium-derived vasodilation is impaired (Merkel et al. 1990).

Endothelial-dependent relaxation is due primarily to the release of prostacyclins and the endothelial-derived relaxing factor, EDRF (Furchgott and Zawadzki 1980). Accordingly, the impaired relaxation encountered during hypercholesterolaemia could involve:
(i)   dysfunction of the endothelial receptors;
(ii) slowed synthesis of EDRF (a Ca^{2+} dependent phenomenon involving a synthase enzyme) (Hiki et al. 1991);
(iii) impaired diffusion of the released EDRF;
(iv) enhanced destruction of the released EDRF;
(v)   altered sensitivity of the smooth muscle cells, and
(vi) the presence of an over-riding constrictor response.

Dissection of these possibilities shows that:
(i)   the vasculature retains its capacity to relax – as shown, for example, by its continued response to sodium nitroprusside (Tagawa et al. 1991), and to the infusion of the EDRF precursor, arginine (Cooke et al. 1991).
(ii) In addition, there is probably an over-riding constrictor effect because:
   a) the vessels are hypersensitive to endothelin-1 (Lopez et al. 1990), and the circulating levels of this polypeptide are raised (Kanno et al. 1990), and
   b) acetylcholine, which normally evokes a dilator response dependent on EDRF release, now provokes constriction (Zeiher et al. 1991).

This means that the most likely cause of this hyperactivity is an increased availability of endothelin-1 (Kanno et al. 1990) coupled with a reduced availability of EDRF. Since the various growth factors promote endothelin-1 production (Yanagisawa and Masaki 1989a; 1989b) it is not too difficult to see why the mRNA for endothelin-1 production is activated. The precise cause of the reduced availability of EDRF is less certain, since impaired production, slowed release or rapid inactivation (Tagawa et al. 1991) may all be involved. The end result is an imbalance between the dilator effect of EDRF on the one hand, and the sustained constrictor effect of endothelin-1 on the other.

Whilst it is a truism to say that a raised plasma cholesterol is all that is needed to achieve this abnormal state of vessel reactivity, the effect is exacerbated in atheromatous arteries (Merkel et al. 1990; Ku et al. 1991) possibly because cholesterol-loaded membranes become hyperpermeable to Ca^{2+} (Kutryk et al. 1991). Under these conditions it is logical to question the usefulness of the calcium antagonists because they do not lower plasma cholesterol. However, there are three reasons why they should improve the situation. Firstly, because they retard the atherogenic process, they should slow the progressive change in vascular reactivity (Tagawa et al. 1991). Secondly, because they attenuate the constrictor activity of endothelin-1 (Chapter 7), they should dampen any over-riding constriction which it provokes at a time when the EDRF "safety net" is malfunctioning. Thirdly, because some of them prevent lipid peroxidation from occurring, they should attenuate the Ca^{2+} hyperpermeability caused by the oxidation of cholesterol-loaded membranes (Kutryk et al. 1991).

In general therefore, as far as coronary atherosclerosis is concerned at least two factors have to be taken into account when considering the efficacy of the calcium antagonists. They are:

(i)   impaired perfusion due to lesion formation and rupture, and
(ii) impaired perfusion (? vasospasms) due to a localized attenuation of the EDRF-mediated dilator response and the raised circulating levels of endothelin-1.

In both instances the calcium antagonists should be of use, both from an immediate and long term point of view. However, once again there is the problem of ensuring sufficient drug is present on a long-term basis. Long-acting, or slow release formulations of shorter acting, drugs may provide the answer, particularly if they are also coronary dilators, lack appreciable negative inotropy and reduce the risk factor of hypertension.

In Summary

1. The formation of an atherogenic plaque is a complex event. The initiating factors involve lipid infiltration through the junctional gaps separating adjacent endothelial cells.
2. Subsequent events include lipid peroxidation, macrophage infiltration and conversion to foam cells, together with smooth muscle cell migration and proliferation.
3. Clinical and laboratory studies have shown that first and second generation calcium antagonists slow the growth of atherogenic lesions.
4. Mechanisms involved in the antiatherogenic effect of these drugs include slow channel Ca^{2+} inhibition, and a direct effect on the biochemical events involved in lesion formation.
5. The use of calcium antagonists to protect against atherogenesis should be considered not only in terms of its long-term effect, because hypercholesterolae-

mia and lipid infiltration render the coronary (and other) vessels hypersensitive to constrictor agents, including endothelin-1. This latter effect may contribute to the occurrence of vasospasm in atherogenic vessels.

6. In terms of the ability of the calcium antagonists to slow atherogenesis on a long-term basis the following mechanisms appear to be involved:
   (i)   reduced monocyte adhesion;
   (ii)   slowed release of growth factors;
   (iii) slowed smooth muscle cell proliferation;
   (iv)   slowed macrophage uptake of cholesterol esters;
   (v)   slowed matrix secretion;
   (vi)   reduced Ca^{2+} availability;
   (vii) protection against lipid-peroxidation, and
   (viii) protection against shear stress-induced damage to the endothelium.

7. There may be an added advantage associated with the use of calcium antagonists under these circumstances, because hypercholesterolaemia renders the coronary vasculature hypersensitive to a variety of constrictor agents – including serotonin, and endothelin-1. This hypersensitivity probably involves impaired relaxation caused by a reduced availability of the endogenous relaxing agent EDRF, together with the presence of excess endothelin-1, a locally-released potent constrictor agent.

Chapter 12

Second Generation Calcium Antagonists:
Their Use in Congestive Heart Failure

"The reason why the blood froze in my veins needs little explanation: the dullest eye could see the delicacy of my position."
From: Aunts Aren't Gentlemen, P.G. WODEHOUSE 1974

Currently there is widespread controversy concerning the wisdom of using calcium antagonists for the long term management of patients with congestive heart failure (Packer et al. 1987; Packer 1990; Francis 1991). This is somewhat surprising, because theoretically, since these drugs "unload" the heart, they might have been expected to be of use under these circumstances (Gorlin 1987), and indeed some investigators have found them to be of benefit (Dunselman et al. 1989; Kassis and Amtorp 1990a; 1990b; Moe et al. 1990; de Cock et al. 1990). Other investigators, however, remain convinced that drugs of this type may "aggravate and unmask heart failure" rather than alleviate it (Francis 1991). As far as the first generation calcium antagonists (nifedipine, verapamil and diltiazem) are concerned this concern is justified. For example, after treating New York Heart Association Class II and III chronic heart failure patients for six weeks with nifedipine, Elkayam et al. (1990) concluded that despite its efficacy as a peripheral dilator, nifedipine was

Table 12.1. Clinical trials showing an unfavourable effect of chronic treatment with first generation calcium antagonists in patients with severely compromised ventricular function

Calcium antagonist	Reference
Verapamil	Chew et al. 1981
	Guazzi et al. 1984
	Ferlinz and Gallo 1984
	Packer et al. 1982
Nifedipine	Elkayam et al. 1985
	Gillmer and Karrk 1980
	Brooks et al. 1980
	Packer et al. 1984
	Anastassiades 1982
Diltiazem	Packer et al. 1985
	Goldstein et al. 1991

There are many other reports in the literature referring to either a lack of effect or a worsening of the condition during long-term treatment with these drugs *despite* the occasional occurence of an apparent immediate beneficial effect

contra-indicated under these circumstances. Nifedipine does not stand alone in this respect, similar conclusions having been reached with respect to diltiazem and verapamil (Table 12.1). Since the use of these agents was based on the physiological-ly sound principle of "unloading the heart" their failure in this respect raises several questions, including:

(i)   why did these first generation antagonists not fulfil their promise in this respect, and

(ii) are the second generation antagonists any better?

To answer these questions it is first necessary to briefly consider the pathophysio-logy of congestive heart failure.

The Pathophysiology of Congestive Heart Failure

Even today, after years of investigations, the pathophysiology of this condition remains relatively poorly defined, possibly because of its complex aetiology (Katz 1990a; 1990b; Morgan and Baker 1991). Valvular heart disease, sustained hyper-tension, myocardial infarction (Fig. 12.1), as well as genetically-determined and drug-induced abnormalities are some of the potential causes. Even the progress of the disease is variable, with hypertrophy appearing as either an early or a late event. By the time hypertrophy has developed, however, the myocardium is already "energy-starved", simply because the proportion of each myocyte which is now occupied by myofibrils is disproportionately large relative to the space occupied by the energy-generating mitochondria (Page and McCalister 1973; Anversa et al. 1980). This, however, is only one of the changes which takes place. Others include:

(i)   impaired Ca^{2+} delivery to the contractile proteins (Limas et al. 1987);

(ii)   a slowed retrieval of Ca^{2+} from the cytosol – due, in part, to a reduced density of the Ca^{2+}-pumping ATPase enzyme of the sarcoplasmic reticulum (Lompré et al. 1988) and not, as happens during overt ischaemia (Chapter 4), to any uncontrolled Ca^{2+} leak;

(iii)   depletion of the endogenous catecholamine stores (Chidsey et al. 1965) – almost certainly because of the accompanying excessive activation of the sympathetic nervous system;

(iv)   β-adrenoceptor density is reduced, resulting in a reduced sensitivity to β-adrenoceptor stimulation (Bristow et al. 1982). By contrast, the density of α-adrenoceptors remains unchanged (Bristow et al. 1985);

(v)   the tissue reserves of ATP and CP fall (Pool et al. 1967);

(vi)   the rate of collagen synthesis is accelerated (Caspari et al. 1977), sometimes resulting in the appearance of abnormally assembled collagen (Weber et al. 1988);

(vii)   abnormal isoforms of the key myocardial proteins appear (Cummins 1982; Mercadier et al. 1987; Izumo et al. 1988) and finally,

(viii) the cytoskeleton, which normally provides a stable scaffold for the various intracellular organelles, becomes disorganized (Schaper et al. 1991).

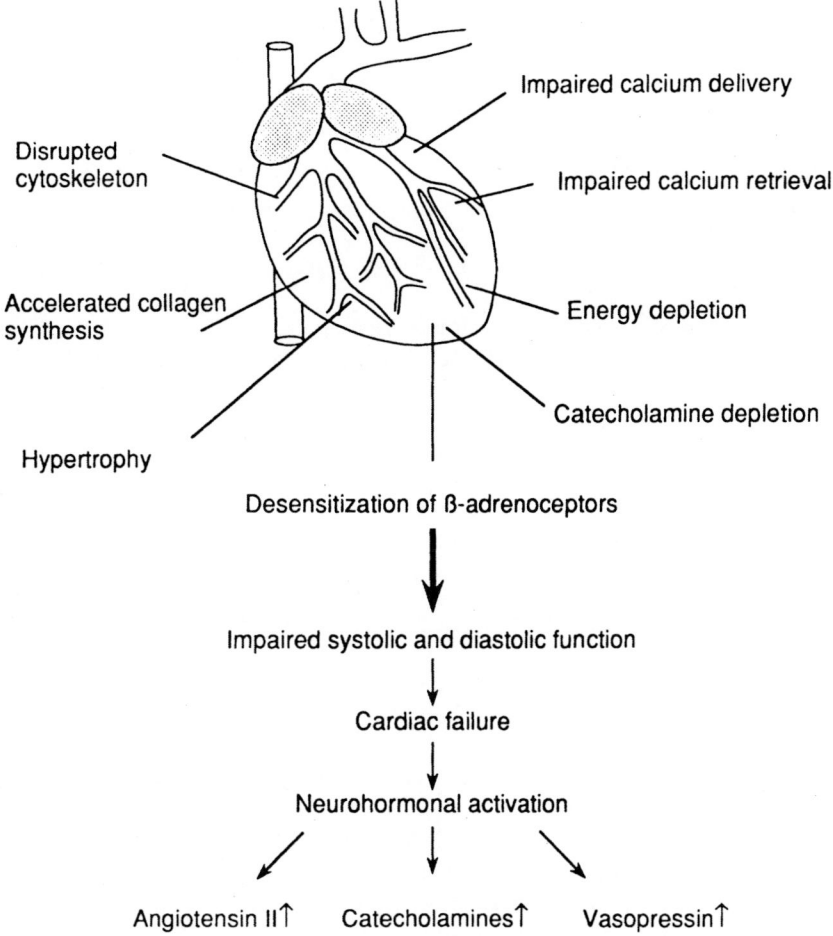

Fig. 12.1. Schematic representation of possible causes of congestive cardiac failure

These changes do not all occur simultaneously but they are progressive and ultimately result in a heart which, because of systolic and diastolic malfunction, can no longer meet the haemodynamic requirements of the circulation. This is when the not so delicate symptoms of congestive cardiac failure begin to appear. The situation is further compounded by the fact that ventricular dysfunction activates the sympathetic nervous system (Cohn, JN 1990). The subsequent neurohumoral changes include:

(i)   activation of the adrenergic and renin – angiotensin systems (Francis and Cohn 1986; Kubo 1990; Cohn, JN 1990);

(ii) raised plasma levels of arginine-vasopressin, and

(iii) excess endothelin-1 production (Margulies et al. 1990; Cavero et al. 1990).

The resultant increases in plasma noradrenaline, angiotensin II, vasopressin and endothelin-1 – may assist in the maintenance of arterial tone and venous return at a

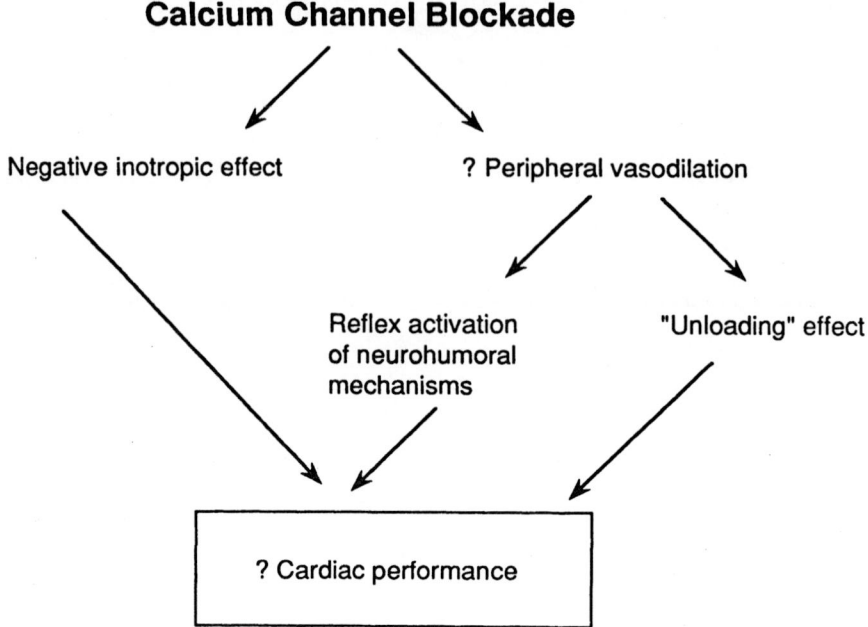

Fig. 12.2. Schematic representation of the factors responsible for the deleterious effects of the first generation calcium antagonists

time when cardiac output does not meet the needs of the circulation, but it imposes an excessive work load on the now failing, energy-starved heart (Fig. 12.2). Moreover, the integrity of the neurohumoral reflex control of the circulation becomes seriously impaired – as indicated by the changes in plasma noradrenaline and renin activity which occur upon orthostatic tilting. Always the response is attenuated in the cardiac failure group (Packer 1988; Marin-Neto et al. 1991; Cohn, JN 1990). The mechanisms involved in this "blunting" of the baroreflex control mechanism are currently under scrutiny. Possibilities include:

(i)   structural distortion of the baroreceptors due to chronic volume overload;
(ii) distortion of the arterial wall underlying the baroreceptors – possibly due to Na^+ accumulation, and
(iii) a secondary consequence of the raised circulating levels of noradrenaline, angiotensin II and arginine vasopressin (Cody and Laragh 1988; Packer 1988).

In general, therefore the pathophysiology of congestive cardiac failure is complex, and involves:

(i)   disturbances of the energy producing and energy utilizing components of the myocytes;
(ii) a limited availability of Ca^{2+} for excitation-contraction coupling and a slowed retrieval of Ca^{2+} from the cytosol – the latter possibly being responsible for the faulty diastolic functioning of these hearts;

(iii) an overactivated autonomic nervous system;
(iv) impaired baroreflex-mediated control of the circulation, and
(v)   the appearance of abnormal myosin isoforms.

The Therapeutic Management of the Failing Heart

Despite it's complex aetiology, there are at least two ways of approaching the pharmacological management of the failing heart. One approach involves the use of positive inotropes, the other, the use of "unloading agents". Whilst a positive inotrope may provide acute relief, that relief is likely to be poorly sustained unless the drug also restores a balance between the rates of energy usage and energy production – otherwise the existing energy deficit (Pool et al. 1967) can only worsen.

By contrast, "unloading" the failing heart by reducing "after load" not only alleviates the symptoms of cardiac failure – it also prolongs survival (Cohn et al. 1986). Why, then, have the first generation calcium antagonists generally not only failed to provide sustained relief from the symptoms of cardiac failure but in some instances have actually caused both haemodynamic and clinical deterioration (Packer et al. 1987; Elkayam et al. 1990; Goldstein et al. 1991; and the Danish DAVIT II and SPRINT trials)? The most obvious, but possibly not the most important explanation involves the negative inotropic activity of these drugs. However, even in patients who have experienced worsening heart failure as the result of the administration of one or other of these first generation calcium antagonists, cardiac performance – measured either in terms of cardiac output or ejection fraction – is often either unchanged, or even improved (Ferlinz and Gallo 1984). This makes it difficult, if not impossible, to account for this calcium antagonist-induced deterioration, which can be life-threatening, simply in terms of their negative inotropy. Instead it seems to be the activation of the sympathetic nervous and renin-angiotensin systems which they trigger which is responsible, simply because this imposes an even greater work load on the already failing heart (Packer 1990).

Hence as far as the first generation calcium antagonists are concerned their potential usefulness in the management of patients with congestive heart failure is limited:
(i)   in part by their negative inotropy, and
(ii) substantially by the vasodilator-induced triggering of the autonomic and renin-angiotensin systems, the activation of which results in:
 (a) an increase in the work load against which the heart now has to pump;
 (b) increased energy expenditure by the heart, because of the stimulation of its adrenergic receptors – particularly the α-adrenoceptors, which mediate a positive inotropic response and coronary vasoconstriction, and
 (c) fluid retention.

Table 12.2. Vascular selectivity of some of the second generation calcium antagonists

Drug	Vascular:Myocardium
Nitrendipine (*)	80:1
Isradipine (**)	15:1
Felodipine (*)	118:1
Nicardipine (*)	300:1
Nisoldipine (*)	>1000:1

Data from Struyker-Boudier et al. (1990) (*) and Ruegg and Hof (1990) (**)

The Second Generation Calcium Antagonists

There are several reasons why some of the second generation antagonists might be more appropriate for use in the management of patients with congestive cardiac failure. The most obvious reason is their relative selectivity for the vasculature (Table 12.2), but there are others, including the ability of some of them, including nisoldipine (Schofer et al, 1990), to restore baroreflex sensitivity.

Isradipine

When given to patients with congestive heart failure isradipine *improves* stroke volume and cardiac index without any change in heart rate, despite a fall in systemic blood pressure (Broudy et al. 1987). Since isradipine is relatively selective for the vasculature the absence of any negative inotropic response is not surprising. However an absence of a reflex-induced increase in heart rate is perhaps unexpected and might provide a clue as to why this particular second generation calcium antagonist provides functional improvement under these circumstances. It could mean that the neurohumoral system has not been unduly activated. Alternatively, since this calcium antagonist also slows conduction (but not so drastically as verapamil), it may be this effect which is responsible for the absence of a positive chronotropic response.

Felodipine

This is another vascular selective second generation calcium antagonist which has negligible negative inotropic activity at therapeutically relevant doses. When given to patients with congestive heart failure it causes a sustained increase in stroke volume and cardiac output, a reduction in afterload, and a *small decline* in heart rate (Kassis and Amtorp 1990b). At the same time, the plasma levels of noradrenaline actually fall – for example, in one study 5.34 ± 1.11 for controls, 4.01 ± 1.14 nmol/l for the felodipine-treated group. This must be indicative of an improved neurohumoral profile. Regional segmental wall motion is improved, as is diastolic function and the clinical status of the patients. The most likely explanation for these findings is that this particular calcium antagonist, as well as causing vasodilation and therefore unloading the heart, restores baroreflex-mediated control without activating the neurohumoral system.

Nicardipine

This is another vascular selective calcium antagonist with relatively little negative inotropic activity, but with selectivity for the coronary and cerebral vasculature (Whiting 1987). In patients with moderately severe heart failure (NYHA Class III and IV) nicardipine has been shown to improve ejection fraction, cardiac output and peak filling rate over a treatment period of four weeks (Lahiri et al. 1990). As with felodipine, diastolic as well as systolic function is improved.

Nisoldipine

This is a well tolerated second-generation calcium antagonist. It is vasoselective, exhibits some selectivity for the coronary vasculature (Serruys et al. 1985) and is useful in the management of patients with myocardial ischaemia (Tzivoni et al. 1991). When given acutely to patients with NYHA class III and IV heart failure it decreases systemic vascular resistance, decreases mean arterial blood pressure and increases stroke volume index without necessarily altering heart rate or pulmonary capillary wedge pressure (Moe et al. 1990; Barjon et al. 1987; Lahiri et al. 1990).

Recently there has been an escalation of interest in the possibility of using nisoldipine in the long-term management of patients with compromised left-ventricular function secondary to ischaemic heart disease (Schofer et al. 1990; Rousseau et al. 1990; De Cock et al. 1990; Moe et al. 1990). A clear distinction should be made between the *acute* use of this antagonist under these conditions, where its beneficial effect is due primarily to its ability to reduce afterload by arteriolar dilation, and its *long-term* beneficial effect which has a complex aetiology (Schofer et al. 1990; Rousseau et al. 1990). In both instances, however, the relevant dose levels must be those which produce arteriolar dilation without evoking a direct negative inotropic effect. For example, Schofer et al (1990) found that 10 mg of nisoldipine given twice daily was a satisfactory dosage whereas others have found higher dose regimes – for example, 40–60 mg per day – to be unsatisfactory for this purpose.

At least two recently completed long-term studies (Schofer et al. 1990; Rousseau et al. 1990) have provided results which indicate that nisoldipine can be used to provide a sustained improvement in left ventricular function (systolic and diastolic) in patients with left ventricular dysfunction. Evidence of this beneficial effect includes:
(i)   improved cardiac and stroke volume index during exercise, accompanied by
(ii)   *an increase in central venous oxygen saturation;*

(iii) an unchanged heart rate;

(iv) a decrease in end-diastolic pressure;

(v) an increase in left ventricular peak filling pressure; and

(vi) a return of the left ventricular diastolic shape towards a more ellipsoid and hence normal geometry. Notably, regional wall function appeared little affected in control zones but was significantly improved in the peri-infarct areas (Rousseau et al. 1990; Schofer et al. 1990).

On the basis of these and other similar observations Rousseau et al (1990) have concluded that "whereas LV function seems to spontaneously deteriorate in a large number of asymptomatic patients with ischaemic heart disease ... nisoldipine not only appears to prevent this effect, but also to improve global and *regional left ventricular function*".

Precisely why nisoldipine produces this sustained improvement in ventricular function is unclear at the moment. The response cannot depend upon a significant and sustained increase in sympathetic drive (Rousseau et al. 1990) since the changes in plasma noradrenaline are insignificant after three months of therapy, as is any change in heart rate. A sustained effect on peripheral vascular resistance has been discounted as a possible cause. Possible mechanisms include:

(i)   improved regional perfusion and metabolism in the affect area (Rousseau et al. 1987);

(ii) a reduction in calcium overload (Lorell and Grossman, 1987);

(iii) a reduction in cardiac hypertrophy secondary to a reduction in afterload;

(iv) an inhibitory effect on ventricular remodelling and associated collagen production (McKay et al. 1986), and

(v)   possibly, a direct effect on the contractile machinery.

Hence, as far as nisoldipine is concerned, clinical trials have now provided data which supports the hypothesis that this vascular-selective calcium antagonist improves left ventricular systolic and diastolic function in patients with sustained left ventricular dysfunction secondary to ischaemic heart disease but who have not yet developed signs of overt heart failure. The interesting concept, therefore, is that maybe low-dose nisoldipine therapy can be used on a prolonged basis not only to prevent mild to severe left ventricular dysfunction progressing to heart failure but also to improve left ventricular function. It is useful to compare the efficacy of nisoldipine in this respect with that of the ACE inhibitors, e.g. captopril (Schofer et al. 1990). Both agents effectively improve diastolic function in patients with left ventricular dysfunction which develops as a secondary consequence of an earlier ischaemic episode, but whereas the prolonged protective effect of the ACE inhibitors is linked to the slowly developing and sustained reduction in afterload caused by such drugs, the beneficial effect of nisoldipine is not dependent simply on the reduction in afterload which develops acutely, then wanes. Instead a direct effect on left ventricular diastolic function seems to be involved and is evident at dose levels which are well below those needed to depress contractility.

In Summary

1. The first generation calcium antagonists are contra-indicated for use in the management of patients with congestive heart failure because:
   (i)   they are all negatively inotropic;
   (ii) they activate the sympathetic nervous system, and
   (iii) in the case of nisoldipine, they have a direct effect on diastolic function.
2. The second-generation antagonists can be used for this purpose although with care. Their improved efficacy relative to their prototypes probably involves:
   (i)   their relative selectivity for the vasculature;
   (ii) in some cases, their ability to restore baroreflex sensitivity, and
   (iii) in the case of nisoldipine, a direct effect on diastolic function.

Chapter 13

Second Generation Calcium Antagonists as Blood Pressure Lowering Agents: The Prevention of Cardiac Hypertrophy

> *"I found it so truly difficult that I almost believed with Fracastorius that it was to be understood by God alone."*
> WILLIAM HARVEY, in De Motu Cordis, 1628

William Harvey was absolutely right. Hypertension is a complex disorder and even now, despite years and years of intensive study, its aetiology and pathophysiology are not fully understood. One thing that is quite certain, however, is that the fundamental feature of hypertension is a raised systemic vascular resistance (Page 1987), and that any change in cardiac output which may occur must be relegated to being a consequence of the raised vascular resistance, and not its cause. It follows as a matter of course, therefore, that any pharmacological intervention which is introduced to normalize blood pressure, should be aimed primarily at either:

(i) the vasculature, or
(ii) any neurohumoral or other mechanisms which may be acting on the vasculature.

Effective antihypertensive regimes should do more than this, however – they should also attenuate some of the secondary consequences of the primary disorder – such as:

(i)   stroke (Chapter 14);
(ii) atherosclerosis (Chapter 11);
(iii) renal damage, and
(iv) ventricular hypertrophy.

The ability of the second generation calcium antagonists to attenuate some of the secondary consequences of hypertension (atherosclerosis and stroke) is discussed elsewhere in this book. This chapter, therefore, is mainly concerned with their efficacy as antihypertensive agents. Theoretically some of these drugs should be extremely useful for this purpose, because of their vascular selectivity and prolonged duration of action. Before discussing their efficacy, however, there may be some point in summarizing:

(i) how Ca^{2+} is involved in smooth muscle contraction, and
(ii) some of the mechanisms which contribute to the hypertensive state.

Calcium and Vascular Smooth Muscle Contraction

Calcium plays a key role in smooth muscle cell contraction, just as it does in cardiac and skeletal muscle. As far as vascular smooth muscle is concerned it derives its "activator Ca^{2+}" from two sources – one extracellular and the other intracellular. The extracellular Ca^{2+} can gain access to the cytosol in several different ways, including:

(i)   by way of calcium antagonist-sensitive, L-type Ca^{2+} channels, and

(ii) to a lesser extent, by way of the $Na^+:Ca^{2+}$ exchanger.

As far as the intracellularly-derived Ca^{2+} is concerned it is released from the sarcoplasmic reticulum (SR) in much the same way as was described in Chapter 4 for cardiac muscle (Hathaway et al. 1991). However, some smooth muscle cells are better supplied with SR than others. For example, the large conduit vessels contain more SR than the small resistance vessels (Somlyo 1985), which may mean that the small resistance vessels rely more on the influx of extracellular Ca^{2+} than their large conduit counterparts.

Although Ca^{2+}-dependent, the physiology of smooth muscle cell contraction is quite different from that of cardiac and skeletal muscle. Even the arrangement of the contractile proteins is different. For instance, whereas the Z band and other components of the cytoskeleton (Schaper et al. 1991) in striated muscle ensure that the major components of the contractile system remain in register, smooth muscle cells operate in an entirely different way because here the contractile proteins can only be described as being in a state of disarray. Nevertheless, in each case, active tension development is a Ca^{2+}-dependent phenomenon (Huxley 1990; Hathaway and Watanabe 1989). In striated muscle the Ca^{2+} interacts with the regulatory protein, troponin, thereby removing its inhibitory effect on the actin-induced activation of the myosin ATPase enzyme. In smooth muscle, including that of the vasculature, the situation is quite different because here it is the phosphorylation of the myosin (or more correctly, the myosin light chain subunits) which activates cross-bridge cycling. This phosphorylation involves:

(i)   the activation of a Ca^{2+}-dependent myosin light chain kinase, and

(ii) the presence of the Ca^{2+}-binding protein, calmodulin (Hathaway and Watanabe 1989; Huxley 1990).

The end result, however, is contraction (Fig. 13.1).

As already stated, the Ca^{2+} that is needed for the sequence of events shown in Figure 13.1 comes from two sources – one extracellular, and the other intracellular. The intracellular source is the SR. It occupies a relatively small proportion of each smooth muscle cell (1.5–7.5 percent, according to Somlyo 1985), its Na^+ and Cl^- content is similar to that of the cytosol, but its calcium content exceeds that of either the cytosol, or the longitudinal section of striated SR (Table 13.1; and Chapter 4). Presumably, therefore, it does have sufficient capacity to supply a significant proportion of the Ca^{2+} that is needed for contraction. In addition, it contains the machinery for controlled Ca^{2+} release by way of SR release channels which are *comparable with those* already described for striated muscle (Chapter 4). There are

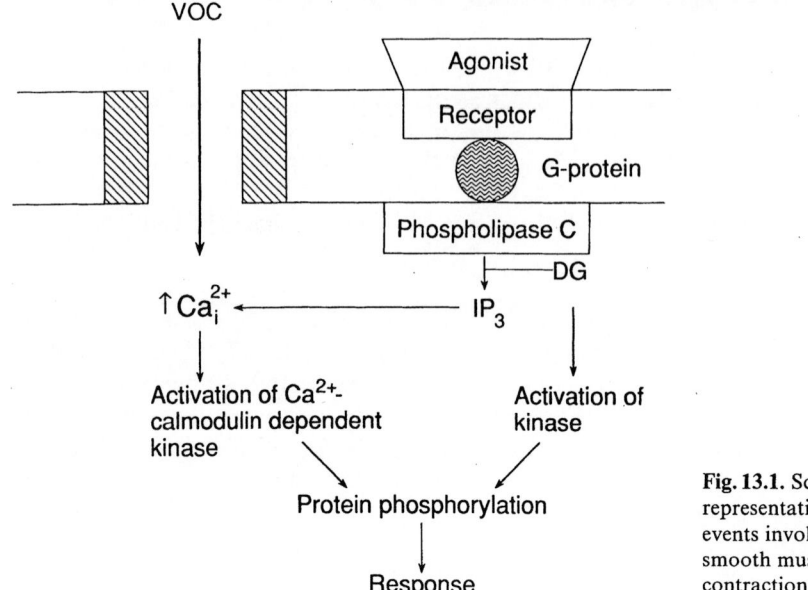

Fig. 13.1. Schematic representation of the events involved in smooth muscle cell contraction

Table 13.1. Calcium content of the sarcoplasmic reticulum in vascular smooth muscle, and striated muscle

Sarcoplasmic reticulum	Calcium content (nmol . dry wt⁻)
Vascular smooth muscle	30–50
Striated Muscle (i) junctional SR	≈ 120
(ii) longitudinal SR	8

Data from Somlyo 1985

at least two trigger mechanisms – one involving Ca^{2+} and the other inositol trisphosphate (IP_3) (Fig. 13.1). Naturally there is a Ca^{2+} ATPase enzyme to pump Ca^{2+} from the cytosol back into the SR – otherwise massive cytosolic overloading would occur in no time at all. However, the aminoacid content of this pump differs from that of either skeletal or cardiac muscle in that the carboxyterminus of the sequence contains an additional forty nine aminoacids (Lytton et al. 1989).

There are other differences between the microphysiology of vascular smooth muscle cells on the one hand and either skeletal or cardiac muscle on the other. Two of these differences are relevant to this chapter because they may contribute to the vascular selectivity which some of the calcium antagonists display. These differences are:

(i) a relatively low transmembrane resting potential (–50 mv for smooth compared with –85–90mv for most striated cells) (Hirst and Edwards 1989), and

(ii)   an unusual aminoacid content of the alpha$_1$ subunit of the Ca^{2+} channel complex (Chapter 3).

In summary, although vascular smooth muscle cells resemble their striated counterparts in requiring Ca^{2+} for excitation-contraction coupling there are marked differences between the two systems, particularly with respect to:
(i)   their ultrastructure;
(ii)   the Ca^{2+}-storing capacity of their SR;
(iii) the Ca^{2+}-mediated events involved in active tension development;
(iv)   their transmembrane resting potentials, and
(v)   the chemical composition of the alpha$_1$ subunit of the channel complex.

The Pathophysiology of Hypertension

According to Shepherd (1990), the major causes of hypertension can be subdivided into four categories:
(i)   humoral vasoconstrictors;
(ii)   pressure-induced structural changes in the resistance vessels;
(iii) sympathetic overdrive, and
(iv)   autocoids, paracoids and mitogens associated with blood vessels.

This list is by no means exhaustive. For example, there are reports of differences in the relative numbers of L- and T-type Ca^{2+} channels which are present in the

Table 13.2. Factors which may be involved in the aetiology of hypertension

---

A. Primary

1. Genetic predisposition

2. Circulating humoral vasoconstrictors
   (i)   angiotensin II
   (ii)   vasopressin
   (iii) digitalis-like factor

3. Excess sympathetic drive
   (i)   increased synthesis of noradrenaline
   (ii)   hypersensitivity to catecholamines

4. Locally released autocoids and paracoids
   (i)   angiotensin II
   (ii)   endothelin-1
   (iii) diminished release of endothelial-derived relaxing factors

5. Abnormal L-type channel function
   (i)   relative increase in L-channel density
   (ii)   sustained activation of L-channels

B. Secondary

Vascular hypertrophy

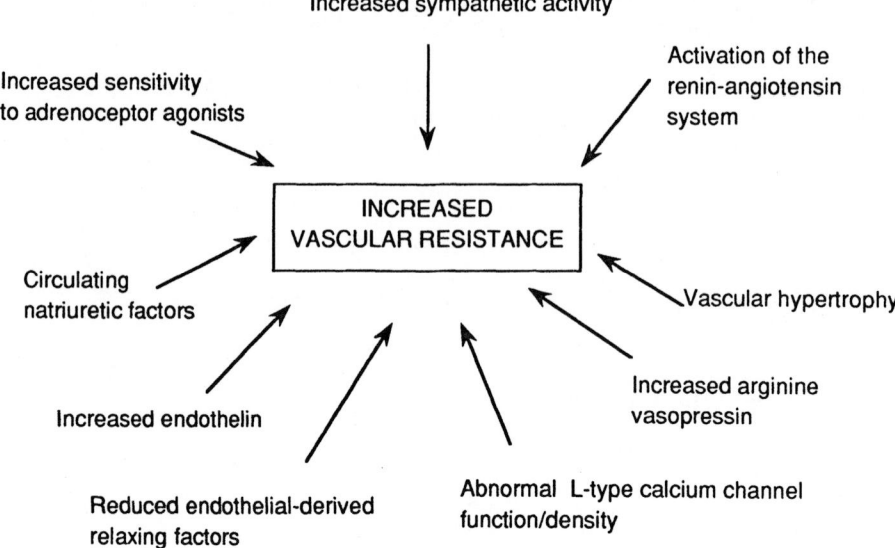

Fig. 13.2. Schematic representation of some of the factors which contribute to the increase in vascular resistance which is fundamental to the hypertensive state

vasculature, with hypertension favouring the predominance of the L-type channels (Rusch and Hermsmeyer 1988). There is also evidence of impaired endothelium-dependent relaxation (Panza et al. 1990), of post-contraction associated with the prolonged activation of the L-type calcium channels (Godfraind et al. 1991) and of hypersensitivity towards agonists which evoke a contractile response (Winquist et al. 1982; Papageorgiou and Morgan 1991). There are many other contributory factors, some of which are listed in Table 13.2 and Figure 13.2; they include structural changes in the resistance vessels, and plasma volume overload.

In general therefore, it is impossible to avoid the conclusion that the aetiology of hypertension at the cellular level is a multifactorial event, with no single cause. However, by turning to the molecular mechanisms which may be involved it is becoming possible to see a clear trend – that of a raised intracellular Ca^{2+} (Ca^{2+}_i) and excessive activation of the protein kinase C enzyme which is involved in the phosphorylation of the myosin light chain – an essential step (Fig. 13.1) in smooth muscle contraction and its response to a wide variety of agonists. Some of the data on which this conclusion is based is listed in Table 13.3.

On balance, therefore, it seems likely that a raised cytosolic Ca^{2+}, accompanied by an over active protein kinase C enzyme, may at least make a substantial contribution to the pathophysiology of essential hypertension. The raised cytosolic Ca^{2+}_i explains why the tissue is hypersensitive to certain agonists, including α-adrenoceptor agonists (Papageorgiou and Morgan 1991). Why cytosolic Ca^{2+} is raised is unknown, at present. Possible factors include:
(i)   enhanced entry of Ca^{2+} in exchange for Na^+;
(ii) enhanced Na^+:H^+ exchange followed by Na^+:Ca^{2+} exchange;

Table 13.3. Evidence supporting the involvement of a raised intracellular Ca^{2+} and excessive activation of the protein kinase C enzyme in the mechanisms involved in the onset of hypertension

Preparation	Reference
A. Raised resting intracellular Ca^{2+} (Ca^{2+}_i)	
Cultured smooth muscle cells from SHR rats	Sugiyama et al. 1986
Smooth muscle cells from hypertensive rats	Papageorgiou and Morgan 1990
Increased L-type Ca channel activity in SHR's	Rush and Hermsmeyer 1988
B. Protein Kinase C activation	
Increased activity in red blood cells of all patients with essential hypertension	Kravtsov et al. 1988
Increased basal PKC activity in SHR's	Murakawa et al. 1988

(For other reference see Morgan and Suematsu 1990)

(iii)   enhanced agonist-induced influx;
(iv)   enhanced agonist-induced release of intracellularly stored Ca^{2+} (e.g. endothelin-1, angiotensin II, arginine-vasopressin);
(v)   enhanced L-type Ca^{2+} channel density;
(vi)   prolonged opening time of each Ca^{2+} channel;
(vii)   impaired SR Ca^{2+} accumulating activity;
(viii)   leakage of Ca^{2+} from the SR, and so on ....

However it is not only the resting cytosolic Ca^{2+} which is raised. Papageorgiou and Morgan have recently shown that vasoconstrictor agents which act by mobilizing intracellular Ca^{2+} produce relatively high levels of Ca^{2+}_i (intacellular Ca^{2+}) in blood vessels from hypertensives, compared with normotensives (Papageorgiou and Morgan 1991).

Calcium Antagonists as Blood Pressure Lowering Agents

First Generation Antagonists

The use of the first generation calcium antagonists (verapamil, nifedipine and diltiazem) to reduce systemic vascular resistance in hypertensive patients was based on three assumptions:
(i)   hypertension is due to an increase in systemic vascular resistance;
(ii)   vascular smooth muscle cells of hypertensives have a raised Ca^{2+}_i, and
(iii)   vascular smooth muscle cells contain functional calcium antagonist-sensitive, voltage-activated channels which admit Ca^{2+} upon depolarization (Bolton et al. 1988).

Since these assumptions are correct, it follows almost without question that the *calcium antagonists are effective blood pressure lowering agents* – along (Table

Table 13.4. Undesirable side effects of other antihypertensive agents

Drug	Disadvantage
Diuretics	*Metabolic* hypokalaemia blood sugar ↑ plasma lipids ↑
β-adrenoceptor antagonists	*Metabolic* fasting blood sugar ↑ glucose tolerance ↓ LDL cholesterol ↑ total cholesterol ↑ *Physiogical* cardiac output ↓ systemic vascular resistance ↑ bronchoconstriction lethargy
α₁-adrenergic antagonists	*Metabolic* sodium and fluid retention *Physiological* Orthostatic hypotension
Centrally acting drugs	*Metabolic* plasma LDL cholesterol ↑ insulin release ↓ *Physiological* mental depression
Angiotensin converting enzyme inhibitors (ACE)	*Metabolic* insulin-mediated glucose disposal ↑ *Physiological* cough

Where ↑ denotes an increase, ↓ denotes a decrease

13.4) with many other drugs. As far as the first generation antagonists are concerned there is a wealth of evidence confirming their efficacy in this respect – particularly for verapamil and nifedipine (Olivari et al. 1979; Pedersen 1981; Buhler 1983; Muller et al. 1984; Agabiti-Rosei et al. 1986). Both of these "first generation" antagonists reduce peripheral vascular resistance without stimulating the renin-aldosterone system (Agabiti-Rosei et al. 1986) and without altering plasma lipids. They are arteriolar dilators, and leave cardiac output either unchanged, or slightly increased (Lund-Johansen 1983; Agabiti-Rosei et al. 1988). Moreover all three of the prototype first generation antagonists (verapamil, diltiazem and nifedipine) cause the hypertension-induced left ventricular hypertrophy to regress (Agabiti-Rosei et al. 1988; Frohlich 1987) – an effect which they share with the converting enzyme inhibitors (Muiesan et al. 1988). As a group, the first generation antagonists have other beneficial effects besides reducing peripheral vascular resistance and causing the regression of left ventricular hypertrophy. For example, they do not have any marked effect on rates of aldosterone secretion, they do not generally cause a sustained rise in plasma renin (as do some other vasodilators, including hydrazaline), and they have an acute diuretic effect. Despite these "plus points" these drugs have some limitations in so far as their use as antihypertensive agents are concerned:

(i)   they are all intrinsically negatively inotropic, verapamil and nifedipine > diltiazem. This precludes their use in patients with left ventricular dysfunction (Chew et al. 1981; Elkayam et al. 1985);

(ii)   the depressant effect of verapamil on sinoatrial and atrioventricular conduction can be responsible for the development of severe bradycardia;

(iii) the rapid fall in blood pressure caused by nifedipine usually precipitates a reflex tachycardia;

(iv)   their relatively short plasma half-lives means that repetitive dosing is essential – unless the newer slow release or GITS formulations are used, and

(v)   at the doses which are needed to produce a sustained decrease in systemic blood pressure side-effects can become troublesome – even for diltiazem.

These side-effects include ankle oedema, headache, facial flushing and, in the case of verapamil, constipation.

Second Generation Calcium Antagonists

As mentioned in the earlier chapters of this book, the chemistry of the second generation calcium antagonists is even more complicated than that of the prototypes. They can be subdivided, however, into the three groups:

(i)   new derivatives of the prototypes;

(ii)   new slow release formulations of the prototypes – including slow release verapamil and nifedipine, and

(iii) new compounds with other receptor blocking activity in addition to that of calcium channel blockade.

Amongst the new prototype derivatives are some which have been used clinically as antihypertensive agents. They include felodipine, nitrendipine, isradipine, amlodipine and nicardipine. As a group, these drugs resemble the prototypes in that:

(i)   they all produce a sustained fall in blood pressure, accompanied by a reduction in peripheral vascular resistance;

(ii)   this reduction in peripheral vascular resistance usually occurs without marked changes in heart rate, or plasma renin;

(iii) plasma lipids either remain unaltered, or there may be a small increase in HDL cholesterol;

(iv)   presumably because of their relative selectivity for the vasculature left ventricular hypertrophy regresses, and

(v)   they have a natriuretic effect and accordingly do not cause Na^+ reabsorption. This is a major plus point.

Table 13.5. Daily doses and plasma levels of second generation calcium antagonists used in the treatment of essential hypertension

Drug	Daily dose	Plasma level
Amlodipine*	$5\text{--}10 \text{ mg} \cdot \text{day}^{-1}$	$2\text{--}12 \text{ ng} \cdot \text{ml}^{-1}$
Felodipine	$20 \text{ mg} \cdot \text{day}^{-1}$	$5\text{--}40 \text{ ng} \cdot \text{ml}^{-1}$
Isradipine	$20 \text{ mg} \cdot \text{day}^{-1}$	$10 \text{ ng} \cdot \text{ml}^{-1}$
Nicardipine	$30 \text{ mg} \cdot \text{day}^{-1}$	$30\text{--}110 \text{ ng} \cdot \text{ml}^{-1}$
Nitrendipine	$5\text{--}40 \text{ mg} \cdot \text{day}^{-1}$	$9\text{--}42 \text{ ng} \cdot \text{ml}^{-1}$

* Amlodipine is an interesting second generation antagonist not only because it has a long-half life (36 hours) but also because of its slow onset of action caused, in part, by the long time (5 hrs) it takes to saturate its binding sites in the alpha$_1$ complex of the channels

There are, however, clear differences between the first and second generation antagonists with respect to their use in the treatment of hypertension. *Firstly*, because the second generation antagonists which are being discussed here are relatively selective for the vasculature, their use in patients with impending or established ventricular dysfunction can be more easily tolerated. *Secondly*, because of their longer half lives, blood pressure can be more easily controlled over a twenty four hour period. *Thirdly*, because of their vascular selectivity, slower onset of action and increased potency, dosage is reduced on a daily basis, resulting in fewer and less dramatic side effects. Some of the commonly used doses are listed in Table 13.5.

Slow Release Formulations

The usefulness of calcium antagonists as blood pressure lowering agents is being extended by incorporating some of them into "slow release" capsules. Thus the extended release formulation of felodipine (FER) allows a once daily treatment regime with only 10mg felodipine to provide effective blood pressure control on a twenty four hour basis (Liedholm and Melander 1989) – as monotherapy. Slow release formulations are not limited to the second generation antagonists, however. Thus the slow release formulation of nifedipine and verapamil, and the nifedipine gastrointestinal therapeutic system (Geizhals et al. 1990) are providing well tolerated and effective monotherapy on a once a day treatment basis. Data from a GITS-nifedipine trial is shown in Figure 13.3.

Mode of Action

Although the primary effect of the calcium antagonists – including the second generation antagonists – is to modulate calcium channel activity, and although this clearly provided the rationale for their use as antihypertensive agents, their blood

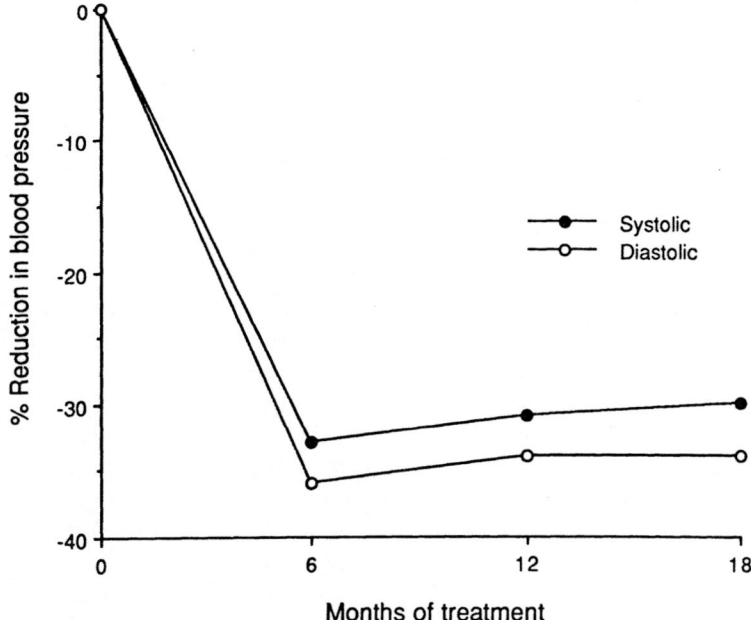

Fig. 13.3. Response of blood pressure to treatment with nifedipine GITS (a slow release formulation) on systolic and diastolic blood pressure over an eighteen month treatment period. (Data from Geizhals et al. 1990

Table 13.6. Effect of second generation calcium antagonists on Na^+ and lipids

	Na^+ Excretion	Plasma lipids	Plasma K^+
Amlodipine	↑	–	–
Felodipine	↑	–	–
Isradipine	↑	–	–
Nitrendipine	↑	–	–

Where ↑ denotes an increase, and – no change

pressure lowering activity may involve actions on other systems in addition to the peripheral vasculature. For example many of these drugs have a direct natriuretic effect (Table 13.6, and Carter et al. 1988; Persson et al. 1989; DiBona 1990) and this may contribute to their blood pressure lowering activity. In contrast to the thiazides, however, this natriuretic effect of the calcium antagonists is not accompanied by a K^+ loss, nor is there any change in plasma lipids. This natriuretic effect persists throughout long-term treatment. It is not the province of the second generation calcium antagonists because a similar effect has been described for nifedipine (Ruilope et al. 1990).

One of the puzzling and as yet not fully understood aspects of the vasodilator activity of the calcium antagonists (including the second generation antagonists) is their greater efficacy in hypertensives, relative to normotensives (MacGregor et al. 1982). Various hypothesis have been put forward to explain this – including cellular abnormalities with respect to Ca^{2+} metabolism and excitation-contraction coupling, and abnormal calcium channel sensitivity – particularly with respect to receptor operated channels (Kazda et al. 1985). Very recently Godfraind and his colleagues (Godfraind et al. 1991) succeeded in showing that the calcium channels of arteries from hypertensive rats have a prolonged activation time which is attenuated by the dihydropyridine-based second generation antagonist, nimodipine (Godfraind et al. 1991). Here then, is an interaction with the calcium channels which is peculiar to the hypertensive state, and which would attenuate Ca^{2+} influx triggered by membrane depolarization – but only in hypertensives.

There are other indirect ways in which the calcium antagonists might attenuate the increase in vascular tone which is so characteristic of hypertension – including their ability to block the vasoconstrictor effect of endothelin-1. Endothelin-1 is a potent vasoconstrictor, and plasma endothelin-1 levels are raised in hypertension (Saito 1990; Shichiri et al. 1990), at a time when the natural defence mechanism – that of the endothelial-derived relaxing factor – seems to be impaired (Shepherd 1990). It is quite possible, therefore that the ability of the calcium antagonists to attenuate the vasoconstrictor effect of endothelin-1 (Chapter 7) contributes to their overall efficacy as blood pressure lowering agents.

Hence, although the calcium antagonists are highly effective antihypertensive drugs which, as well as decreasing peripheral vasculature also have a beneficial effect on the associated left ventricular hypertrophy, their mode of action may be more complex than was first imagined. Other actions, including an ability to "normalize" abnormally functioning calcium channels, and a direct diuretic effect which involves inhibition of Na^+ reabsorption are undoubtedly involved.

In Summary

1. Calcium antagonists provide effective therapy for the control of hypertension.
2. Their blood pressure lowering activity is accompanied by a reduction in other known risk factors – including atherosclerosis and left ventricular hypertrophy.
3. The newer formulations of the prototype calcium antagonists, and the vascular selective second generation calcium antagonists with relatively long half lives, are effective antihypertensive agents which produce less marked side-effects than their prototypes.
4. The second generation antagonists have retained the natriuretic activity of the prototypes and therefore do not cause Na^+ accumulation.

Chapter 14

Second Generation Calcium Antagonists and the Management of Cerebral Ischaemia

> *"This apoplexy is a kind of lethargy, a kind of sleeping in the blood, a whoreson tingling."*
> SHAKESPEARE: Henry IV, Part 2

Another way of demonstrating the advantages the second generation calcium antagonists have relative to their prototypes is to consider their use in the management of patients with cerebral ischaemia – because their use under these circumstances depends largely upon their tissue selectivity. Even a cursory search of the literature on this subject shows that the antagonists which are most effective in this regard share two properties:

(i)   vasoselectivity, but with heightened specificity for the cerebral vasculature, and
(ii) an ability to cross the blood-brain barrier.

The compounds which exhibit these properties are nimodipine (Gelmers and Hennerici 1990), and isradipine (Sauter and Ruden 1990a; 1990b), both of which are dihydropyridine derivatives, and the more recently developed phenylalkylamine-derivative (S)-emopamil (Morikawa et al. 1991). (S)-emopamil is the combined 5-hydroxytryptamine-calcium antagonist compound already referred to in Chapter 2. Of these three compounds (nimodipine, isradipine and (S)-emopamil) only nimodipine has been subjected to extensive clinical testing relative to it's use in the management of patients with cerebral ischaemia. Nimodipine was actually the first of the calcium antagonists to be identified as having some specificity for the cerebral vasculature (Towart and Kazda 1979; Kazda and Towart 1982). This is an important property when considered in the context of the management of patients with cerebral ischaemia, because it facilitates improved cerebral perfusion without any accompanying precipitous fall in systemic perfusion pressure – an effect which, if allowed to occur, could exacerbate the damage caused by the initial ischaemic event, simply because of the resultant fall in perfusion pressure.

The Ischaemic Brain

As a prelude to exploring why these particular calcium antagonists attenuate injury associated with cerebral ischaemia, it is necessary to consider briefly how the brain responds to an inadequate blood supply. The consequences are remarkably similar to those which occur in other organs – including the heart – but they appear more rapidly – presumably because the brain lacks any appreciable energy reserves. Nevertheless, as with any other part of the body, the brain requires an uninterrupted

Table 14.1. Effect of cerebral blood flow on brain function

Cerebral blood flow	Response
50 ml/100 g tissue/minute	Normal function
15–17 ml/100 g tissue/minute	Electrical instability
< 10 ml/100 g tissue/minute	Cell death

Data from Spetzler and Hadley (1989)

supply of energy (as ATP) to maintain its structure and function. The necessary ATP is generated by oxidative metabolism, resulting in an average cerebral oxygen consumption of around 3.5ml/100g/minute. A cerebral blood flow of about 50ml/ 100g tissue/minute (Fieschi et al. 1990) is needed to satisfy this requirement. If cerebral blood flow falls below this level, to around 15–17ml/100g tissue/minute, then electroencephalographic evidence of impaired cellular electrical activity becomes apparent, but the affected tissue remains viable – presumably because sufficient energy is still being generated to maintain membrane ultrastructure and selective ionic permeability. Reducing cerebral blood flow even further, until it falls below 10ml/100g tissue/minute typically results in loss of cellular integrity, in ion pump failure and finally in cell death, Ca^{2+} overloading and tissue necrosis (Table 14.1) (Astrup et al. 1977).

Causes of Cerebral Ischaemia

Cerebral ischaemia can occur for a variety of reasons including:
(i)   a precipitous fall in systemic blood pressure,
(ii)   emboli originating from thrombi, or from ulcerated or ruptured atherogenic plaques;
(iii) sustained cerebral vasospasm, and
(iv)   cerebral haemorrhage – which can occur anywhere, including the cerebrum, cerebellum and brain stem.

A precipitous fall in blood pressure is, more often than not, a "one-off" event – caused, perhaps by an overambitious blood pressure lowering regime, severe haemorrhage – irrespective of its cause (trauma, aneurysm etc.) – or cardiac arrest. The embolitic and cerebral haemorrhagic-induced episodes, however, have a far more complex aetiology. As already stated, cerebral haemorrhages can occur anywhere in the brain, and can vary in size from a small to a massive event. Usually the haemorrhages are the sequelae of untreated hypertension. If a thrombus has triggered the ischaemic episode it may, if the patient is lucky, spontaneously lyse; alternatively additional thromboemboli may form – the latter event resulting in a stepwise progression of the occlusion and the attendant cellular injury. As far as cerebral vasospasm is concerned there are many potential causes – including excess secretion of, or hypersensitivity to, a host of vasoconstrictor agents including thomboxane A_2, 5-hydroxytryptamine (serotonin), endothelin-1 (de Aguilera et al. 1990; Yoshimoto et al. 1991) and noradrenaline.

Ischaemic "Stroke" and Subarachnoid Haemorrhage

Ischaemic "stroke" is obviously an acute event, and the resultant damage to the brain is immediate. This condition should not be confused with that caused by a subarachnoid haemorrhage (Fig. 14.1), since patients who suffer this latter fate appear to recover from the initial haemorrhage only to develop delayed brain damage (Ljunggren et al. 1984), the most likely cause of which is cerebral ischaemia *triggered by secondary vasospasm* (Tettenborn and Dycka 1990). Delayed, vaso-spasm-induced ischaemia is not an infrequent event – it occurs in between fifty and seventy percent of patients who suffer a subarachnoid haemorrhage, with fatal consequences in approximately fifteen percent of the cases. In some ways the sequelae of subarachnoid haemorrhage can be likened to the condition encountered in the hibernating heart (Chapter 9), where underperfusion causes sustained cardiac dysfunction. In the brain, however, the hypoperfusion is caused by sustained cerebral vasospasm.

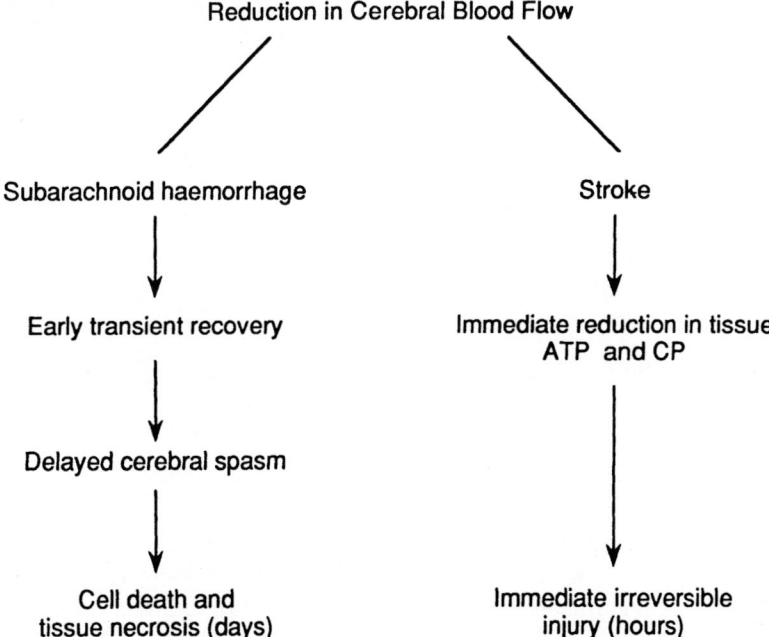

Fig. 14.1. Schematic representation of the time-courses associated with cerebral ischaemia caused by subarachnoid haemorrhage, or "stroke". Note that the irreversible injury caused by "stroke" is an immediate event, whereas the damage caused by subarachnoid haemorrhage is delayed, sometimes for days

Aetiology of Acute Cerebral Ischaemia (Stroke) and Subarachnoid Haemorrhage

Acute Cerebral Ischaemia

As already stated cerebral ischaemia can be triggered by acute but severe systemic hypotension, an intracerebral haemorrhage, or occlusion. Known risk factors include hypertension. It is not too difficult to see why sustained hypertension might evoke an intracerebral haemorrhage, nor is it difficult to imagine how either the rupturing of an atherosclerotic plaque or the trapping of microemboli might precipitate an occlusive event. The link between systemic hypotension and cerebral ischaemia is equally obvious.

Subarachnoid Haemorrhage-Induced Ischaemia

This has an entirely different history from that outlined for acute cerebral ischaemia. Usually it begins with the rupturing of a cerebral arterial aneurysm (Solomon and Correll 1988). A temporary seal then develops, leaving the residual risk of a fatal recurrence and the almost certain onset of a delayed ischaemia. Usually this delayed phase occurs in three stages:
(i) an *early* stage, caused by a fall in cerebral perfusion pressure due to:
    (a) the accompanying increase in intracranial pressure, and
    (b) the introduction of blood pressure lowering regimes;
(ii) an *intermediate* stage, which involves an acute but *transient* constriction of the intracranial arteries, and
(iii) a *late* stage, which may take days to develop and often persists for weeks. This late stage is almost certainly triggered by locally-released vasoactive agents including:
    (a) thromboxane A_2,
    (b) the polypeptide, endothelin-1 (Chapter 7),
    (c) 5-hydroxytryptamine,
    (d) prostaglandin $F_{2\alpha}$,
    (e) histamine, and
    (f) noradrenaline.

As far as cerebral arteries are concerned the constrictor effect of thromboxane $A_2 >$ endothelin $>$ 5-hydroxytryptamine $>$ prostaglandin $F_{2\alpha} >$ histamine $>$ noradrenaline (Asano et al. 1990). However, when considering the relative potencies of these agents it is their *combined* effects which should be taken into account. For example (Chapter 7), endothelin-1 potentiates the constrictor effect of noradrenaline, and stimulates thromboxane A_2 formation (Reynolds and Mok 1990). Nevertheless, it is endothelin which evokes a *long-lasting* constrictor response in cerebral arteries – including human cerebral arteries (Fig. 14.2) (Hardebo et al. 1989; de Aguilera et al. 1990).

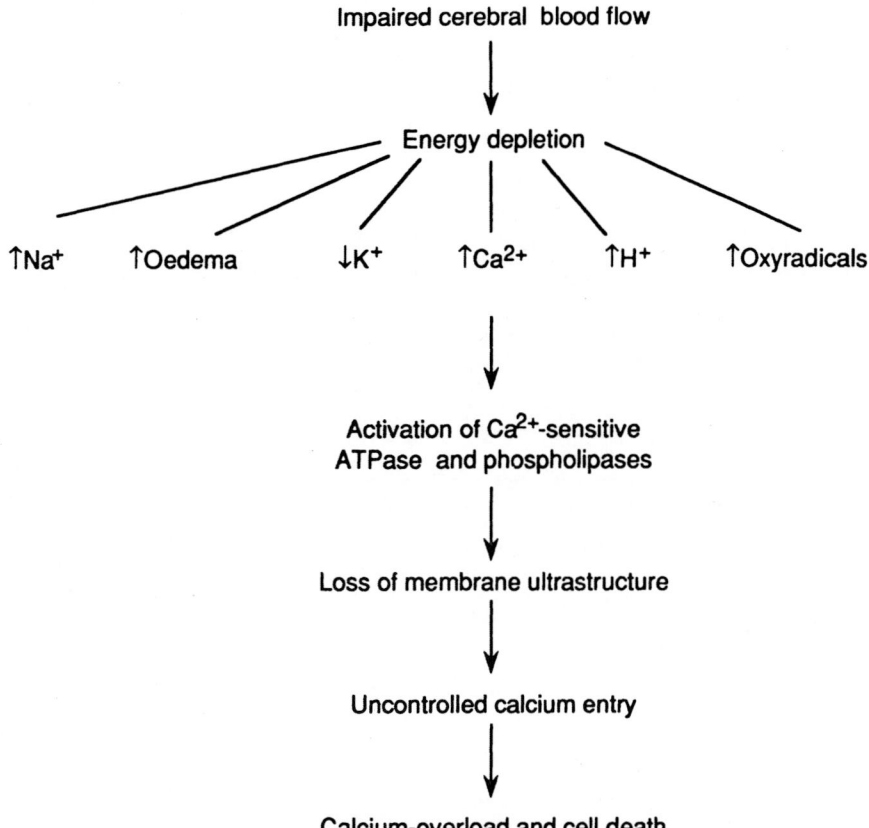

Fig. 14.2. Effect of endothelin-1 on human cerebral arteries. Note that tension development is measured in g. Nimodipine (10^{-6}M) attenuated ($p < 0.001$) the constrictor effect of endothelin-1

Consequences of Cerebral Ischaemia

Irrespective of whether the initiating event is a sudden occlusion, severe hypotension, a primary intracerebral haemorrhage, an embolus or a subarachnoid haemorrhage followed by prolonged vasospasm the end result is disturbed energy metabolism (Siesjo and Bengtsson 1989). As the affected area switches from aerobic to anaerobic metabolism extracellular and intracellular acidosis develops – mainly because of the accumulation of lactate ions. K^+ ions also accumulate in the extracellular space, Na^+ accumulates intracellularly, and the tissue stores of ATP (adenosine triphosphate) and CP (creatine phosphate) disappear. In addition, oxyradicals are generated and accumulate (Siesjo et al. 1989), oedema develops and – exactly as happens in the myocardium (Chapter 10) – cytosolic Ca^{2+} rises (Greenberg et al. 1990). The finale (Fig. 14.3) is Ca^{2+} overload, cell death and tissue necrosis in the affected zone. Catastrophic as this sequence of events may be, other potentially hazardous changes are also taking place. For example, various

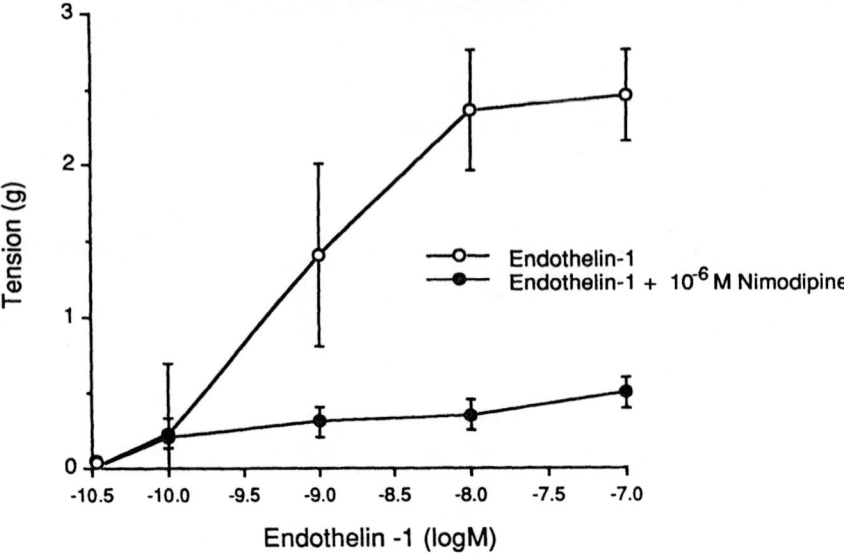

Fig. 14.3. Schematic representation of the effect of impaired cerebral blood flow on brain metabolism. Note that a rise in cytosolic Ca^{2+} (Ca^{2+}_i) precedes Ca^{2+} overload and cell death. ↑ denotes an increase, and ↓ a decrease

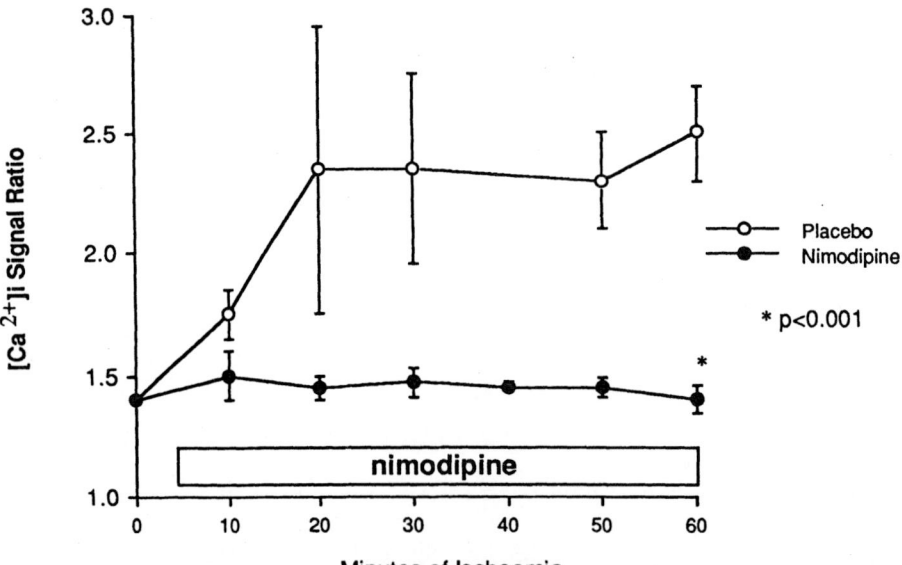

Fig. 14.4. Effect of nimodipine given as an infusion starting ten minutes before the initiation of the occlusive event on brain cytosolic Ca^{2+} measured with the Ca^{2+}-indicator indo-1-AM (see Greenberg et al. 1990 for methodology). Occlusion was of the middle cerebral artery in cats (data from Greenberg et al. 1990). Nimodipine was infused at a rate of 1µg/kg/minute

neurotransmitters, including noradrenaline, are released, and the accumulating thrombi and released platelet-derived growth factor signal further endothelin-1 production – effects which can only progressively augment the area affected by the initial event.

In general, therefore, irrespective of whether the condition is that of acute "stroke" or the delayed injury associated with subarachnoid haemorrhage, the ultimate scenario involves energy depletion, loss of ionic homeostasis, a raised cytosolic Ca^{2+} followed by Ca^{2+} overload, cell death and tissue necrosis (Fig. 14.3). The brain, therefore, resembles the heart in so far as its response to an ischaemic episode is concerned (Chapter 10), with a raised cytosolic Ca^{2+} being a relatively early event (Fig. 14.4).

Protection of the Ischaemically-Injured Brain

Theoretically, if acute cerebral ischaemia reflects an imbalance between the metabolic requirements of the individual cells and the amount of substrate available to them, then cerebral protection could involve:
(i)   improving cerebral blood flow in the affected area;
(ii) reducing the energy requirements of the affected cells;
(iii) ameliorating the consequences of the switch to anaerobic metabolism (thereby reducing lactate accumulation and reducing oedema formation), and
(iv) preventing, or attenuating:
    (a)   the excessive rise in cytosolic Ca^{2+} (Greenberg et al. 1990 and Fig 14.4), and
    (b)   oxyradical generation and accumulation, or oxyradical-mediated injury (Siesjo et al. 1989 and Chapter 6).

Potential therapies include surgical interventions (embolectomy, endoarterectomy and extracranial to intracranial bypass), reduction in energy usage (barbiturates), manoeuvres designed to maintain membrane integrity (barbiturates, corticosteroids and dimethylsulphoxide), interventions designed to augment cerebral blood flow in the affected area (calcium antagonists), agents designed to prevent or minimize the damage caused by newly generated oxyradicals (free radical scavengers, and calcium antagonists), and agents which will attenuate the ischaemia-induced Ca^{2+} overload (calcium antagonists).

Efficacy of Second Generation Calcium Antagonists in the Management of Acute Cerebral Ischaemia

Animal Studies

Surgical occlusion of the middle cerebral artery in rats (Sauter and Rudin 1990a; 1990b) provides a useful model for studying embolic stroke, because in this model

Table 14.2. Effect of second generation calcium antagonists (isradipine, nimodipine and nicardipine) on cerebral infarct size in rats

Calcium antagonist	Dose (mg/kg s.c.)	% Reduction in infarct size
1st Generation Antagonists		
Nifedipine	30	<10
2nd Generation Antagonists		
Isradipine	60	25
Nimodipine	40	50
Nitrendipine	40	10
Nicardipine	15	20

From Sauter and Rudin (1990a). Drugs were given intravenously immediately after coronary artery occlusion

Table 14.3. Evidence of a protective effect of the second generation calcium antagonists in acute cerebral ischaemia

Calcium antagonist	Species	Reference
Nimodipine	Rats	Hara et al. 1990
	Rats	Welsch et al. 1990
	Rats	Bielenberg et al. 1990
	Rats	Teasdale et al. 1990
	Dog	Steen et al. 1983
	Rabbit	Lazarewicz et al. 1990
	Cat	Uematsu et al. 1989
	Gerbil	Fujisawa et al. 1986
	Baboon	Hadley et al. 1987
Isradipine	Rat	Sauter and Rudin 1990a
		Sauter and Rudin 1990b

neuronal cell death and necrosis develop rapidly and can be easily quantitated. This model has already been used to determine whether calcium antagonists – including some of the second generation calcium antagonists – have a beneficial effect in terms of reducing infarct size under these conditions. In the studies which have been undertaken so far the calcium antagonists have mainly been given subcutaneously, immediately after the occlusive event, and their efficacy has been quantitated (Sauter and Rudin 1990a) by magnetic resonance imaging, reduction in neurological deficit, and reduction in infarct size, as determined histologically at postmortem. The results are impressive, with isradipine and nimodipine causing substantial reductions in infarct size (Table 14.2). Other experimental studies which support the hypothesis that these two second generation calcium antagonists ameliorate the damage caused by acute cerebral ischaemia are listed in Table 14.3.

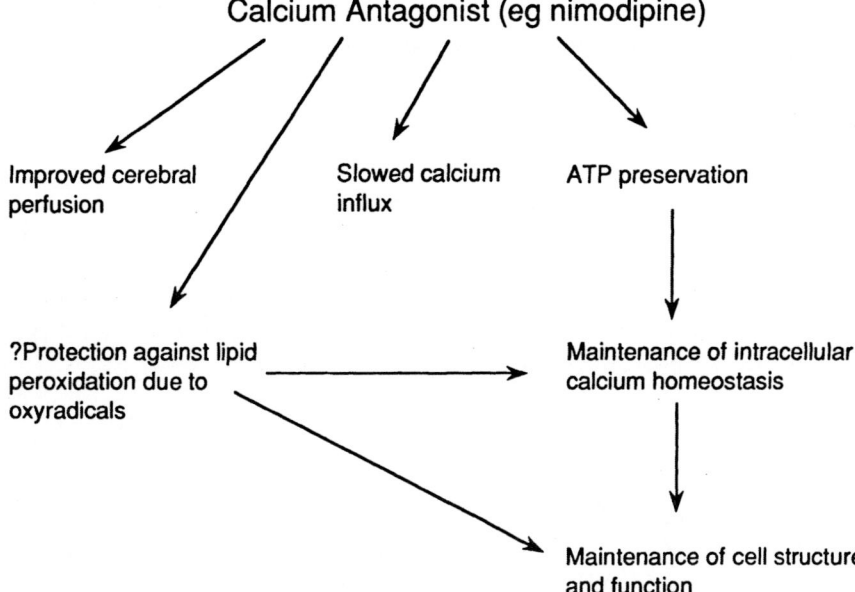

Fig. 14.5. Schematic representation of the mechanisms involved in the ability of certain calcium antagonists (nimodipine, isradipine and (S)-emopamil) to attenuate ischaemia-induced injury to the brain

Nimodipine, nicardipine and isradipine all penetrate the blood-brain barrier and accordingly can gain access to the cells in the affected area. In addition they exhibit some selectivity for the cerebral vasculature, where they are potent dilators. This specificity for the cerebral vasculature is particularly well documented for nimodipine (Towart and Kazda 1979). Maybe nimodipine should be classified as the prototype of the cerebrovascular-specific antagonists! However (S)-emopamil, the combined 5-hydroxytryptamine-phenylalkylamine-based calcium antagonist (Chapter 2), also crosses the blood-brain barrier (Morikawa et al. 1991), and like nimodipine, nicardipine and isradipine, is a potent cerebral dilator, capable of increasing cerebral blood flow by as much as fifty percent without altering local glucose utilization (Szabo 1989).

Probably the ability of these compounds to reduce cerebral infarct size depends upon at least four facets of their pharmacology. As Figure 14.5 shows, this encompasses:

(i)   an ability to slow Ca^{2+} influx through the voltage-activated channels in the membranes of the flow-deprived cells, prompting protection against Ca^{2+} overloading at the cellular levels in cells which contain L-type and hence calcium antagonist-sensitive Ca^{2+} channels;

(ii) an "energy-sparing" effect,

(iii) a *direct* calcium antagonist-dependent dilation of the relevant cerebral vessels, *and*

(iv) inhibition of any locally-mediated, Ca^{2+}-dependent constriction of the cerebral blood vessels – as caused, for example, by endothelin-1, or histamine, or prostaglandin $F_{2\alpha}$.

In the case of (S)-emopamil it's 5-hydroxytryptamine antagonist effect may provide an added benefit, and could explain why the beneficial effect of this compound is still evident even when the drug is not administered until one or two hours *after* the initiation of the ischaemic event – and hence at a time when secondary cerebrovasospasm is occurring.

   As far as nimodipine is concerned it has another property which may contribute to its ability to protect under these circumstances – that is, as described in Chapter 6, an ability to protect against oxyradical-induced lipid-peroxidation.

Clinical Data

Clinical trials relating to the efficacy of calcium antagonists in the management of patients with cerebral ischaemia have been largely restricted to the use of nimodipine, but undoubtedly other trials are either being contemplated or are in progress. One such trial is the ASCLEPIOS trial on isradipine (Azcona and Lataste 1990). Pooled data from the five double-blind placebo-controlled studies of nimodipine in acute ischaemic stroke which have been completed so far (Gelmers and Hennerici 1990) has confirmed – albeit on a small sample number – that nimodipine therapy is beneficial for stroke patients. Neurological impairment was found to be reduced in favour of the nimodipine-treated patients, with a fifty one percent reduction in mortality, again in favour of the nimodipine treatment group.

Mode of Action

As already mentioned, as far as focal cerebral ischaemia is concerned, the calcium antagonist which has been most thoroughly investigated is nimodipine. This applies to its efficacy and its mode of action (Scriabine et al. 1989). Factors which contribute to its protective effect include (Fig. 14.5):
(i)   a slowed ischaemia-induced decline in brain ATP (Heffez and Passonneau 1985);
(ii) an attenuation of the ischaemia-induced fall in intracellular pH (Meyer et al. 1986; Meyer 1990);
(iii) a reduction in the ischaemia-induced rise in cytosolic Ca^{2+} (Greenberg et al. 1990, and Fig. 14.4);
(iv) an increased blood flow to the ischaemic area (Meyer et al. 1986); this may involve a direct vasodilator effect and an attenuation of the constriction caused by locally-released constrictor substances, including endothelin-1, and
(v)   an attenuation of the ischaemia-induced oedema (Bielenberg et al. 1990; Uematsu et al. 1989).

Probably the *slowed rise in cytosolic Ca²⁺* (Fig. 14.4) *is the critical event* at the cellular level since this will attenuate the activation of the various endogenous Ca^{2+}-activated phospholipases and proteases and in so doing ensure the maintenance of membrane structure and function. It will also have an energy sparing effect, as less ATP will now be needed to maintain ionic homeostasis with respect to Ca^{2+}, and other ions. Of course it is possible that it is *because* these drugs have an energy sparing effect on brain metabolism (Heffez and Passonneau 1985) that they facilitate the maintenance of a low cytosolic Ca^{2+}, particularly since neuronal cells contain predominantly N-type Ca^{2+} channels which are insensitive to the calcium antagonists, and since there are other routes of Ca^{2+} entry, including entry in exchange for Na^{+}. As far as (S)-emopamil is concerned, its additional ability to antagonize 5-hydroxytryptamine receptors may provide an extra advantage, since 5-hydroxytryptamine is a relatively potent constrictor of cerebral blood vessels. However the relevance of this effect will depend entirely on the nature of the locally-released vasoconstrictor agent. If it is endothelin-1, then nimodipine is just as effective as (S)-emopamil in attenuating the response.

Subarachnoid Haemorrhage

This condition differs from that of acute ischaemic haemorrhage (stroke), although the end-result is the same – energy depleted cells which rapidly become overloaded with Ca^{2+}, die and necrose (Robinson and Teasdale 1990). The difference lies in the time-course of the events. In occlusive stroke, or stroke caused by a large intracerebral bleed, the major injury to the brain occurs early, at the time of the "stroke". By contrast, many patients with subarachnoid haemorrhage recover from the initial bleed, but subsequently develop brain damage (Robinson and Teasdale 1990). Several mechanisms may contribute to this delayed adverse response:

(i) cerebral perfusion pressure may fall. This may be caused by:
  (a) an increase in intracranial pressure – due either to an acute hydroencephalus or a space-occupying intracranial haematoma, or
  (b) systemic hypotension – often associated with a deliberate reduction in systemic hypertension. Alternatively,
(ii) the cerebral vascular resistance vessels may become vasospastic – due, perhaps to 5-hydroxytryptamine-induced constriction, or endothelin-1 (Fig. 14.2). Endothelin-1 production is substantially enhanced under these conditions (Masaoka et al. 1989) and it is a potent constrictor, but this does not necessarily mean that endothelin-1 is primarily responsible for this delayed vasoconstriction. Many other vasoactive substances have been incriminated, including catecholamines, serotonin, histamine, haemoglobin, and even K^{+} ions. Nevertheless it is pertinent to remember that the end-result – cerebral vasoconstriction – is a Ca^{2+}-dependent event, involving Ca^{2+} entry through voltage-sensitive L-type Ca^{2+} channels.

Table 14.4. Use of nisoldipine in the clinical management of subarachnoid haemorrhage as assessed by residual neurological deficit

Year	Neurological deficit	Sig	Reference
1983	Reduced	p = 0.03	Allen et al. 1983
1986	Reduced	p = 0.03	Philippon et al. 1986
1987	Reduced	p = 0.04	Neil-Dwyer et al. 1987
1988	Reduced	p = 0.05	Petruk et al. 1988
1989	Reduced	p > 0.001 (34%)	Pickard et al. 1989 (BRANT study)

The BRANT study is of particular interest. It showed a 34% reduction in the neurological deficit. Treatment was 60 mg nimodipine every four hours. This repetitive dosing probably prevented the large swings in plasma levels which occur if the intervals between doses is large. Maybe nimodipine should be produced as a GITS formulation

Effect of Second Generation Calcium Antagonists on Recovery After Subarachnoid Haemorrhage

Robinson and Teasdale (1990) recently reviewed the currently available data relating to the efficacy of nimodipine in the management of patients with proved subarachnoid haemorrhage. The details of these trials are listed in Table 14.4. Robinson and Teasdale concluded that "nimodipine reduces the occurrence of delayed ischaemic deficit and hence improves clinical outcome" (Robinson and Teasdale 1990). These clinical trials were undertaken because of the results obtained from experimental studies which showed that this calcium antagonist prevents vasoconstriction of human cerebral arteries induced by a wide variety of constrictor agents. Such an effect is not altogether surprising, because central to the constrictor response is an enhanced influx of Ca^{2+} by way of the voltage-activated L-type Ca^{2+} channels (Fleckenstein-Grun and Fleckenstein 1990). Hence, at least four factors may be responsible for the ability of nimodipine (and presumably other drugs) to attenuate the cerebral injury caused by subarachnoid haemorrhage. These are:

(i)   a general ability to increase cerebral blood flow;
(ii) an ability to cross the blood-brain barrier;
(iii) a direct protective effect at the cellular level, as described for the acute "stroke" syndrome (Fig. 14.5), and
(iv) an ability to attenuate the secondary vasoconstrictor· response to locally released vasoactive agents.

In Summary

1. The second-generation calcium antagonists nimodipine, isradipine and (S)-emopamil, show evidence of being useful in the management of cerebral

ischaemia, irrespective of whether the ischaemia is due to acute "stroke" or subarachnoid haemorrhage.

2. These drugs share some common characteristics – including their potency as calcium antagonists, relative selectivity for the cerebral vasculature, and an ability to cross blood-brain barrier, and hence to gain access to the jeopardized cells.

3. Clinical trials undertaken with nimodipine confirm that the protection seen in animal models of cerebral ischaemia also applies to naturally occurring cerebral ischaemia in man.

4. At the cellular level these drugs protect by:
   (i)   increasing cerebral blood flow – thereby reducing the perfusion deficit;
   (ii) preserving the metabolic status of the affected cells, so that tissue ATP is spared, cytosolic Ca^{2+} remains low, and the fall in intracellular pH is attenuated.

5. Acting on the vasculature these drugs improve flow to the ischaemic area by:
   (i)   a direct dilator effect associated with their ability to inhibit the L-type Ca^{2+} channel in the vasculature, and
   (ii) attenuating the vasoconstrictor response to locally-released vasoconstrictor agents.

Chapter 15

Second Generation Calcium Antagonists and the Coronary Circulation

> *"There ain't nothing more to write about, and I am rotten glad of it, because if I'd a knowed what a trouble it was to make a book I wouldn't a tackled it..."*
> Huckleberry Finn, in Tom Sawyer, by MARK TWAIN.

Fortunately Huckleberry Finn was not even contemplating writing about calcium antagonists or the coronary circulation when he uttered this now famous sentence, because of course much remains to be written on both topics. Here we are concerned with the relative value of second generation calcium antagonists (including the slow release formulations of the prototypes) in the management of patients with impaired or inadequate coronary circulation. Patients with vasospastic angina, with effort or rest induced angina pectoris, and patients with silent myocardial ischaemia are therefore the target group.

The potential benefits which might result from calcium antagonist therapy in this population of patients needs to be considered in terms of:
(i)   long-term benefit, and
(ii) short-term relief.

The factors which contribute to the long-term benefit include:
(i)   a slowed progression of atheromatous lesions (Chapter 11);
(ii) a reduction in cardiac hypertrophy (Chapter 13), and
(iii) a reduced afterload (Chapter 13).

As far as the immediate effects are concerned they centre around three facets of the response to these drugs:
(i)   the *direct* dilator effect on the coronary vasculature, coupled with an increase in coronary reserve (Cohn, PF 1990). The dilator response involves the large conductive as well as the small resistance vessels (Chew et al. 1980);
(ii) the attenuation of vasoconstriction caused by locally-released and circulating constrictor agents – including endothelin-1 (Luscher 1991, and Chapter 7), noradrenaline and 5-hydroxytryptamine, and
(iii) improved diastolic functioning (Fujibashi et al. 1985; Applegate et al. 1987).

The application of the second generation calcium antagonists to this sphere of medicine does not mean that the prototype drugs – verapamil, nifedipine and diltiazem – are ineffective. To the contrary, all three of these prototypes have been shown to be highly effective – as gauged by the restoration of coronary flow, recruitment of coronary vasodilator reserve and improved left ventricular function (Schwartz and Bache 1988; Fujibayashi et al. 1985; Heusch et al. 1987). However, there are several reasons why the second-generation antagonists might be even more suitable for this task:

(i)   the absence of any marked negative inotropy should reduce the likelihood of "pushing" an already compromised left ventricle into cardiac failure;

(ii) a long duration of action should ensure adequate calcium channel blockade on a twenty four hour basis – an important property bearing in mind the circadian patterns of ischaemia (Fox et al. 1989);

(iii) at least in the case of nisoldipine, and possibly nicardipine, selective vasodilation of the coronary vasculature is advantageous (Kazda et al. 1980; Pepine 1989);

(iv) because of the relative increase in potency, fewer side-effects should occur, and

(v)   the slower rate of onset of calcium channel blockade when induced either by the slow release formulations of the prototypes, including slow release nifedipine (Waller and Challenor 1990) or the new slow acting derivatives, should reduce the incidence of reflex-induced tachycardia caused by the accompanying vasodilation, because the baroreceptors have a longer time to reset.

Coronary Spasm

Maseri et al. (1989), have recently concluded that coronary vasospasm occurs whenever the coronary constriction is:

(i)   focal;

(ii) sufficiently profound as to cause transient episodes of coronary occlusion, and

(iii) responsible for causing reversible attacks of angina at rest.

Fortunately it is a relatively rare condition, except (Table 15.1) in patients who develop angina at rest. The most likely cause is believed to be hyperreactivity to locally released constrictor agents, including endothelin-1 (Luscher 1991). Whatever the cause of the sustained increase in vasomotor tone which gives rise to vasospastic angina, there is ample proof of its sensitivity to the second generation calcium antagonists – including the slow release formulations of some of the prototypes (Table 15.2). Evidence of efficacy usually reflects a reduced incidence of

Table 15.1. Incidence of vasospastic angina – as indicated by the occurrence of ergonovine-induced spasm

Patient type	%
Atypical chest pain	2
Chronic stable angina	4
Old myocardial infarctions	6
Recent myocardial infarctions	20
Angina at rest	38

Data from Maseri et al. 1989

Table 15.2. Second generation calcium antagonists and the management of vasospastic angina

Calcium antagonist	Dose	Reference
Slow-release nifedipine	20 mg at 10 p.m. or twice daily	Yasue and Morikami 1990
Amlodipine	10 mg, once daily	Taylor 1989
		Chahine et al. 1989
Nisoldipine	20 mg (ergometric provocation)	Lablanche et al. 1990
Nicardipine	40–160 mg . day	Gelman et al. 1985

anginal episodes – apart from the ergometrine provocation test used by Lablanche et al. (1990). One way of emphasising just how effective these second generation antagonists are – and particularly amlodipine, nisoldipine and slow-release nifedipine – is to compare the doses used in the studies listed in Table 15.2 with the doses of the original formulations of the prototype drugs that have also been used for this same purpose. These range between 120–360mg.day^{-1} for diltiazem, 40–80mg.day^{-1} for nifedipine, and 120–360mg.day^{-1} for verapamil (Kloner and Przyklenk 1990). It follows, therefore that the newer vascular-selective, dihydropy-ridine based antagonists are more effective on a weight basis in controlling vasospastic angina than the prototypes. The use of the newer long-acting (amlodipine) antagonists or slow-release formulations of the prototypes (e.g. slow release nifedipine, Yasue and Morikama 1990) is also advantageous, because attacks of variant angina most often occur from midnight to early morning, and hence at a time when, following the administration of the conventional form of the prototypes, the plasma levels will have fallen below the level needed to suppress the attacks. Nisoldipine, which is relatively selective for the vasculature, is effective at the same dose as slow-release nifedipine (Table 15.2).

Angina Pectoris

Calcium antagonists are widely used for this condition, and, as with vasospastic angina, their efficacy involves their ability to relax contracted coronary arteries, thereby improving coronary perfusion. Dose-related increases in epicardial coro-nary blood flow have been described for each of the prototypes (Bache 1989), the effect being more pronounced when coronary vasoconstriction has been deliberate-ly invoked – as by the hand grip test, for example. Myocardial blood flow, however, is normally controlled by the vasomotor activity of the coronary resistance vessels. It is these vessels which regulate blood flow in response to the changing metabolic needs of the myocardium, and it is these vessels which are largely responsible for maintaining a normal distribution of perfusion across the ventricular wall. Fortunately the prototype calcium antagonists dilate these coronary resistance vessels (Bache 1989).

If the prototype calcium antagonists are so effective in improving coronary blood flow and hence attenuating anginal episodes, then the question arises as to whether the second generation antagonists need to be investigated for this purpose? To answer this question it is only necessary to recall some of the limitations of the first generation antagonists, which are:

(i) they are all negatively inotropic;
(ii) their relatively short duration of action makes effective therapy on a twenty four hour basis problematical;
(iii) in the case of standard nifedipine, the accompanying fall in peripheral vascular resistance can enhance the problem of underperfusion, and even increase the frequency of anginal episodes because of the attendant reflex-induced tachycardia. By contrast,
(iv) in the case of verapamil the attendant bradycardia can be undesirable.

These problems have largely been circumvented by the development of the second generation antagonists – including the slow release formulations of the prototypes.

Nifedipine – Retard

This slow release tablet formulation provides a relatively steady plasma level of nifedipine. That it has a beneficial effect on patients with angina pectoris is shown by its ability to increase maximum exercise in patients for up to 8 hours after the last dose. Moreover the onset of anginal episodes is delayed (Gibelli et al. 1983; Waller and Challenor 1990).

Amlodipine

This long-acting second generation antagonist has been shown to be efficacious in reducing anginal attacks (as assessed by formal exercising and patient information) in doses of 2.5–10mg given as a single daily dose (Kinnard et al. 1988; Taylor et al. 1989). There seem to be a large number of studies which relate to the effectiveness of amlodipine under these circumstances (Table 15.3). Three conclusions can be drawn from them:

Table 15.3. Efficacy of amlodipine in the management of angina pectoris

Condition	Daily dose	Result	Reference
Stable angina pectoris	2.5–10 mg	Positive	Deedwania et al. 1989
Stable angina pectoris	7.7 mg	Positive	Singh et al. 1989
Angina pectoris	10 mg	Positive	Kinnard et al. 1989
			Thadani et al. 1989
Exertional angina	10 mg	Positive	Taylor et al. 1989

Efficacy assayed in terms of increased exercise duration and reduced incidence of anginal episodes

(i)   amlodipine is effective at a relatively low dose (10mg.day^{-1});
(ii) the side effects are minimal, and
(iii) the beneficial effect extends over a twenty four hour period.

Felodipine

The primary effect of felodipine is on the peripheral vasculature (Ljung and Nordlander 1987). Accordingly, it's use is largely directed towards controlling hypertension, and since it lacks any effect on atrioventricular conduction, β-adrenoceptor antagonist therapy often has to be added, to avoid reflex tachycardia. It's use as an antianginal agent is probably based on its afterload reducing activity, rather than a direct and selective dilator effect on the coronary vasculature (Emanuelsson et al. 1986), and in many cases necessitates ancillary β-blockade.

Isradipine

This is another vascular selective second generation antagonist which lacks appreciable negative inotropic activity, and primarily targets the peripheral vasculature. It's side-effect profile resembles that of nifedipine and the other dihydropyridines (ankle oedema and facial flushing). Compared with some of the other second generation antagonists its antianginal efficacy is relatively short-lived – for example 7.5mg provides protection for only nine hours (Parker et al. 1988).

Nicardipine

Nicardipine is very like nifedipine except that:
(i)   it has less negative inotropy,
(ii) it is more selective for the coronary vasculature, and
(iii) side effects *appear* to be less severe.

Table 15.4. Efficacy of nisoldipine

Condition	Daily dose	Result	Reference
Stable angina	5–10 mg*	Positive	Rousseau et al. 1987
Stable angina	10–20 mg	Positive	Klein et al. 1987
Stable angina	10 mg	Positive	Reicher-Reiss et al. 1987
Effort angina	10 mg	Positive	Von Arnim et al. 1987
Effort angina	20 mg	Positive	Marra et al. 1990
Effort angina	10 mg	Positive	Tzivoni et al. 1990

* Plus β-blockade
This table only lists a small proportion of the trials undertaken with nisoldipine

However treatment of effort angina with nicardipine requires as much as 30–40mg, three times daily (Scheidt et al. 1986). Its use in chronic effort angina requires 40mg three times daily (Thomassen et al. 1987).

Nisoldipine

In effort-induced angina nisoldipine is effective, despite an accompanying but relatively small increase in heart rate and rate-pressure product (Lam et al. 1985). A daily dose of 10mg is as effective as 10mg nifedipine, given three times daily (Reicher-Reiss et al. 1987). It's efficacy (Tzivoni et al. 1990) has been established in terms of:
(i)   increased exercise duration (16%);
(ii)   increased time to 1mm ST depression (49%), and
(iii) time to develop pain (37%).

Similar results have been obtained in other trials – for example Deeg et al. (1987) reported a sixty one percent reduction in anginal attacks per week with an eighteen percent increase in exercise duration.

Silent Ischaemia

Silent ischaemia is not uncommon in high risk patients, and can often be identified by non-invasive stress testing and ambulatory ECG monitoring. Nifedipine is certainly effective in reducing the incidence of these painless episodes of ischaemia (Nesto 1990) presumably because of its ability to restore the balance between the oxygen supply to and utilization by the heart. This may involve its coronary dilator effect as well as its ability to reduce the work load on the heart. Nisoldipine, however, is equally effective (Salmasi 1990; Glasser et al. 1987) and, presumably because of its relative selectivity for the vasculature, at a dose level which does not cause any significant change in heart rate.

In Summary

1. The second generation calcium antagonists provide effective therapy for the management of patients with vasospastic angina, angina pectoris and silent ischaemia.
2. New formulations of the prototypes, and new derivatives are effective.
3. The increased potency of some of the newer derivatives avoids some of the unwanted reflex changes associated with the use of standard formulations of the prototypes.
4. The efficacy of these drugs depends upon their ability to restore the oxygen supply: oxygen usage balance by:
   (i)   dilating the coronary vasculature, and
   (ii)   reducing cardiac work

Chapter 16

The Second Generation Calcium Antagonists

> *"There is something in this more than natural, if philosophy could find it out."*
> W. SHAKESPEARE, in Hamlet

At the very beginning of this book the question was raised as to whether the second generation calcium antagonists are different from their prototypes in terms of their usefulness as therapeutic agents. Throughout the subsequent chapters clear differences have emerged, based predominantly on:
(i) improved tissue selectivity;
(ii) longer duration of action, and
(iii) less bothersome side-effects.

Improved Tissue Selectivity

A variety of factors contribute to the tissue selectivity of the calcium antagonists. The main factors include:

(i) *The Source of Origin of the Activator Ca^{2+} in a Specific Tissue*
For example (Chapter 4) skeletal muscle relies predominantly on Ca^{2+}-release from the SR, and the activation of the release mechanism is not Ca^{2+} dependent. By contrast, vascular and cardiac muscle rely to a great extent on Ca^{2+} entry by way of the L-type Ca^{2+} channels to activate SR Ca^{2+} release. Modulation of L-type Ca^{2+} channel activity, therefore, will have a profound effect on cardiac and smooth, but not on skeletal muscle function.

(ii) *Ca^{2+}-Channel Distribution*
Calcium antagonists interact with L-type Ca^{2+} channels (which contain the alpha$_1$ binding subunit) (Chapter 3). Tissues which rely on Ca^{2+} entry by other routes – including the T- and N-type Ca^{2+} channels – cannot therefore be expected to be sensitive to the calcium antagonists – irrespective of whether they are "first" or "second" generation drugs.

(iii) *State-Dependent Interactions*
L-type Ca^{2+} channels exhibit state-dependent interactions such that increasing depolarization and increased frequency of stimulation increase pharmacological activity. For example, increasing membrane depolarization favours dihydropyridine binding (Glossmann and Striessnig 1990). This may explain

why the dihydropyridine-based calcium antagonists are vascular selective, because the potential difference of the vascular smooth muscle cells is suited to dihydropyridine binding. Similarly drugs of the verapamil and diltiazem class exhibit frequency-dependent interactions, whereby their activity increases with increasing frequency of depolarization (Talajic et al. 1989). One explanation for this is that the charged and more hydrophilic verapamil and diltiazem-type calcium antagonists may only have access to their binding sites in the alpha$_1$ subunit when the channel is open, whereas the hydrophobic dihydropyridines have continuous access through the lipid phase of the membrane.

(iv) *Tissue-Specific Chemistry of the Alpha$_1$ Subunit of the Ca^{2+} Channel Complex*
This was described in Chapter 3. Clearly, if there are subtle differences between the chemical composition of the alpha$_1$ subunits in different tissues – for example, there are differences between skeletal muscle on the one hand, and vascular smooth muscle on the other, – this almost certainly will influence the ability of certain chemical configurations to interact with the binding sites in the subunit.

(v) *The Pathological State of the Tissue*
Clinical disease states – including hypertension, ischaemia and hyperthyroidism are just a few of the conditions which modify the number of calcium channels – and hence the number of alpha$_1$ subunits which are available for interaction with the calcium antagonists (Chapter 5). There are other conditions which can be expected to modify calcium antagonist sensitivity – as for example, cardiomyopathy, or the ingestion of excess alcohol. Even age influences the density of the binding sites (Chapter 5) – and therefore, presumably, the sensitivity of the tissue.

(v) *Chemistry of the Various Compounds*
Obviously this is important, given that the chemistry of the alpha$_1$ subunit with which they interact is tissue specific.

Relevance of Improved Tissue Selectivity

There can be no doubt as to the relevance of this because:
(i) as a group the second generation calcium antagonists are less negatively inotropic than their prototypes, which means that they can be used (admittedly with care) under conditions in which impending or already existent left ventricular dysfunction would prevent the use of their prototypes. The use of some of the second generation antagonists to "unload" the heart in patients with congestive cardiac failure (e.g. nisoldipine) provides an example of the benefit gained from the improved tissue specificity of the newer drugs. Likewise, the use of calcium antagonists which are relatively selective for the cerebral circulation (e.g. nimodipine) for the management of patients with cerebral ischaemia (Chapter 14) depends upon their tissue selectivity, since a

Table 16.1. Preferred sites of action of second generation calcium antagonists

Drug	Preferred tissue
Amlodipine	Peripheral vasculature (conduit and resistance vessels)
Anipamil	Peripheral vasculature (conduit and resistance vessels)
Felodipine	Peripheral vasculature (conduit and resistance vessels)
Isradipine	Peripheral vasculature (conduit and resistance vessels)
Nitrendipine	Peripheral vasculature (conduit and resistance vessels)
Nicardipine	Peripheral vasculature (conduit and resistance vessels)
Nimodipine	Cerebral vasculature
Nisoldipine	Coronary vasculature

Table 16.2. Dose, plasma levels and primary target site of second generation antagonists

Compound	Daily dose (mg)	Peak plasma levels (ng/ml)	Uses (major)
Amlodipine	10	2–12	Hypertension
Felodipine	17.5–30	5–40	Hypertension
Isradipine	5–20	10	Hypertension
Nicardipine	90	30–110	Hypertension
Nimodipine	90–120	80	Cerebral ischaemia
Nisoldipine	20	1–4	1. Coronary heart disease 2. Congestive cardiac failure
Nitrendipine	21–40	9–42	Hypertension

(Data from Opie 1990)

decrease in overall perfusion pressure could worsen the situation. Even the increasing use of these newer calcium antagonists as blood pressure lowering agents in patients with raised peripheral vascular resistance (Chapter 13, and Tables 16.1 and 16.2) takes account of tissue selectivity, so that the vascular beds can be dilated without compromising ventricular function or atrioventricular conduction. The preferred sites of action of some of those second generation antagonists are summarized in Table 16.1.

Duration of Action

The second generation antagonists have other benefits, in addition to improved tissue selectivity. They include:
(i) their slower onset of activity, and
(ii) a prolonged duration of action.

Slowed Onset of Action

This has been achieved in two ways – the use of slow release formulations (e.g. slow release felodipine, nifedipine and verapamil, as well as the GITS formulation of nifedipine) and the development of drugs which only slowly associate with their receptors or have a slow absorption rate (e.g. amlodipine). The advantage of this slowed onset of action is clearly manifest in the use of these drugs for the management of patients with essential hypertension, where the slowed rate of onset of the vasodilator response allows time for the resetting of the baroreceptors so that marked reflex-induced changes in heart rate are avoided (Chapter 13), but without losing the beneficial effect these drugs exert on the regression of left ventricular hypertrophy.

Prolonged Duration of Action

Again there are two reasons for this:
(i)   some of the drugs (e.g. amlodipine, Nayler and Gu 1991), once bound, dissociate slowly, and
(ii) the slow release formulations facilitate treatment on a once a day basis. This has the added advantage of avoiding surges in blood levels, with a consequent reduction in the intensity of the side-effects – including reflex-induced tachycardia, and non-cardiac oedema.

Future Directions

The use of the calcium antagonists in cardiovascular medicine is probably in its infancy. The development of tissue selective, long-acting drugs has removed, to a large extent, unwanted side-effects. At the same time, new uses for these drugs are emerging, including their use to slow the growth of atherosclerotic plaques (Lichtlen et al. 1990; Waters et al. 1990, and Chapter 11). Such use depends upon the availability of long-acting drugs which do not become useless because of the development of tachyphylaxis. So far as the first or second generation antagonists are concerned tachyphylaxis has not been observed to any marked extent – which is fortunate. In addition, recognition of the complex manner in which these drugs interrupt the atherosclerotic mechanisms has drawn attention to their ancillary properties – as, for example, their ability to slow smooth muscle cell migration and proliferation. The future, therefore, may be even more exciting than the past – because not only will tissue-selective antagonists be available – some of them will have clinically important ancillary properties – including, as in the case of (S)-emopamil, an ability to interact with other receptors at the same dose level needed to achieve effective calcium channel blockade. Hence, even the pessimists can no longer doubt that the development of the second generation calcium antagonists represents a significant and clinically relevant advance.

References

Agabiti-Rosei E, Muiesan ML, Romanelli G, Beschi M, Castellano M, Muiesan G (1988) Reversal of cardiac hypertrophy by long-term treatment with calcium antagonists in hypertensive patients. J Cardiovasc Pharmacol 12 (Suppl 6):S75–S78

Agabiti-Rosei E, Muiesan ML, Romanelli G, Castellano M, Beschi M, Corea L, Muiesan G (1986) Similarities and differences in the antihypertensive effect of two calcium antagonist drugs, verapamil and nifedipine. J Am Cell Cardiol 7:916–926

Agnew WS (1989) Cloning of the SR foot. Nature 339:422–423

Agnew WS, Levinson SR, Brabson JS, Raftery MA (1978) Purification of the tetrodotoxin-binding component associated with the voltage-sensitive sodium channel from Electrophorus electricus electroplax membrane. Proc Natl Acad Sci USA 75:2606–2610

Akins CW, Pohost GM, DeSanctis RW, Block PC (1980) Selection of angina-free patients with severe left ventricular dysfunction after myocardial revascularization. Am J Cardiol 46:695–699

Allen GS, Ahn HS, Preziosi TJ, Battye R, Boone SC, Chou SN, Kelly DL, Weir BK, Crabbe RA, Lavik PJ, Rosenbloom SB, Dorsey FC, Ingram CR, Mellits DE, Bertsch LA, Boisvert DPJ, Hundley MB, Johnsson RK, Strom JA, Transou CR (1983) Cerebral arterial spasm a controlled trial of nimodipine in patients with subarachnoid hemorrhage. N Eng J Med 308:619–624

Allen DG, Orchard CH (1984) Measurements of intracellular calcium concentration in heart muscle; the effects of inotropic interventions and hypoxia. J Mol Cell Cardiol 16:117–128

Almers W, McCleskey EW, Palade PT (1985) The mechanism of ion selectivity in calcium channels of skeletal muscle membranes. Prog Zool 33:61–73

Ambrosio G, Jacobus WE, Bergman CA, Weisman HF, Becker LC (1987) Preserved high energy phosphate metabolic reserve in globally 'stunned' hearts despite reduction of basal ATP content and contractility. J Mol Cell Cardiol 19:953–964

American Heart Association (1990) Heart and Stroke Facts. American Heart Association, Dallas, Texas, 1989

Anastassiades C (1982) Nifedipine and beta-blockade as a cause of cardiac failure. Br Med J 284:506

Anderson JL, Marshall HW, Bray BE, Lutz JR, Frederick PR, Yanowitz FG, Datz FL, Klausner SC, Hagan AD (1983) A randomized trial of intracoronary streptokinase treatment of acute myocardial infarction. N Eng J Med 308:1313–1318

Anversa P, Olivetti G, Melissari M, Loud AU (1980) Stereological measurement of cellular and subcellular hypertrophy and hyperplasia in the papillary muscle of adult rat. J Mol Cell Cardiol 12:781–795

Applegate RJ, Walsh RA, O'Rourke RA (1987) Effects of nifedipine on diastolic function during brief episodes of flow-limiting ischemia in the conscious dog. Circulation 76:1409–1421

Apstein CS, Wexler LF, Vogell WM, Weinberg EO, Ingwall JS (1988) Comparative effects of ischemia and hypoxia on ventricular relaxation in isolated perfused hearts. In: Grossman W, Lorell BH (eds) Diastolic Relaxation of the Heart. Nijhoff, Boston pp169–184

Arai H, Hori S, Aramori I, Ohkubo H, Nakanishi S (1990) Cloning and expression of a cDNA encoding an endothelin receptor. Nature 348:730–732

Arnold G, Kosche F, Meissner E, Neitzert A, Lochner W (1968) The importance of the perfusion pressure in the coronary arteries for the contractility and oxygen consumption of the heart. Pflugers Arch 299:339–356

Arnold JMO, Braunwald E, Sandor T, Kloner RA (1985) Inotropic stimulation of reperfused myocardium with dopamine: effects on infarct size and myocardial function. J Am Coll Cardiol 6:1026–1034

Asano T, Ikegaki I, Satoh S, Suzuki Y, Shibuya M, Sugita K, Hidaka H (1990) Endothelin: a potential modulator of cerebral vasospasm. Eur J Pharmacol 190:365–372

Ascher EK, Stauffer JC, Barchi RL (1983) Biochemical studies of the excitable membrane sodium channel. J Neurochem 40:1377–1385

Ascher EK, Stauffer JC, Gaasch WH (1988) Coronary artery spasm, cardiac arrest, transient electrocardiographic Q waves and stunned myocardium in cocaine-associated acute myocardial infarction. J Am Coll Cardiol 11:744–751

Astrup J, Symon L, Branston NM, Lassen NA (1977) Cortical evoked potential and extracellular K^+ and H^+ levels of brain ischaemia. Stroke 8:51–57

Azcona A, Lataste X (1990) Isradipine in patients with acute ischaemic cerebral infarction: an overview of the ASCLEPIOS programme. Drugs 40 (Suppl 2):52–57

Bache RJ (1989) Effects of calcium entry blockade on myocardial blood flow. Circulation 80 (Suppl IV):IV-40–IV-46

Bagchi D, Prasad R, Das DK (1989) Direct scavenging of free radicals by captopril, an angiotensin converting enzyme inhibitor. Biochem Biophys Res Comm 158:52–57

Ballantyne CM, Vernai MS, Short HD, Hyatt C, Noon GP (1987) Delayed recovery of severely 'stunned' myocardium with the support of a left ventricular assist device after coronary artery bypass surgery. J Am Coll Cardiol 10:710–712

Banka VS, Bodenheimer MM, Shah R, Helfant RH (1976) Intervention ventriculography: comparative value of nitroglycerin, post-extrasystolic potentiation and nitroglycerin plus post-extrasystolic potentiation. Circulation 53:632–637

Barchi RL (1983) Biochemical studies of the excitable membrane sodium channel. J Neurochem 40:1377–1385

Barjon J-N, Rouleau JL, Bichet D, Juneau C, De Champlain J (1987) Chronic renal and neurohumoral effects of the calcium entry blocker nisoldipine in patients with congestive heart failure. J Am Coll Cardiol 9:622–630

Barrett RJ, Appell KC, Kilpatrick BF, Proakis AG, Nolan JC, Walsh DA (1991a) AHR-16303B, a novel antagonist of 5-HT$_2$ receptors and voltage-sensitive calcium channels. J Cardiovasc Pharmacol 17:41–53

Barrett RJ, Wright KF, Allen AD, Taylor DR (1991b) Cardiovascular and renal actions of AHR-16303B, and antagonist of 5-HT$_2$ receptors and calcium channels, in hypertensive and normotensive rats. J Cardiovasc Pharmacol 17:134–144

Beam KG, Knudson CM, Powell JA (1986) A lethal mutation in mice eliminates the slow calcium current in skeletal muscle cells. Nature 320:168–170

Bean BP (1989) Classes of calcium channels in vertebrae cells. Annu Rev Physiol 51:367–384

Becker LC, Levine JH, Dipaula AT, Guarnieri T, Aversano T (1986) Reversal of dysfunction in postischaemic stunned myocardium by epinephrine and postextrasystolic potentiation. J Am Coll Cardiol 7:580–589

Berbinschi A, Ketelslegers JM (1989) Endothelin in urine. Lancet ii: 46

Bernier M, Hearse DJ (1988) Reperfusion-induced arrhythmias: mechanisms of protection by glucose and mannitol. Am J Physiol 254:H862–H870

Betocchi S, Bonow RO, Cannon RO, Lesko LJ, Ostrow HG, Watson RM, Rosing DR (1988) Relation between serum nifedipine concentration and hemodynamic effects in non-obstructive hypertrophic cardiomyopathy. Am J Cardiol 61:830–835

Bielenberg GW, Burniol M, Rosen R, Klaus W (1990) Effects of nimodipine on infarct size and cerebral acidosis after middle artery occlusion. Stroke 21 (Suppl IV): IV-90–IV-92

Blanchard EM, Solaro RJ (1984) Inhibition of the activation and troponin calcium binding of dog cardiac myofibrils by acidic pH. Circ Res 55:382–391

Blaustein AS, Schine L, Brooks WW, Fanburg BL, Bing OHL (1986) Influence of exogenously generated oxidant species on myocardial function. Am J Physiol 250:H595–H599

Bloch KD, Friedrich SP, Lee ME, Eddy RL, Shows TB, Quertermous T (1989) Structural organization and chromosomal assignment of the gene encoding endothelin. J Biol Chem 264:10851–10857

Blumein S, Sievers R, Kidd P, Parmley WW (1984) Mechanisms of protection from atherosclerosis by verapamil in cholesterol-fed rabbit. Am J Cardiol 54:884–889

Bodenheimer MM, Banka VS, Hermann GA, Trout RG, Pasdar H, Helfant RH (1976) Reversible asynergy. Histopathologic and electrographic correlations in patients with coronary artery disease. Circulation 53:792–796

Bodenheimer MM, Banka VS, Fooshee C, Hermann GA, Helfant RH (1978) Relationship between regional myocardial perfusion and the presence, severity and reversibility of asynergy in patients with coronary heart disease. Circulation 58:789–795

Bolger GT, Basile AS, Janowsky AJ, Paul SM, Skolnick P (1987) Regulation of dihydropyridine calcium antagonist binding sites in the rat hippocampus following neurochemical lesions. J Neurol Res 17:285–290

Bolli R (1990) Mechanism of myocardial 'stunning'. Circulation 82:723–738

Bolli R, Jeroudi MO, Patel BS, DuBose CM, Lai EK, Roberts R, McCay PB (1989) Direct evidence that oxygen-derived free radicals contribute to postischemic myocardial dysfunction in the intact dog. Proc Natl Acad Sci USA 86:4695–4699

Bolli R, Zhu WX, Hartley CJ, Michael LH, Repine JE, Hell ML, Kukreia RC, Roberts R (1987) Attenuation of dysfunction in postischemic 'stunned' myocardium by dimethylthiourea. Circulation 76:458–468

Bolli R, Zhu WX, Myers ML, Hartley CJ, Roberts R (1985) Beta-adrenergic stimulation reverses post-ischemic myocardial dysfunction without producing subsequent function deterioration. Am J Cardiol 56:964–968

Bolli R, Zhu WX, Thornby JI, O'Neill PG, Roberts R (1988) Time-course and determinants of recovery of function after reversible ischemia in conscious dogs. Am J Physiol 254:H102–H114

Bolton TB, MacKenzie I, Aaronson PI (1988) Voltage-dependent calcium channels in smooth muscle cells. J Cardiovasc Pharmacol 12 (Suppl 6):S3–S7

Borhani NO, Brugger SB, Byington RP (1990) Multicenter study with isradipine and diuretics against atherosclerosis. J Cardiovasc Pharmacol 15 (Suppl 1):S23–S29

Borsotto M, Barhanin J, Norman RI, Lazdunski M (1984) Purification of the dihydropyridine receptor of the voltage-dependent Ca^{2+} channel from skeletal muscle transverse tubules using (+)-[^{3}H]PN200-110. Biochem Biophys Res Commun 122:1357–1366

Bossaller C, Habib GB, Yamamoto H, Williams C, Henry PD (1987) Impaired muscarinic endothelium-dependent relaxation and cyclic guanosine 5'-monophosphate formation in atherosclerotic human coronary artery and rabbit aorta. J Clin Invest 79:170–174

Boulanger CM, Tanner FC, Hahn AWA, Luscher TF (1990) Release of endothelin from the porcine aortic endothelium by oxidized low-density lipoproteins. J Vasc Med Biol 2:185

Braunwald E, Kloner RA (1982) The stunned myocardium: prolonged postischemic ventricular dysfunction. Circulation 66:1146–1149

Braunwald E, Rutherford JD (1986) Reversible ischemic left ventricular dysfunction: evidence for the 'hibernating myocardium'. J Am Coll Cardiol 8:1467–1470

Breisblatt WM, Brown DL, Weiland FL (1986) Reversibility of long-standing left ventricular aneurysm predicted by thallium–201 imaging. J Am Coll Cardiol 7:1162–1168

Breisblatt WM, Stein KL, Wolfe CJ, Follansbee WP, Capozzi J, Armitage JM, Hardesty RL (1990) Acute myocardial dysfunction and recovery: a common occurrence after coronary bypass surgery. J Am Coll Cardiol 15:1261–1269

Brennan CH, Guppy LJ, Littleton JM (1989) Chronic exposure to ethanol increases dihydropyridine-sensitive calcium channels in excitable cells. Proc Natl Acad Sci USA 560:467–479

Bristow MR, Ginsburg R, Minobe W, Cubicciotti RS, Sageman WS, Lurie K, Billingham ME, Harrison DC, Stinson EB (1982) Decreased catecholamine sensitivity and β-adrenergic receptor density in failing human hearts. New Eng J Med 307:205–211

Bristow MR, Minobe W, Rasmussen R (1985) Differential regulation of alpha and beta-adrenergic receptor in the failing human heart. Circulation 72 (Suppl III):III-329

Brooks N, Cattell M, Pidgeon J, Balcon R (1980) Unpredictable response to nifedipine in severe cardiac failure. Br Med J 281:1324

Broudy DR, Greenberg BH, Siemienczuk D (1987) Beneficial effects of the calcium antagonist PN200-110 in patients with congestive heart failure. J Cardiovasc Pharmacol 10:190–195

Brown G, Albers JJ, Fisher LD, Schaefer SM, Lin JT, Kaplan C, Zhao XQ, Bisson BD, Fitzpatrick VF, Dodge HT (1990) Regression of coronary artery disease as a result of intensive lipid-lowering therapy in man with high levels of apolipoprotein B. N Eng J Med 323:1289–1298

Brundage BH, Massie BM, Botvinick EH (1984) Improved regional ventricular function after successful surgical revascularization. J Am Coll Cardiol 3:902–908

Buchwald A, Klein HH, Lindert S, Pich S, Nebendahl K, Wiegand V, Kreuzer H (1989) Effect of intracoronary superoxide dismutase on regional function in stunned myocardium. J Cardiovasc Pharmacol 13:258–264

Buhler FR (1983) Age and cardiovascular response adaptation. Determination of an antihypertensive treatment concept primarily based on beta blockers and calcium entry blockers. Hypertension 5 (Suppl III): III-94–III-100

Burton KP, McCord JM, Ghai G (1984) Myocardial alterations due to free radical generation. Am J Physiol 246:H776–H783

Cade C, Lumma WC, Mohan R, Rubanyi GB, Parker-Botelho LH (1990) Lack of biological activity of preproendothelin (110–130) in several endothelin assays. Life Sci 47:2097–2103

Camici P, Araujo LI, Spinks T, Lammertsma AA, Kaski JC, Shea MJ, Selwyn AP, Jones T, Maseri A (1986) Increased uptake of ^{18}F-fluorodeoxyglucose in postischemic myocardium of patients with exercise-induced angina. Circulation 74:81–88

Carew TE, Schwenke DC, Steinberg D (1987) Antiatherogenic effect of probucol unrelated to its hypocholesterolemic effect: evidence that antioxidants in vivo can selectively inhibit low density lipoprotein degradation in macrophage-rich fatty streaks slowing the progression of atherosclerosis in WHHL rabbits. Proc Natl Acad Sci USA 84:7725–7729

Carter AJ, Gardiner DG, Burges RA (1988) Natriuretic activity of amlodipine, diltiazem, and nitrendipine in saline-loaded anesthetized dogs. J Cardiovasc Pharmacol 12 (Suppl 7):S34–S38

Caspari PG, Newcomb M, Gibson K, Harris P (1977) Collagen in normal and hypertrophied human ventricle. Cardiovasc Res 11:554–558

Castelli WP (1984) Epidemiology of coronary heart disease: the Framingham Study. Am J Med 76(2A):4–12

Catapano AL, Maggi FM, Cicerano U (1988) The antiatherosclerotic effect of anipamil in cholesterol-fed rabbits. Ann NY Acad Sci 522:519–521

Catterall WA, Seagar MJ, Takahashi M, Nunoki K (1989) Molecular properties of dihydropyridine-sensitive calcium channels. Ann NY Acad Sci 560:1–14

Cavero PG, Miller WY, Heublein DM, Margulies KB, Burnett JC (1990) Endothelin in experimental congestive heart failure in anesthetized dogs. Am J Physiol 259:F312–F317

Cernacek P, Stewart DJ (1989) Immunoreactive endothelin in human plasma: marked elevations in patients in cardiogenic shock. Biochem Biophys Res Commun 161:562–567

Chabrier PE, Auget M, Roubert P, Onchampt MO, Gillard V, Guillon JM, Delaflotte S, Braquet P (1989) Vascular mechanisms of action of endothelin-1: Effects of Ca^{2+}-antagonists. J Cardiovasc Pharmacol 13 (Suppl 5):218–219

Chahine RA, Feldman RL, Giles TD, Raizner AE, Weiss RJ, Nicod P, and the Investigators of Study 160 (1989) Efficacy and safety of amlodipine in vasospastic angina: an interview report of a multicenter placebo-controlled trial. Am Heart J 118:1128–1129

Charney RH, Takahashi S, Zhao M, Sonnenblick EH, Factor SM, Eng C (1989) Collagen loss in the stunned myocardium. Circulation 80 (Suppl II):II-99 (abstract)

Chatelain P, Demol D, Roba J (1984) Comparison of [^{3}H]nitrendipine binding to heart membranes of normotensive and spontaneously hypertensive rats. J Cardiovasc Pharmacol 6:220–223

Chatterjee K, Swan HJC, Parmley WW, Sustaita H, Marcus H, Matloff J (1972) Depression of left ventricular function due to acute myocardial ischemia and its reversal after aortocoronary saphenous vein bypass. N Engl J Med 286:1117–1122

Chatterjee K, Swan HJC, Parmley WW, Sustaita H, Marcus HS, Matloff J (1973) Influence of direct myocardial revascularization on left ventricular asynergy and function in patients with coronary heart disease. Circulation 47:276–286

Chew CYC, Brown BG, Singh BN, Hecht HS, Schnugg SJ, Wong M, Shah PM, Dodge HT (1980) Mechanism of action of verapamil in ischemic heart disease: observations on changes in systemic and coronary hemodynamics and coronary vasomobility. Clin Invest Med 3:151–158

Chew CYC, Hecht HS, Collett JT, McAllister RG, Singh BN (1981) Influence of severity of ventricular dysfunction on hemodynamic responses to intravenously administered verapamil in ischemic heart disease. Am J Cardiol 47:917–922

Chidsey CA, Braunwald E, Morrow AG (1965) Catecholamine excretion and cardiac stores of norepinephrine in congestive heart failure. Am J Med 39:442–451

Chierchia S, Lazzari M, Freeman B, Brunell B, Maseri A (1983) Impairment of myocardial perfusion and function during painless myocardial ischemia. J Am Coll Cardiol 1:924–930

Christian TF, Behrenbeck T, Pellika PA, Huber KC, Chesebro JH, Gibbons RJ (1990) Mismatch of left ventricular function and infarct size demonstrated by technetium-99m isonitrile imaging after reperfusion therapy for acute myocardial infarction: identification of myocardial stunning and hyperkinesia. J Am Coll Cardiol 16:1632–1638

Chuang DM, Kinnier WJ, Farber L, Costa E (1980) A biochemical study of receptor internalization during β-adrenergic receptor desensitization in frog erythrocytes. Mol Pharmacol 18:348–355

Clarke JG, Benjamin N, Larkin SW, Webb DJ, Davies GJ, Maseri A (1989) Endothelin is a potent long-lasting vasoconstrictor in men. Am J Physiol 257:H2033–H2035

Cleemann L, Morad M (1991) Role of Ca^{2+} channel in cardiac excitation-contraction coupling in the rat: evidence from Ca^{2+} transients and contraction. J Physiol 432:283–312

Clozel JP, Banken L, Osterrieder W (1989) Effects of R040-5967, a novel calcium antagonist, on myocardial function during ischemia induced by lowering coronary perfusion pressure in dogs: comparison with verapamil. J Cardiovasc Pharmacol 14:713–721

Cody RJ, Laragh JH (1988) The renin angiotensin aldosterone system in chronic heart failure. Pathophysiology and implications for treatment. In: Cohn JN (ed) Drug Treatment of Heart Failure, New Jersey Advanced Therapeutic Communications Inc, pp79–104

Cohn JN (1990) Abnormalities of peripheral sympathetic nervous system control in congestive heart failure. Circulation 82(Suppl I):I-59–I-67

Cohn JN, Archibald DG, Ziesche S, Franciosa JA, Hartson WE, Tristani FE, Dunkman WB, Jacobs W, Rancis GS, Flohr KH, Goldman S, Cobb FR, Shah PM, Saunders R, Fletcher RD, Loeb HS, Hughes VC, Baker B (1986) Effect of vasodilator therapy on mortality in chronic congestive heart failure. Results of a Veterans Administrative Cooperative Study (V-HEFT). N Eng J Med 314:1547–1558

Cohn PF (1990) Effects of calcium channel blockers on the coronary circulation. Am J Hypertens 3:299S–304S

Cook NS, Rudin M, Zerwes HG, Pally C, Lekoape K, Tschopp K, Peter J, Hof R (1991) Antiproliferative effect of spirapril and isradipine following balloon catheter injury of the rat carotid artery. Abstract 81: 2nd International Symposium on Calcium Antagonists in Cardiovascular Care. Basel, Switzerland, 1991

Cooke JP, Andon NA, Girerd XJ, Hirsch AT, Creager MA (1991) Arginine restores cholinergic relaxation of hypercholesterolemic rabbit thoracic aorta. Circulation 83:1057–1062

Cooper CL, Vandaele S, Barhanin J, Fosset M, Lazdunski M, Hosey MM (1987) Purification and characterization of the dihydropyridine-sensitive voltage-dependent calcium channel from cardiac tissue. J Biol Chem 262:509–512

Corr PB, Shayman JA, Kramer JB (1981) Increased α adrenergic receptors in ischemic cat myocardium. J Clin Invest 67:1232–1236

Cummins P (1982) Transition in human atrial and ventricular myosin light-chain isoenzymes in response to cardiac pressure-overload-induced hypertrophy. Biochem J 205:195–204

Curtis BM, Catterall WA (1983) Solubilization of the calcium antagonist receptor from rat brain. J Biol Chem 258:7280–7283

Curtis BM, Catterall WA (1984) Purification of the calcium antagonist receptor of the voltage-sensitive calcium channel from skeletal muscle transverse tubules. Biochemistry 23:2113–2118

Curtis BM, Catterall WA (1986) Reconstitution of the voltage-sensitive calcium channel purified from skeletal muscle transverse tubules. Biochemistry 25:3077–3083

Daemen MJAP, Lombardi DM, Bosman FT, Schwartz SM (1991) Angiotensin II induces smooth muscle cell proliferation in the normal and injured rat arterial wall. Circ Res 68:450–456

Daugherty A, Rateri DL, Schonfeld G, Sobel BE (1987) Inhibition of cholesteryl ester deposition in macrophages by calcium entry blockers: an effect dissociable from calcium entry blockade. Br J Pharmacol 91:113–118

Davenport AP, Nunez DJ, Hall JA, Kaumann AJ, Brown MJ (1989) Autoradiographical localization of binding sites for porcine [^{125}I]endothelin-1 in humans, pigs and rats: functional relevance in humans. J Cardiovasc Pharmacol 13 (Suppl 5):S166–S170

Davies KJA (1987) Protein damage and degradation by oxygen radicals. 1. General aspects. J Biol Chem 262:9895–9901

Davies MJ (1990) A macro and micro view of coronary vascular insult in ischaemic heart disease. Circulation 82 (Suppl II):II-38–II-46

De Aguilera ME, Irurzun A, Vila JM, Aldasoro M, Galeote MS, Lluch S (1990) Role of endothelium and calcium channels in endothelin-induced contraction of human cerebral arteries. Br J Pharmacol 99:439–440

De Cock CC, Visser FC, Peels KH, Van Eenige MJ, Roos JP (1990) Nisoldipine in patients with reduced left ventricular function following myocardial infarction. A randomized double-blind, placebo-controlled study. In: Lichtlen PR, Krayenbuhl HP (eds) New Aspects of Nisoldipine, Schattauer Press, Stuttgart, pp85–94

De Jongh KS, Merrick DK, Catterall WA (1989) Subunits of purified calcium channels: a 212 kDa form of α_1 and partial amino acid sequence of a phosphorylation site of an independent β subunit. Proc Natl Acad Sci USA 86:8585–8589

De Jongh KS, Warner C, Catterall WA (1990) Subunits of purified calcium channels α_2 and δ are encoded by the same gene. J Biol Chem 265:14738–14741

De Meis L, Inesi G (1982) The transport of calcium by sarcoplasmic reticulum and various microsomal preparations. In: Carafoli E (ed) Membrane Transport of Calcium, Academic Press, London, pp141–186

De Nucci G, Thomas R, D'Orleans-Juste P, Walder C, Antune SE, Warner D, Vane JR (1988) Pressor effects of circulating endothelin are limited by its removal in the pulmonary circulation and by the release of prostacyclin and endothelium-derived relaxing factor. Proc Natl Acad Sci USA 85:9797–9800

Deedwania P, Cheitlin M, Das S, Pool P, Singh J, Pasternak R, Carabello B (1989) Double-blind crossover comparison of amlodipine at three dose levels and placebo in chronic stable angina. Am Heart J 118 (Suppl 5):1132–1133

Deeg P, Weiss KH, Schmitz H (1987) Anti-ischemic effect of nisoldipine in patients with stable angina pectoris. In: Hugenholtz PG, Meyer J (eds) Nisoldipine. Springer-Verlag, Berlin, pp244–248

Defeudis FV (1989) The Ca^{2+} channel and 5-HT$_2$ receptor antagonists (s)-emopamil in cerebral ischaemia. Trends Pharmacol Sci 10:215–223

Demopoulos HB, Flamm ES, Pietronigro DD, Seligman ML (1980) The free radical pathology and the microcirculation in the major central nervous system disorders. Acta Physiol Scand (Suppl) 492:91–120

Diaz-Munoz M, Hamilton SL, Kaetzel MA, Hazarika P, Dedman JR (1990) Modulation of Ca^{2+} release channel activity from sarcoplasmic reticulum by annexin VI (67-kDa calcimedin). J Biol Chem 265:15894–15899

DiBona GF (1990) Renal effects of felodipine: A review of experimental evidence and clinical data. J Cardiovasc Pharmacol 15 (Suppl 4):S29–S32

Dillon JS, Gu XH, Nayler WG (1989) Effect of age and hypertrophy on cardiac Ca^{2+} antagonist binding sites. J Cardiovasc Pharmacol 14:233–240

Dillon JS, Nayler WG (1987) [^{3}H]Verapamil binding to rat cardiac sarcolemmal membrane fragments: an effect of ischaemia. Br J Pharmacol 90:99–109

Dillon JS, Nayler WG (1988) The Ca^{2+}-antagonist and binding properties of the phenylalkylamine, Anipamil. Br J Pharmacol 94:253–263

Dolin S, Little H, Hudspith M, Pagonis C, Littleton J (1987) Increased dihydropyridine-sensitive calcium channels in rat brain may underlie ethanol physical dependence. Neuropharmacology 26:275–279

Downing SE, Chen V (1990) Myocardial hibernation in the ischaemic neonatal heart. Circ Res 66:763–772

Dulhunty AF (1989) Feet, bridges, and pillars in triad junctions of mammalian skeletal muscle: the possible relationship to calcium buffers in terminal cisternae and T-tubules and to excitation contraction coupling. J Membr Biol 109:73–83

Dunselman PHJM, Edgar B, Scaf AHJ, Kuntze CEE, Van Bruggen A, Lie KI, Wesseling H (1989) Plasma concentration-effect relationship of felodipine intravenously in patients with congestive heart failure. J Cardiovasc Pharmacol 14:438–443

Dyke SH, Cohn PF, Gorlin R, Sonnenblick EH (1974) Detection of residual myocardial function in coronary artery disease using post-extrasystolic potentiation. Circulation 50:694–699

Elkayam U, Amin J, Mehra A, Vasquez J, Weber L, Rahimtoola SH (1990) A prospective, randomized, double-blind crossover study to compare the efficacy and safety of chronic nifedipine therapy with that of isosorbide dinitrate and their combination in the treatment of chronic congestive heart failure. Circulation 82:1954–1961

Elkayam U, Weber L, McKay C, Rahimtoola S (1985) Spectrum of acute hemodynamic effects of nifedipine in severe congestive heart failure. Am J Cardiol 56:560–566

Elliot H, Meredith PA, Reid JL, Faulkner JK (1988) A comparison of the disposition of single oral doses of amlodipine in young and elderly subjects. J Cardiovasc Pharmacol 12 (Suppl 7):S64–S66

Ellis SG, Henschke CI, Sandor T, Wynne J, Braunwald E, Kloner RA (1983) Time course of functional and biochemical recovery of myocardium salvaged by reperfusion. J Am Coll Cardiol 1:1047–1055

Ellis SB, Williams ME, Ways NR, Brenner R, Sharp AH, Leung AT, Campbell KP, McKenna E, Koch WJ, Hui A, Schwartz A, Harpold MM (1988) Sequence and expression of mRNA's encoding the α_1 and α_2 subunits of a DHP-sensitive calcium channel. Science 241:1661–1664

Emanuelsson H, Hjalmarson A, Holmberg S, Waagstein F (1986) Effects of felodipine on pacing-induced angina pectoris. J Cardiovasc Pharmacol 8:500–506

Engler RL, Covell JW (1987) Granulocytes cause reperfusion ventricular dysfunction after 15 minutes ischaemia in the dog. Circ Res 61:20–28

Eskinder H, Hillard CJ, Gross GJ (1989) Effect of KT-362, a new intracellular calcium antagonist, on norepinephrine-induced contraction and inositol monophosphate accumulation in canine femoral artery. J Cardiovasc Pharmacol 13:502–507

Fabiato A (1983) Calcium-induced release of calcium from the cardiac sarcoplasmic reticulum. Am J Physiol 245:C1–C14

Fabiato A (1985) Time and calcium dependence of activation and inactivation of calcium-induced release of calcium from the sarcoplasmic reticulum of a skinned canine cardiac Purkinje cell. J Gen Physiol 85:247–289

Fabiato A, Fabiato F (1978) Effects of pH on the myofilaments and the sarcoplasmic reticulum of skinned cells from cardiac and skeletal muscles. J Physiol 276:233–255

Fabiato A, Fabiato F (1979) Calcium and cardiac excitation-contraction coupling. Annu Rev Physiol 41:473–484

Farber NE, Gross GJ (1989) Collateral blood flow following acute coronary artery occlusion: comparison of a new intracellular calcium antagonist (KT-362) and diltiazem. J Cardiovasc Pharmacol 14:66–72

Farber NE, Vercellotti GM, Pieper GM, Gross GJ (1987) Enhancement of postischemic metabolic and functional recovery in the stunned canine myocardium by desferrioxamine (DF). Circulation 76 (Suppl IV):IV-230 (abstract)

Feher J, Csomos G, Vereckei A (1987) Free Radical Reactions in Medicine. Springer Verlag, Berlin, p138–140

Feher JJ, LeBolt WR, Manson NH (1989) Differential effect of global ischemia on the ryanodine-sensitive and ryanodine-insensitive calcium uptake of cardiac sarcoplasmic reticulum. Circ Res 65:1400–1408

Ferlinz J, Gallo CT (1984) Responses of patients in heart failure to long-term oral verapamil administration. Circulation 70 (Suppl II):II-305 (abstract)

Fernandes VB, Freedman B, Allman KC, Bautovich GJ, Hutton BF, McLaughlin AF, Whitehead EK, Kelly DT, Harris PJ, Morris JG (1991) Detection of myocardial viability in stunned or hibernating myocardium by delayed emptying on radionuclide ventriculography. Am J Cardiol 67:529–532

Ferrante J, Triggle DJ (1990) Drug and disease-induced regulation of voltage-dependent calcium channels. Pharmacol Rev 42:29–44

Ferrari R, Alferi O, Curello S, Ceconi C, Cargnoni A, Marzollo P, Pardini A, Caradonna E, Visioli O (1990) Occurrence of oxidative stress during reperfusion of the human heart. Circulation 81:201–211

Ferrari R, Ceconi C, Curello S, Guarnieri C, Caldarera CM, Albertini A, Visioli O (1985) Oxygen mediated myocardial damage during ischaemia and reperfusion. Role of the cellular defence against oxygen toxicity. J Mol Cell Cardiol 17:937–945

Fieschi C, Piero VD, Lenzi GL, Pantano P, Giubilei F, Buttinelli C, Carolei A (1990) Pathophysiology of ischemic brain disease. Stroke 21 (Suppl IV):IV-9–IV-11

Fill M, Coronado R (1988) Ryanodine receptor channel of sarcoplasmic reticulum. Trends Neurosci 11:453–457

Fill M, Ma J, Knudson CM, Imagawa T, Campbell KP, Coronado R (1989) Role of the ryanodine receptor of skeletal muscle in excitation-contraction coupling. Ann NY Acad Sci 560:155–162

Fine DG, Clements IP, Callahan MJ (1989) Myocardial stunning in hypertrophic cardiomyopathy: recovery predicted by single photon emission computed tomographic thallium-201 scintigraphy. J Am Coll Cardiol 13:1415–1418

Finkel MS, Marks ES, Patterson RE, Speir EH, Steadman KA, Keiser HR (1987a) Correlation of changes in cardiac calcium channels with hemodynamics in Syrian hamster cardiomyopathy and heart failure. Life Sci 41:153–159

Finkel MS, Marks ES, Patterson RE, Speir EH, Steadman KA, Keiser HR (1987b) Increased cardiac calcium channels in hamster cardiomyopathy. Am J Cardiol 57:1205–1206

Finkel MS, Patterson RE, Roberts WC, Smith TD, Keiser HR (1988) Calcium channel binding characteristics in the human heart. Am J Cardiol 62:1281–1284

Fleckenstein A (1983) History of calcium antagonists. Circ Res 52 (Suppl I):I3–I16

Fleckenstein A, Frey M, Thimm F, Fleckenstein-Grun G (1990) Excessive mural calcium overload – a predominant causal factor in the development of stenosing coronary plaques in humans. Cardiovasc Drugs Ther 4:1005–1014

Fleckenstein-Grun G, Fleckenstein A (1990) Prevention of cerebrovascular spasm with nimodipine. Stroke 21 (Suppl IV):IV-64–IV-71

Flockerzi V, Oeken HJ, Hofmann F, Pelzer D, Cavalie A, Trautwein W (1986) Purified dihydropyridine-binding site from skeletal muscle T-tubules is a functional calcium channel. Nature 323:66–68

Fosset M, Jaimovich E, Delpont E, Lazdunski M (1983) [³H]Nitrendipine receptors in skeletal muscle. Properties and preferential localization in transverse tubules. J Biol Chem 258:6086–6092

Fowler MB, Schroeder JS, Gao S-Z, Valantine HA, Alderman EA, Hunt SA, Stinson EB (1991) Vascular protection: influence of diltiazem on accelerated graft atherosclerosis in heart transplantation. Abstract 62: 2nd International Symposium on Calcium Antagonists in Cardiovascular Care. Basel, Switzerland 1991

Fox K, Mulcahy D, Keegan J, Wright C (1989) Circadian patterns of myocardial ischaemia. Am Heart J 118:1084–1086

Francis GS (1991) Calcium channel blockers and congestive heart failure. Circulation 83:336–338

Francis GS, Cohn JN (1986) The autonomic nervous system in congestive heart failure. Annu Rev Med 37:235–247

Franzini-Armstrong C (1970) Studies of the triad.11. Penetration of tracers into the junctional gap. J Cell Biol 47:488–499

Franzini-Armstrong C, Wunzi C (1983) Junctional feet and particles in the triads of a fast-twitch muscle fibre. J Muscle Res Cell Motil 4:233–252

Frohlich ED (1987) Correction of physiological alterations of hypertension. Cardiovasc Drugs Therap 1:345–348

Fronek K (1988) Effects of nisoldipine on diet-induced atherosclerosis in rabbits. Ann NY Acad Sci 522:525–526

Fujibayashi Y, Yamazaki S, Chang BL, Rajagopalan RE, Meerbaum S, Corday E (1985) Comparative echocardiographic study of recovery of diastolic versus systolic function after brief periods of coronary occlusion: differential effects of intravenous nifedipine administered before and during occlusion. J Am Coll Cardiol 6:1289–1298

Fujisawa A, Matsumoto M, Matsuyama T, Ueda H, Wanaka A, Yoneda S, Kimura K, Kamada T (1986) The effect of the calcium antagonist nimodipine on the gerbil model of experimental cerebral ischaemia. Stroke 17:748–752

Furchgott RF, Zawadzki JV (1980) The obligatory role of endothelial cells in the relaxation of arterial smooth muscle by acetylcholine. Nature 288:373–376

Fuster V, Stein B, Ambrose JA, Badimon L, Badimon JJ, Chesbro JH (1990) Atherosclerotic plaque rupture and thrombis: evolving concepts. Circulation 82 (Suppl II):II-47–II-59

Gaab MR, Haubitz I, Brawanski A, Korn A, Czech TH (1985) Acute effects of nimodipine on the cerebral blood flow and intracranial pressure. Neurochirurgia 28:93–99

Ganote CE, Vander Heide RS (1987) Cytoskeletal lesions in anoxic myocardial injury. A conventional and high-voltage electronmicroscopic and immunofluorescence study. Am J Pathol 129:327–344

Garlick PB, Davies MJ, Hearse DJ, Slater TF (1987) Direct detection of free radicals in the reperfused rat heart using electron spin resonance spectroscopy. Circ Res 61:757–760

Geizhals M, Phillips RA, Ardeljan M, Krakoff LR (1990) Sustained calcium channel blockade in the treatment of severe hypertension. A two year experience. Am J Hypertens 3:313S–317S

Gelman JS, Feldman RL, Scott E, Pepine CJ (1985) Nicardipine for angina pectoris at rest and coronary arterial spasm. Am J Cardiol 56:232–236

Gelmers HJ, Corter K, De Weerdt CJ, Wiezer HJA (1988) A controlled trial of nimodipine in acute ischemic stroke. N Eng J Med 318:203–207

Gelmers HJ, Hennerici M (1990) Effect on nimodipine on acute ischemic stroke: pooled results from five randomized trials. Stroke 21 (Suppl IV):IV-81–IV-84

Gengo P, Bowling N, Wyss VL, Hayes JS (1988a) Effects of prolonged phenylephrine infusion on cardiac adrenoceptors and calcium channels. J Pharmacol Exp Ther 244:100–105

Gengo P, Skattebol A, Moran JF, Gallant S, Hawthorn M, Triggle DJ (1988b) Regulation by chronic drug administration of neuronal and cardiac calcium channel, beta-adrenoceptor and muscarinic receptor levels. Biochem Pharmacol 37:627–633

Gibelli G, Carnovali M, Orvieni C (1983) Effect and duration of action of nifedipine 20mg tablets: double blind ergometric evaluation versus placebo. Curr Ther Res 33:244–245

Gillmer D, Karrk P (1980) Pulmonary oedema precipitated by nifedipine. Br Med J 280:1420–1421

Ginsburg R, Davis K, Bristow MR, McKennett K, Kodsi SR, Billingham EM, Schroeder JS (1983) Calcium antagonists suppress atherogenesis in aorta but not in the intramural coronary arteries of cholesterol-fed rabbits. Lab Invest 49:154–158

Glasser SP, Arce-Weston B, Clark PI (1987) Improvement in silent myocardial ischemia with nisoldipine. In: Hugenholtz PG, Meyer J (eds) Nisoldipine. Springer-Verlag, Berlin, pp296–298

Glossmann H, Ferry DR, Boschek, CB (1983) Purification of the putative calcium channel from skeletal muscle with the aid of [^{3}H]–nimodipine binding. Naunyn Schmiedebergs Arch Pharmacol 323:1–11

Glossmann H, Striessnig J (1990) Molecular properties of calcium channels. Rev Physiol Biochem Pharmacol 114:1–105

Glower DD, Spratt JA, Newton JR, Wolfe JA, Ranking JS, Swain JL (1987) Dissociation between early recovery of regional function and purine nucleotide content in postischaemic myocardium of conscious dogs. Cardiovasc Res 21:328–336

Godfraind T, Kazda S, Wibo M (1991) Effects of a chronic treatment by nisoldipine, a calcium antagonistic dihydropyridine, on arteries of spontaneously hypertensive rats. Circ Res 68:674–682

Goldstein RE, Boccuzzi SJ, Cruess D, Nattel S (1991) Diltiazem increases late-onset congestive heart failure in postinfarction patients with early reduction in ejection fraction. Circulation 83:52–60

Golino P, Ashton JH, Buja LM, Rosolowsky M, Taylor AL, McNatt A, Campbell WB, Willerson JT (1989) Local platelet activation causes vasoconstriction of large epicardial canine coronary arteries in vivo. Thromboxane.A2 and serotonin are possible mediators. Circulation 79:154–166

Gordon EE, Morgan HE (1986) Principles of metabolic regulation. In: Fozzard HA, Haber E, Jennings RB, Katz AM, Morgan HE (eds) The Heart and Cardiovascular System: Scientific Foundations. Raven Press, New York, pp51–60

Gorlin R (1987) Treatment of congestive heart failure: where are we going. Circulation 75 (Suppl IV): IV108–IV111

Gottlieb SO, Brinker JA, Mellits ED, Achuff SC, Baughman KL, Traill TA, Weiss JL, Reitz BA, Weisfeldt ML, Gerstenblith G (1989) Effect of nifedipine on the development of coronary bypass graft stenosis in high-risk patients: a randomized double-blind, placebo-controlled trial. Circulation 80 (Suppl 2):II-228 (abstract 0909)

Grassegger A, Striessnig J, Weiler M, Knaus HG, Glossmann H (1989) [^{3}H]HOE166 defines a novel calcium antagonist drug receptor – distinct from the 1,4 dihydropyridine binding domain. Naunyn-Schmiedebergs Arch Pharmacol 340:752–759

Greenberg JH, Uematsu D, Araki N, Hickey WF, Reivich M (1990) Cytosolic free calcium during focal cerebral ischemia and the effects of nimodipine on calcium and histological damage. Stroke 21 (Suppl IV):IV-72–IV-77

Greenfield RA, Swain JL (1987) Disruption of myofibrillar energy use: dual mechanism that may contribute to postischemic dysfunction in stunned myocardium. Circ Res 60:283–289

Gross GJ, Farber NE, Hardman HF, Waritier DC (1986) Beneficial actions of superoxide dismutase and catalase in stunned myocardium in dogs. Am J Physiol 250:H372–377

Grover GJ, Dzwonczyk S, Sleph PG (1990) Ruthenium red improves postischemic contractile function in isolated rat hearts. J Cardiovasc Pharmacol 16:783–789

Grum CM, Gallagher KP, Kirsh MM, Shlafer M (1989) Absence of detectable xanthine oxidase in human myocardium. J Mol Cell Cardiol 21:263–267

Gu XH, Dillon JS, Nayler WG (1989a) The effect of hypoxia and energy depletion on 1,4 dihydropyridine binding sites in rat cardiac membranes. Biochem Pharmacol 38:1897–1907

Gu XH, Liu JJ, Dillon JS, Nayler WG (1989b) The failure of endothelin to displace radioactively labelled calcium antagonists (PN200-110, D888 and diltiazem). Br J Pharmacol 96:262–264

Guarnieri C, Flamigni F, Caldarera CM (1980) Role of oxygen in the cellular damage induced by re-oxygenation of hypoxic heart. J Mol Cell Cardiol 12:797–805

Guazzi MD, Cipolla C, Bella PD, Fabbiocchi F, Montorsi P, Sganzerla P (1984) Disparate unloading efficacy of the calcium channel blockers, verapamil and nifedipine, on the failing hypertensive left ventricle. Am Heart J 108:116–123

Habib JB, Bossaller C, Henry PD (1986a) Suppression of atherogenesis in cholesterol-fed rabbit with low-dosed calcium antagonist (PN200-110). J Am Coll Cardiol 7:58A (abstract)

Habib JB, Bossaller C, Wells S, Williams C, Morrissett JD, Henry PD (1986b) Preservation of endothelium-dependent vascular relaxation in cholesterol-fed rabbits by treatment with the calcium channel blocker PN200-110. Circ Res 58:305–309

Hadley MN, Spetzler RF, Fitfield MS, Bichard WD, Hodak JA (1987) Nimodipine reduced intracranial pressure. Volume-pressure studies in primate model. N Neurosurg 678:387–393

Hammond B, Hess ML (1985) The oxygen free radical system: Potential mediator of myocardial injury. J Am Coll Cardiol 6:215–220

Hara H, Nagagawa H, Kogure K (1990) Nimodipine prevents postischemic brain damage in the early phase of focal cerebral ischemia. Stroke 21 (Suppl IV):IV-102–IV-105

Hardebo JE, Kahrstrom J, Owman C, Salford LG (1989) Endothelin is a potent constrictor of human intracranial arteries and veins. Blood Vessels 26:249–255

Harder S, Thurmann P, Siewert M, Blume H, Huber TH, Reitbrock N (1991) Pharmacodynamic profile of verapamil in relation to absolute bioavailability: investigations with a conventional and a controlled-release formulation. J Cardiovasc Pharmacol 17:207–212

Hartshorne RP, Catterall WA (1981) Purification of the saxitoxin receptor of the sodium channel from rat brain. Proc Natl Acad Sci USA 78:4620–4624

Hathaway DR, March KL, Lash JA, Adam LP, Wilensky RL (1991) Vascular smooth muscle. A review of the molecular basis of contractility. Circulation 83:382390

Hathaway DR, Watanabe AM (1989) Biochemical basis for cardiac and vascular smooth muscle contraction. In: Kelly WN (ed) Textbook of Internal Medicine, Philadelphia, Harper and Row

Hatjis, CG, McLaughlin MK (1982) Identification and ontogenesis of beta-adrenergic receptors in fetal and neonatal rabbit myocardium. J Dev Physiol 4:327–338

Hawthorn M, Gengo P, Wei XY, Rutledge A, Moran JF, Gallant S, Triggle D (1988) Effect of thyroid status on beta-adrenoceptor and calcium channels in rat cardiac and vascular tissue. Naunyn-Schmiedebergs Arch Pharmacol 337:539–544

Headrick JP, Armiger LC, Willis RJ (1990) Behaviour of energy metabolites and effects of allopurinol in the 'stunned' isovolumic rat heart. J Mol Cell Cardiol 22:1107–1116

Heffez DS, Passonneau JV (1985) Effect of nimodipine on cerebral metabolism during ischemia and recirculation in the mongolian gerbil. J Cereb Blood Flow Metab 5:523–528

Heinecke JW, Baker L, Rosen H, Chart A (1986) Superoxide-mediated modification of low density lipoprotein by arterial smooth muscle cells. J Clin Invest 77:757–761

Heistad DD, Breese K, Armstrong ML (1987) Cerebral vasoconstrictor responses to serotonin after dietary treatment of atherosclerosis: implications for transient ischemic attacks. Stroke 18:1068–1073

Helfant RH, Pine R, Meister SG, Feldman MS, Trout RG, Banka VS (1974) Nitroglycerin to unmask reversible asynergy. Correlation with post-coronary bypass ventriculography. Circulation 50:108–113

Henry PD (1990a) Calcium antagonists as antiatherosclerotic agents. Atherosclerosis 10:963–965

Henry PD (1990b) Atherogenesis, calcium and calcium antagonists. Am J Cardiol 66:3I–7I

Henry TD, Archer SL, Nelson D, Weir EK, From AHL (1990) Enhanced chemiluminescence as a measure of oxygen-derived free radical generation during ischemia and reperfusion. Circ Res 67:1453–1461

Henry PD, Bentley KI (1981) Suppression of atherogenesis in cholesterol-fed rabbits treated with nifedipine. J Clin Invest 68:1366–1369

Hess ML, Okabe E, Kontos HA (1981) Proton and free oxygen radical interaction with the calcium transport system of cardiac sarcoplasmic reticulum. J Mol Cell Cardiol 13:767–772

Hess P (1990) Calcium channels in vertebrate cells. Ann Rev Neurosci 13:337–356

Heusch G, Guth BD, Seitelberger R, Ross J Jr (1987) Attenuation of exercise-induced myocardial ischemia in dogs with recruitment of coronary vasodilator reserve by nifedipine. Circulation 75:482–490

Heyndrickx GR, Millard RW, McRitchie RJ, Maroko PR, Vatner SF (1975) Regional myocardial function and electrophysiological alterations after brief coronary artery occlusion in conscious dogs. J Clin Invest 56:978–985

Hiki K, Yui Y, Hattori R, Eizawa H, Kosuga K, Kawai C (1991) Three regulation mechanisms of nitric oxide synthase. Eur J Pharmacol 206:163–164

Himmel HM, Glossmann H, Ravens U (1991) Naftopidil, a new α adrenoceptor blocking agent with calcium antagonistic properties: characterization of Ca^{2+} antagonistic effects. J Cardiovasc Pharmacol 17:213–221

Hinshaw DB, Burger JM, Armstrong BC, Hyslop PA (1989) Mechanism of endothelial cell shape change in oxidant injury. J Surg Res 46:339–349

Hirata Y, Takagi Y, Fukuda Y, Marumo F (1989) Endothelin is a potent mitogen for rat vascular smooth muscle cells. Atherosclerosis 78:225–228

Hirst GDS, Edwards FR (1989) Sympathetic neuroeffector transmission in arteries and arterioles. Physiol Rev 69:546–604

Hittinger L, Shannon RP, Kohin S, Manders WT, Kelly P, Vatner SF (1990) Exercise-induced subendocardial dysfunction in dogs with left ventricular hypertrophy. Circ Res 66:329–343

Hoberg E, Kubler W (1991) Prevention of restenosis after PTCA: the role of calcium antagonists. 2nd International Symposium on Calcium Antagonists in Cardiovascular Care, Basel, Switzerland, 1991 (abstract 21)

Hof RP (1987) Comparison of cardiodepressant and vasodilator effects of PN200-110 (isradipine), nifedipine and diltiazem in anesthetized rabbits. Am J Cardiol 59:37B–42B

Hof RP, Hof A, Scholtysik G, Menninger K (1984) Effects of the new calcium antagonist PN200-110 on the myocardium and the regional peripheral circulation in anesthetized cats and dogs. J Cardiovasc Pharmacol 6:407–416

Hof RP (1987) Comparison of cardiodepressant and vasodilator effects of PN200-110 (isradipine), nifedipine and diltiazem in anesthetized rabbits. Am J Cardiol 59:37B–42B

Hoffmeister HM, Mauser M, Schaper W (1985) Effect of adenosine and AICaribinose on ATP content and regional contractile function in reperfused canine myocardium. Basic Res Cardiol 80:445–458

Holmberg SRM, Williams AJ (1989) Single channel recordings from human cardiac sarcoplasmic reticulum. Circ Res 65:1445–1449

Horn HR, Teichholz LE, Cohn PF, Herman MU, Gorlin R (1974) Augmentation of left ventricular contraction pattern in coronary artery disease by inotropic catecholamines. The epinephrine ventriculogram. Circulation 49:1063–1071

Howlett SE, Gordon T (1987) Calcium channels in normal and dystrophic hamster cardiac muscle: [³H]nitrendipine binding studies. Biochem Pharmacol 36:2653–2659

Huxley H (1990) Sliding filaments and molecular motile systems. J Biol Chem 265:8347–8350

Hymel L, Inui M, Fleischer S, Schmaler H (1988a) Purified ryanodine receptor of skeletal muscle sarcoplasmic reticulum forms Ca^{2+}-activated oligomeric channels in planar bilayers. Proc Natl Acad Sci USA 85:441–445

Hymel L, Striessnig J, Glossmann H, Schindler H (1988b) Purified skeletal muscle 1,4-dihydropyridine receptor forms phosphorylation-dependent oligomeric calcium channels in planar lipids. Proc Nat Acad Sci USA 85:4290–4294

Iaizzo PA, Klein W, Lehmann-Horn F (1988) Fura-2 detected myoplasmic calcium and its correlation with contracture force in skeletal muscle from normal and malignant hyperthermia-susceptible pigs. Pflugers Arch 411:648–653

Imagawa T, Smith JS, Coronado R, Campbell KP (1987) Purified ryanodine receptor from skeletal muscle sarcoplasmic reticulum is the Ca^{2+}-permeable pore of the calcium release channel. J Biol Chem 262:16636–16643

Insel PA (1989) Structure and function of the alpha-adrenergic receptors. Am J Med 87 (Suppl 2A):12S–18S

Inui M, Saito A, Fleischer S (1987) Purification of the ryanodine receptor and identity with feet structures of junctional terminal cisternae of sarcoplasmic reticulum from fast skeletal muscle. J Biol Chem 262:1740–1747

Inui M, Wang S, Saito A, Fleischer S (1988) Characterization of junctional and longitudinal sarcoplasmic reticulum from heart muscle. J Biol Chem 263:10843–10850

Ishi K, Kano T, Ando J, Yoshida H (1986) Binding of [³H]nitrendipine to cardiac and cerebral membranes from normotensive and renal deoxycorticosterone/NaCl and spontaneously hypertensive rats. Eur J Pharmacol 123:271–278

Ito BR, Tate H, Kobayashi M, Schaper W (1987) Reversibly injured, post ischaemic canine myocardium retains normal contractile reserve. Circ Res 61:834–846

Izumo S, Nadal-Ginard B, Mahdavi V (1988) Prooncogene induction and reprogramming of cardiac gene expression produced by pressure overload. Proc Natl Acad Sci USA 85:339–343

Jackson CV, Mickelson JK, Pope TK, Rao PS, Lucchesi BR (1986) O_2 free radical-mediated myocardial and vascular dysfunction. Am J Physiol 251:H1225–H1231

Janero DR, Burghardt B (1989) Antiperoxidant effects of dihydropyridine calcium antagonists. Biochem Pharmacol 38:4344–4348

Jay M, Kojima S, Gillespie MN (1986) Nicotine potentiates superoxide anion generation by human neutrophils. Toxicol Appl Pharmacol 86:484–487

Jay SD, Ellis SB, McCue AF, Williams ME, Vedvick T, Harpold MM, Campbell KP (1989) Primary structure of the subunit of the DHP-sensitive calcium channels from skeletal muscle. Science 248:490–492

Jayakody RF, Senaratne MPJ, Thomson ABR, Kappagoda CT (1985) Cholesterol feeding impairs endothelium-dependent relaxation of rabbit aorta. Can J Physiol Pharmacol 63:1206–1209

Jennings RB, Reimer KA (1981) Lethal myocardial ischemic injury. Am J Pathol 102:241–255

Jennings RB, Schaper J, Hill ML, Steenbergen C Jr, Reimer KA (1985) Effect of reperfusion late in the phase of reversible ischemic injury. Circ Res 56:262–278

Jennings RB, Murry CE, Steenbergen C Jr, Reimer KA (1990) Development of cell injury in sustained acute ischaemia. Circulation 82 (Suppl II):II-2–II-12

Jeremy RW, Stahl L, Gillinov M, Litt M, Aversano TR, Becker LC (1989) Preservation of coronary flow reserve in stunned myocardium. Am J Physiol 256:H1303–H1310

Jeroudi MO, Triana FJ, Patel BS, Bolli R (1990) Effect of superoxide dismutase and catalase, given separately, on myocardial 'stunning'. Am J Physiol 259:H889–H901

Jones E, Joy M (1988) Acute myocardial infarction after a wasp sting. Br Heart J 59:506–508

Kageyama M, Nishimura K, Takada T, Miyawaki N, Yamauchi H (1991) SD-3211, a novel benzothiazine calcium antagonist alone and in combination with a beta-adrenoceptor antagonist, produces antihypertensive effects without affecting heart rate and atrioventricular conduction in conscious renal hypertensive dogs. J Cardiovasc Pharmacol 17:102–107

Kanazawa T, Morita T, Harada K, Iwamoto T, Ohtaka H, Sukamoto T, Ito K, Nurimoto S (1990) Selective effect of KB 2796, a new calcium entry blocker, on cerebral circulation: a comparative study of the effects of calcium entry blockers on cerebral and peripheral arterial blood flows. J Cardiovasc Pharmacol 16:430–437

Kaneko M, Beamish RE, Dhalla NS (1989) Depression of heart sarcolemmal Ca^{2+} pump activity by oxygen free radicals. Am J Physiol 256:H368–H374

Kannel WB (1989) Detection and management of patients with silent myocardial ischemia. Am Heart J 117:221–226

Kanno K, Hirata Y, Numano F, Emori T, Ohta K, Shichiri M, Murumo F (1990) Endothelin and vasculitis. J Am Med Ass 264:2868

Kantelip JP, Talmant JM, Marullaz PD (1988) Effects of diproteverine, a new calcium antagonist on sinoatrial node and atrioventricular conductions in conscious unsedated dogs. J Cardiovasc Pharmacol 12:432–437

Kassis E, Amtorp O (1987) Cardiovascular and neurohumoral postural responses and baroreceptor abnormalities during a course of adjunctive vasodilator therapy with felodipine for congestive heart failure. Circulation 75:1204–1213

Kassis E, Amtorp O (1990a) Short and long-term controlled studies of felodipine in patients with congestive heart failure. J Cardiovasc Pharmacol 15 (Suppl 4):S26

Kassis E, Amtorp O (1990b) Long term clinical, hemodynamic angiographic and neurohumoral responses to vasodilation with felodipine in patients with chronic congestive heart failure. J Cardiovasc Pharmacol 15:347–352

Katz AM (1990a) Cardiomyopathy of overload. A major determinant of prognosis in congestive heart failure. New Eng J Med 322:100–110

Katz AM (1990b) Future perspectives in basic science understanding of congestive heart failure. Am J Cardiol 65:468–471

Kawachi Y, Tomoike H, Kikuchi Y, Araki H, Ishii Y, Tanaka Y, Nakamaura M (1984) Selective hypercontraction caused by ergonovine in the canine coronary artery under conditions of induced atherosclerosis. Circulation 69:441–450

Kawamoto RM, Brunschwig JP, Kim KC, Caswell AH (1986) Isolation, characterization, and localization of the spanning protein from skeletal muscle triads. J Cell Biol 103:1405–1414

Kazazoglou T, Schmid A, Renaud JF, Lazdunski M (1983) Ontogenic appearance of Ca^{2+} channels characterized as binding sites for nitrendipine during development of nervous, skeletal and cardiac muscle systems in the rat. FEBS Lett 164:75–79

Kazda S, Garthoff B, Knorr A (1985) Interference of the calcium antagonist nisoldipine with the abnormal response of vessels from hypertensive rats to α–adrenergic stimulation. J Cardiovasc Pharmacol 7:S61–S65

Kazda S, Garthoff B, Meyer H, Schlossmann K, Stoepel K, Towart R, Vater W, Wehinger E (1980) Pharmacology of a new calcium antagonistic compound, isobutyl methyl 1, 4 – dihydro – 2, 6 – dimethyl – 4 – (2 – nitrophenyl) – 3, 5 – pyridinedicarboxylate (Nisoldipine, BayK5552). Arzneimittel-Forschung Drug Res 30:2144–2162

Kazda S, Towart R (1982) Nimodipine, a new calcium antagonist drug with a preferential cerebrovascular action. Acta Neurochir 63:259–265

Kenny BA, Kilpatrick AT, Spedding M (1986) Changes in [³H]nitrendipine binding in gerbil cortex following ischaemia. Br J Pharmacol 89:858P

Kentish JC (1986) The effects of inorganic phosphate and creatine phosphate in skinned muscles from rat ventricle. J Physiol 370:585–604

Kentish JC, Barsotti RJ, Lea TJ, Mulligan IP, Patel JR, Ferenczi MA (1990) Calcium release from cardiac sarcoplasmic reticulum induced by photorelease of calcium or Ins(1,4,5)P₃. Am J Physiol 258:H610–H615

Keung EC (1989) Calcium current is increased in isolated adult myocytes from hypertrophied rat myocardium. Circ Res 64:753–763

Kinnard DR, Harris M, Hossack KF (1988) Endurance testing for evaluation of antianginal therapy with amlodipine, a calcium channel blocking agent. J Am Coll Cardiol 12:791–796

Kinnard DR, Harris M, Hossack KF (1989) Amlodipine in angina pectoris: Effect on maximal and submaximal exercise performance. Am Heart J 118 (Suppl 5):1136

Kiowski W, Luscher TF, Linder L, Buhler FR (1991) Endothelin-1-induced vasoconstriction in humans. Reversal by calcium channel blockade but not by nitrovasodilators or endothelium-derived relaxing factor. Circulation 83:469–475

Kita T, Nagano Y, Yokode M, Ishii K, Kume N, Ooshima A, Yoshida H, Kawai C (1987) Probucol prevents the progression of atherosclerosis in Watanabe heritable hyperlipidemic rabbit, an animal model for familial hypocholesterolemia. Proc Natl Acad Sci USA 84:5928–5931

Kitakaze M, Marban E (1989) Cellular mechanism of the modulation of contractile function by coronary perfusion pressure in ferret hearts. J Physiol (Lond) 414:455–472

Kitakaze M, Weisman HF, Marban E (1987) Contractile dysfunction and ATP depletion after transient calcium overload in perfused ferret hearts. Circulation 77:685–695

Klausner SC, Ratshin RA, Tybert JV, Lappin HA, Chatterjee K, Parmley WW (1976) The similarity of changes in segmental contraction patterns induced by post-extrasystolic potentiation and nitroglycerin. Circulation 54:615–623

Klein W, Brandt D, Fluch N, Sterz F (1987) Nisoldipine versus mononitrate in stable angina. In: Hugenholtz PG, Meyer J (eds) Nisoldipine. Springer-Verlag, Berlin, pp228–232

Kloner RA, Ellis SG, Lange R, Braunwald E (1983) Studies of experimental coronary artery reperfusion: effects on infarct size, myocardial function, biochemistry, ultrastructure and microvascular damage. Circulation 68 (Suppl):I-8–I-15

Kloner RA, Przyklenk K (1990) Progress in cardioprotection: The role of calcium antagonists. Am J Cardiol 66:2H–9H

Kloner RA, Pryzklenk K, Patel B (1989) Altered myocardial states: the stunned and hibernating myocardium. Am J Med 86 (Suppl A):A14–A22

Knudson CM, Chaudhari N, Sharp AH, Powell JA, Beam KG, Campbell KP (1989) Specific absence of the α_1 subunit of the dihydropyridine receptor in mice with muscular dysgenesis. J Biol Chem 264:1345–1348

Knudson CM, Imagawa T, Kahl SD, Gauer MG, Leung AT, Sharp AH, Jay SD, Campbell KP (1988) Evidence for physical association between junctional sarcoplasmic reticulum ryanodine receptor and junctional transverse tubular dihydropyridine receptor. Biophys J 53:605a (abstract)

Kober G, Schneider W, Kaltenbach M (1989) Can the progression of coronary sclerosis be influenced by calcium antagonists? J Cardiovasc Pharmacol 13 (Suppl 4):S2–6

Koch WJ, Ellinor PT, Schwartz A (1990) cDNA cloning of a dihydropyridine-sensitive calcium channel from rat aorta. J Biol Chem 265:17786–17791

Koch WJ, Hui A, Shull G, Ellinor P, Schwartz A (1989) Characterization of cDNA clones encoding two putative isoforms of the α_1 subunit of the dihydropyridine-sensitive calcium channel isolated from rat brain and rat aorta. FEBS Lett 250:386–388

Koener JE, Anderson BA, Dage RC (1991) Protection against postischemic myocardial dysfunction in anesthetized rabbits with scavengers of oxygen-derived free radicals: superoxide dismutase plus catalase, N-2-mercaptopropionyl glycine and captopril. J Cardiovasc Pharmacol 17:185–191

Kojima M, Ishima T, Taniguchi N, Kimura K, Sada H, Sperelakis N (1990) Developmental changes in β-adrenoceptors, muscarinic cholinoceptors and Ca^{2+} channels in rat ventricular muscles. Br J Pharmacol 99:334–339

Koller PT, Bergmann SR (1989) Reduction of lipid peroxidation in reperfused isolated rabbit hearts by diltiazem. Circ Res 65:838–846

Koolen JJ, Visser CA, David GK, Hoedemaker G, Van Wezel H, Dunning AJ (1990) Effects of nisoldipine and nifedipine on ischemic tolerance during coronary angioplasty. In: Lichtlen PR, Krayenbuhl HP (eds) New Aspects of Nisoldipine Therapy, Schattauer Press, Stuttgart, pp139–148

Koretsune Y, Marban E (1990a) Relative roles of Ca^{2+}-dependent and Ca^{2+}-independent mechanisms in hypoxic contractile dysfunction. Circulation 82:528–535

Koretsune Y, Marban E (1990b) Mechanisms of ischemic contracture in ferret hearts: relative roles of $[Ca^{2+}]_i$ elevation and ATP depletion. Am J Physiol 258:H9–H16

Korthuis RJ, Granger DN, Townsley MI, Taylor AE (1985) The role of oxygen-derived free radicals in ischemia-induced increases in canine skeletal muscle vascular permeability. Circ Res 57:599–609

Kramer JH, Mak IT, Weglicki WB (1984) Differential sensitivity of canine cardiac sarcolemmal and microsomal enzymes to inhibition by free radical-induced lipid peroxidation. Circ Res 55:120–124

Kramer K, Rademaker B, Rozendal WHM, Timmerman H, Bast A (1986) Influence of lipid peroxidation on β-adrenoceptors. FEBS Lett 198:80–84

Krause SM (1990) Effect of global myocardial stunning on Ca^{2+}-sensitive myofibrillar ATPase activity and creatine kinase kinetics. Am J Physiol 259:H813–H819

Krause SM, Hess ML (1985) Characterization of cardiac sarcoplasmic reticulum dysfunction during short-term normothermic global ischaemia. Circ Res 55:176–184

Krause SM, Jacobus WE, Becker LC (1986) Alterations in sarcoplasmic reticulum Ca^{2+} transport in the post-ischemic 'stunned' myocardium. Circulation 74 (Suppl II):II-67 (abstract)

Krause SM, Jacobus WE, Becker LC (1989) Alterations in sarcoplasmic reticulum calcium transport in the postischemic 'stunned' myocardium. Circ Res 65:526–530

Kravtsov GM, Dulin NO, Postnov IUV (1988) Activity of protein kinase C in erythrocytes in primary hypertension. Hypertension 11:853–857

Krukenkamp IB, Silverman NA, Sorlie D, Pridjian A, Feinberg H, Levitsky S (1986) Characterization of post-ischemic myocardial oxygen utilization. Circulation 74 (Suppl III):III-125–III-129

Ku DD, Caulfield JB, Kirklin JK (1991) Endothelium-dependent responses in long-term human coronary artery bypass grafts. Circulation 83:402–411

Kubo SH (1990) Neurohormonal activation and the response to converting enzyme inhibitors in congestive heart failure. Circulation 81 (Suppl III):III-107–III-114

Kusuoka H, Koretsune Y, Chacko VP, Weisfeldt ML, Marban E (1990) Excitation-contraction coupling in postischemic myocardium. Circ Res 66:1268–1276

Kusuoka H, Porterfield JK, Weisman HF, Weisfeldt ML, Marban E (1987) Pathophysiology and pathogenesis of stunned myocardium. J Clin Invest 79:950–961

Kusuoka H, Weisfeldt ML, Zweier JL, Jacobus WE, Marban E (1986) Mechanism of early contractile failure during hypoxia in intact ferret heart: evidence for modulation of maximal Ca^{2+}-activated force by inorganic phosphate. Circ Res 59:270–282

Kutryk MJB, Maddaford TG, Ramijiawan B, Pierce GN (1991) Oxidation and membrane cholesterol alters active and passive transsarcolemmal calcium movement. Circ Res 68:18–26

Lablanche J-M, Fourrier J-L, Gommeaux A, Griener L, Bertrand ME (1990) Prevention of coronary artery spasm by nisoldipine. In: Lichtlen PR, Krazenbuhl HP (eds) New Aspects on Nisoldipine. Schattauer Press, Stuttgart, Germany, pp61–68

Lahiri A, Rodriques EA, Carboni GP, Raftery EB (1990) Effects of long-term treatment with calcium antagonists on left ventricular diastolic function in stable angina and heart failure. Circulation 81 (Suppl III):III-130–III-138

Lai FA, Erikson HP, Rousseau E, Meissner G (1988) Purification and reconstruction of the calcium release channel from skeletal muscle. Nature 331:315–319

Lai FA, Meissner G (1989) The muscle ryanodine receptor and its intrinsic Ca^{2+} channel activity. J Bioenerg Biomembr 21:227–245

Lam J, Chaitman BR, Crean P, Blum R, Waters DD (1985) A dose-ranging placebo-controlled, double-blind trial of nisoldipine in effort angina: duration and extent of antianginal effects. J Am Coll Cardiol 6:447–452

Lamping KA, Gross GJ (1985) Improved recovery of myocardial segment function following a short coronary occlusion in dogs by nicorandil, a potential new antianginal agent, and nifedipine. J Cardiovasc Pharmacol 7:158–166

Lamping KG, Dole WP (1987) Acute hypertension selectively potentiates constrictor responses of large coronary arteries to serotonin by altering endothelin function in vivo. Circ Res 61:904–913

Lange R, Ingwall J, Halle SL, Alker KJ, Kloner RA (1984) Preservation of high energy phosphates by verapamil in reperfused myocardium. Circulation 70:734–741

Langer GA, Nudd LM (1983) Effects of cations, phospholipases, and neuraminidase on calcium binding to 'gas-dissected' membranes from cultured cardiac cells. Circ Res 53:482–490

Laster SB, Becker LC, Ambrosio G, Jacobus WE (1989) Reduced aerobic metabolic efficiency in globally 'stunned' myocardium. J Mol Cell Cardiol 21:419–426

Lazarewicz JW, Pluta R, Puka M, Salinska E (1990) Diverse mechanisms of neuronal protection by nimodipine in experimental rabbit brain ischemia. Stroke 21 (Suppl IV):IV-108–IV-110

Lee HC, Mohabir R, Smith N, Franz MR, Clusin WT (1988) Effect of ischemia on calcium-dependent fluorescence transients in rabbit hearts containing indo I. Circulation 78:1047–1059

Lette J, Gagnon A, Water D (1989) Acute pulmonary edema caused by prolonged myocardial stunning after dipyridamole-thallium imaging. Am J Med 87:461–463

Leung AT, Imagawa T, Campbell KP (1987) Structural characterization of the 1,4-dihydropyridine receptor of the voltage-dependent Ca^{2+} channel from rabbit skeletal muscle. J Biol Chem 262:7943–7946

Levine JH, Moore EN, Weisman HF, Kadish AH, Becker LC, Spear JF (1987) Depression of action potential characteristics and a decreased space constant are present in postischaemic, reperfused myocardium. J Clin Invest 79:107–116

Lewis MS, Whatley RE, Cain P, McIntyre TM, Prescott SM, Zimmerman GH (1988) Hydrogen peroxide stimulates the synthesis of platelet-activating factor by endothelium and induces endothelial-cell dependent neutrophil adhesion. J Clin Invest 82:2045–2055

Lichtlen PR, Hugenholtz PG, Rafflenbeul W, Hecker H, Jost S, Deckers JW (1990) Retardation of angiographic progression of coronary artery disease by nifedipine. The Lancet 335:1109–1113

Liedholm H, Melander A (1989) A placebo-controlled dose-response study of felodipine extended release in hypertensive patients. J Cardiovasc Pharmacol 14:109–113

Liedtke AJ, De Maison L, Eggleston AM, Cohen LM, Nellis SH (1988) Changes in substrate metabolism and effects of excess fatty acids in reperfused myocardium. Circ Res 62:535–542

Limas CJ, Olivari MT, Goldenberg IF, Levine TB, Benditt DG, Simon A (1987) Calcium uptake by cardiac sarcoplasmic reticulum in human dilated cardiomyopathy. Cardiovasc Res 21:601–605

Limbruno U, Zucchi R, Ronca-Teston S, Galbani P, Ronca G, Mariani M (1989) Sarcoplasmic reticulum function in the 'stunned' myocardium. J Mol Cell Cardiol 21:1063–1072

Litvack F, Grundfest WS, Papaioannoo T, Mohr FW, Jakubowski AT, Forrester JS (1988) Role of laser and thermal ablation devices in the treatment of vascular diseases. Am J Cardiol 61:81G–86G

Liu J, Chen J, Casley DJ, Nayler WG (1990) Ischemia and reperfusion increase ^{125}I-labelled endothelin-1 binding in rat cardiac membranes. Am J Physiol 258:H829–H835

Ljung B, Nordlander M (1987) Pharmacological properties of felodipine. Drugs 34 (Suppl 3):7–15

Ljunggren B, Saveland H, Brandt L, Uski T (1984) Aneurysmal subarachnoid haemorrhage. Surg Neurol 22:435–438

Loaldi A, Polese A, Montorsi P, De Cesare N, Fabbiocchi F, Ravagnani P, Guazzi M (1989) Comparison of nifedipine, propranolol and isosorbide dinitrate on angiographic progression and regression of coronary arterial narrowing in angina pectoris. Am J Cardiol 64:433–439

Lombet A, Lazdunski M (1984) Characterization, solubilization, affinity labelling and purification of the cardiac Na^+ channel using Tityus toxin gamma. Eur J Biochem 141:651–660

Lompré A-M, Levitsky D, De La Bastie D, Mercadier J-J, Rappaport L, Schwartz K (1988) Function of the sarcoplasmic reticulum and expression of its Ca^{2+} ATPase gene in pressure overloaded rat myocardium. Circulation 78 (Suppl II):II-535 (abstract)

Lopez JAG, Armstrong ML, Piegors DJ, Heistad DD (1990) Vascular responses to endothelin-1 in atherosclerotic primates. Arteriosclerosis 10:1113–1118

Lorell BH, Grossman W (1987) Cardiac hypertrophy; consequences of diastole. J Am Coll Cardiol 9:1189–1193

Lucchesi BR (1990) Myocardial ischaemia, reperfusion and free radical injury. Am J Cardiol 65:14I–23I

Lucchi L, Govoni S, Battaini F, Pasinetti G, Trabucchi M (1985) Ethanol administration in vivo alters calcium ion control in rat striatum. Brain Res 332:376–379

Lullmann H, Mohr K (1987) High and concentration proportional accumulation of ^{3}H-nitrendipine by intact cardiac tissue. Br J Pharmacol 90:567–573

Lund-Johansen P (1983) Decrease in cardiac output vs reduction in vascular resistance. Hypertens 5 (Suppl III):III-49–III-57

Luria MH, Erel J, Sapoznikov D, Gotsman MS (1991) Cardiovascular risk factor clustering and ratio of total cholesterol to high-density lipoprotein cholesterol in angiographically documented coronary artery disease. Am J Cardiol 67:31–36

Luscher TF (1991) Endothelin: key to coronary vasospasm. Circulation 83:701–703

Luscher TF, Yang Z, Tschudi M, Von Segesser L, Stulz P, Boulanger C, Siebenmann R, Turina M, Bühler FR (1990) Interaction between endothelin-1 and endothelium-derived relaxing factor in human arteries and veins. Circ Res 66:1088–1094

Lytton J, Zarain-Herzberg A, Periasamy M, MacLennan DH (1989) Molecular cloning of the mammalian smooth muscle sarco (endo) plasmic reticulum Ca^{2+}-ATPase. J Biol Chem 264:7059–7065

MacGregor GA, Rotellar C, Markandu ND, Smith SJ, Saguella GA (1982) Contrasting effects of nifedipine, captopril and propranolol in normotensive and hypertensive subjects. J Cardiovasc Pharmacol 4 (Suppl 3):S358–S362

MacLennan DH, Brandl CJ, Korczak B, Green NM (1985) Amino acid sequence of a Ca^{2+}- and Mg^{2+}-dependent ATPase from rabbit muscle sarcoplasmic reticulum, deduced from its complementary DNA sequence. Nature 316:696–700

MacLennan DH, Holland PC (1975) Calcium transport in sarcoplasmic reticulum. Annu Rev Biophys Bioengin 4:377–403

Magnoni MS, Govoni S, Battaini F, Trabucchi M (1988) L-Type calcium channels are modified in rat hippocampus by short-term experimental ischemia. J Cereb Blood Flow Metab 8:96–99

Maisel AS, Motulsky HJ, Insel PA (1986) Propranolol treatment externalizes β-adrenergic receptors in guinea pig myocardium and prevents further externalization by ischemia. Circ Res 60:108–112

Mak IT, Weglicki WB (1990) Comparative antioxidant activities of propranolol, nifedipine, verapamil, and diltiazem against sarcolemmal membrane lipid peroxidation. Circ Res 66:1449–1452

Malis CD, Bonventre JV (1986) Mechanism of calcium potentiation of oxygen free radical injury to renal mitochondria. J Biol Chem 261:14201–14208

Marangos PJ, Sperelakis N, Patel J (1984) Ontogeny of calcium antagonist binding sites in chick brain and heart. J Neurochem 42:1338–1342

Marban E (1991) Myocardial stunning and hibernation. The physiology behind the colloquialisms. Circulation 83:681–688

Marban E, Kitakaze M, Koretsune Y, Yue OT, Chacko VP, Pike MM (1990) Quantification of [Ca^{2+}]$_i$ in perfused hearts: Critical evaluation of the 5F-BAPTA and nuclear magnetic resonance method as applied to the study of ischaemia and reperfusion Circ Res 66:1255–1267

Marban E, Kitakaze M, Kusuoka H, Porterfield JK, Yue DT, Chacko VP (1987) Intracellular free calcium concentration measured with ^{19}FNMR spectroscopy in intact ferret hearts. Proc Natl Acad Sci USA 84:6005–6009

Margulies KB, Hildebrand FL, Lerman A, Perrella MA, Burnett JC (1990) Increased endothelin in experimental heart failure. Circulation 82:2226–2230

Marin-Neto JA, Pintya AO, Gallo L, Maciel BC (1991) Abnormal baroreflex control of heart rate in decompensated congestive heart failure and reversal after compensation. Am J Cardiol 67:604–610

Marra S, Picciotto G, Varetto T, Blengino S, Montagna L, Alberti A, Defilippi PG, Casaccia M (1990) Radionuclide left ventricular ejection fraction and antianginal effects of oral nisoldipine in patients with stable effort angina. In: Lichtlen PR, Krayenbuhl HP (eds) New Aspects on Nisoldipine, Schattauer, Stuttgart, pp119–130

Marsden PA, Danthuluri NR, Brenner BM, Ballermann BJ, Brock TA (1989) Endothelin action on vascular smooth muscle involves inositol triphosphate and calcium metabolism. Biochem Biophys Res Commun 158:86–92

Marshall JC, Waxman HL, Sauerwein A, Gilchrist I, Kurnik PB (1990) Frequency of low-grade residual coronary stenosis after thrombolysis during acute myocardial infarction. Am J Cardiol 66:773–778

Masaki T, Yanagisawa M, Goto K, Kimura S (1990) Role of endothelin in mechanisms of local blood pressure control. J Hypertens 8 (Suppl 7):S107–S112

Masaoka H, Suzuki R, Hirata Y, Emori T, Marumo F, Hirakawa K (1989) Raised plasma endothelin in subarachnoid haemorrhage. Lancet ii:1402

Maseri A, Newman C, Davies G (1989) Coronary vasomotor tone: a heterogeneous entity. Eur Heart J 10 (Suppl F):2–5

Massie B, Botvinick EH, Brundage BH, Greenberg B, Shames D, Gelberg H (1978) Relationship of regional myocardial perfusion to segmental wall motion. Physiological basis for understanding the presence and the reversibility of asynergy. Circulation 58:1154–1163

Mathias P, Kerin NZ, Blevins RD, Cascade P, Rubenfire M (1987) Coronary vasospasm as a cause of stunned myocardium. Am Heart J 113:383–385

Matucci R, Bennardini F, Sciammarella ML, Baccaro C, Stendardi I, Franconi F, Giotti A (1987) [^{3}H]Nitrendipine binding in membranes obtained from hypoxic and reoxygenated heart. Biochem Pharmacol 36:1059–1062

Mayoux E, Callens F, Swynghedauw B, Charlemagne D (1988) Adaptational process of the cardiac Ca^{2+} channels to pressure overload: biochemical and physiological properties of the dihydropyridine receptors in normal and hypertrophied rat hearts. J Cardiol Pharmacol 12:390–396

McAnulty JH, Hattenhauer MT, Rosch J, Kloster FE, Rahimtoola SH (1975) Improvement in left ventricular wall motion following nitroglycerin. Circulation 51:140–145

McCord JM (1983) The biochemistry and pathophysiology of superoxide. Physiologist 26:165–169

McCord JM (1985) Oxygen-derived free radicals in postischemic tissue injury. N Eng J Med 312:159–163

McKay RG, Pfeffer MA, Pasternak RC, Markis JE, Come PC, Nakao S, Alderman JD, Ferguson JJ, Safian RD, Grossman W (1986) Left venticular remodelling after myocardial infarction; a corollary to infarct expansion. Circulation 74:693–702

McKenna E, Koch WJ, Slish DF, Schwartz A (1990) Toward an understanding of the dihydropyridine-sensitive calcium channel. Biochem Pharmacol 39:1145–1150

McPherson PS, Campbell KP (1990) Solubilization and biochemical characterization of the high affinity [^{3}H]ryanodine receptor from rabbit brain membranes. J Biol Chem 265:18454–18460

Meerson FZ, Kagan VE, Kozlov YP, Belkina LM, Arkhipenko YV (1982) The role of lipid peroxidation in the pathogenesis of ischaemic damage and the antioxidant protection of the heart. Basic Res Cardiol 77:465–485

Meissner G (1975) Isolation and characterization of two types of sarcoplasmic reticulum vesicles. Biochem Biophys Acta 389:51–68

Meissner G (1986) Ryanodine activation and inhibition of the Ca^{2+} release channel of sarcoplasmic reticulum. J Biol Chem 261:6300–6306

Mentzer RM, Van Wylen DGV, Sodhi J, Weiss RJ, Lasley RD, Willis J, Bunger R, Habil DR, Fnint LM (1989) Effect of pyruvate on regional ventricular function and stunned myocardium. Ann Surg 209:629–634

Mercadier JJ, De La Bastie D, Menasche P, Cao A, Bouvert P, Lorente P, Pinnica A, Slama R, Schwartz K (1987) Alpha myosin heavy chain isoform and atrial size in patients with various types of mitral valve dysfunction: a quantitative study. J Am Coll Cardiol 9:1024–1030

Merkel LA, Rivera LM, Bilder GE, Perrone MH (1990) Differential alteration of vascular reactivity in rabbit aorta with modest elevation of serum cholesterol. Circ Res 67:550–555

Meyer FB (1990) Intracellular brain pH and ischemic vasoconstriction in the White New Zealand rabbit. Stroke 21 (Suppl IV):IV-117–IV-119

Meyer FB, Anderson RE, Yaksh TL, Sundt TM Jr (1986) Effect of nimodipine on intracellular brain pH, cortical blood flow, and EEG in experimental focal cerebral ischemia. J Neurosurg 64:617–626

Midtbø KA (1990) Effects of long-term verapamil therapy on serum lipids and other metabolic parameters. Am J Cardiol 66:13I–15I

Mikami A, Imoto K, Tanabe T, Niidome T, Mori Y, Takeshima H, Narumiya S, Numa S (1989) Primary structure and functional expression of the cardiac dihydropyridine-sensitive calcium channel. Nature 340:230–233

Milei J, Boveris A, Llesuy S, Molina HA, Storino R, Ortega D, Milei SE (1986) Amelioration of adriamycin-induced cardiotoxicity in rabbits by prenylamine and vitamins A and E. Am Heart J 111:95–102

Miller R (1987) Multiple calcium channels and neuronal function. Science 235:46–52

Miyauchi T, Yanagisawa M, Tomizawa T, Sugishita Y, Suzuki N, Fujino M, Ajisaka R, Goto K, Masaki T (1989) Increased plasma concentrations of endothelin-1 and big endothelin-1 in acute myocardial infarction. Lancet i:53

Moe GW, Karlinsky SJ, Frankel D, Armstrong PW (1990) Intravenous nisoldipine in severe congestive failure. In: Lichtlen PR, Krayenbuhl HP (eds) New Aspects on Nisoldipine, Schattauer Press, Stuttgart, Germany, pp95–106

Morgan HE, Baker KM (1991) Cardiac hypertrophy. Mechanical, neural and endocrine dependence. Circulation 83:12–25

Morgan KG, Suematsu E (1990) Effects of calcium on vascular smooth muscle tone. Am Heart J 3:291S–298S

Morikawa E, Ginsberg MD, Dietrich D, Duncan RC, Busto R (1991) Postischemic (S)-emopamil therapy ameliorates focal ischemic brain injury in rats. Stroke 22:355–360

Morton M, McAnulty J, Rahimtoola SH (1978) Ventricular function curve from a single diagnostic left ventriculogram: technique, results and value. Am J Cardiol 41:710–717

Mossakowski MJ, Gadamski R (1990) Nimodipine prevents delayed neuronal death of sector CA, pyramidal cells in short-term forebrain ischemia in mongolian gerbils. Stroke 21 (Suppl IV):IV-120–IV-122

Muiesan ML, Agabiti-Rosei E, Romanelli G, Castellano M, Beschi M, Muiesan G (1988) One year treatment with captopril has beneficial effects on left ventricular anatomy and function in hypertensive patients with left ventricular hypertrophy. Am J Med 84 (Suppl 3A):129–132

Muller FB, Bolli P, Erne P, Kiowski W, Buhler FR (1984) Use of calcium channel blockers as monotherapy of hypertension. Am J Med 77 (Suppl IIB):1–5

Murakawa K, Kohno M, Yasunari K, Yokokawa K, Horio T, Takeda T (1988) Possible involvement of protein kinase C in the maintenance of hypertension in spontaneously hypertensive rats. J Hypertens 6 (Suppl): S157–S159

Murata S, Kikkawa K, Yabana H, Nagao T (1988) Cardiovascular effects of a new 1,5-benzothiazepine calcium antagonist in anesthetized dogs. Arzneim Forsch/Drug Res 38:521–527

Myers ML, Bolli R, Lekich RF, Hartley CJ, Roberts R (1985) Enhancement of recovery of myocardial function by oxygen free radical scavengers after reversible regional ischemia. Circulation 77:915–921

Myers ML, Bolli R, Lekich RF, Hartley CJ, Roberts R (1986) N-2-mercaptopropionyl glycine improves recovery of myocardial function following reversible regional ischemia. J Am Coll Cardiol 8:1161–1168

Nabauer M, Callewaert G, Cleemann L, Morad M (1989) Regulation of calcium release is gated by calcium current, not gating charge, in cardiac myocytes. Science 244:800–803

Nabauer M, Morad M (1990) Ca^{2+}-induced Ca^{2+} release as examined by photolysis of caged Ca^{2+} in single ventricular myocytes. Am J Physiol 258:C189–C193

Nabel EG, Selwyn AP, Ganz P (1990) Large coronary arteries in humans are responsive to changing blood flows: an endothelium-dependent mechanism that fails in patients with atherosclerosis. J Am Coll Cardiol 16:349–356

Nagao T, Matlib, MA, Franklin D, Millard RW, Schwartz A (1980) Effects of diltiazem, a calcium antagonist, on regional myocardial function and mitochondria after brief coronary occlusion. J Mol Cell Cardiol 12:29–43

Nagasaki K, Fleischer S (1988) Ryanodine sensitivity of the calcium release channel of sarcoplasmic reticulum. Cell Calcium 9:1–7

Nakao I, Ito H, Ooyama T, Chang WC, Murota S (1983) Calcium dependency of aortic smooth muscle cell migration induced by 12-L-hydroxy-5,8,10,14-eicosatetraenoic acid. Atherosclerosis 46:309–319

Nakayama N, Kirley TL, Vaghy PL, McKenna E, Schwartz A (1987) Purification of a putative Ca^{2+} channel protein from rabbit skeletal muscle. J Biol Chem 262:6572–6576

Nathan CV (1987) Secretory products of macrophages. J Clin Invest 79:319–326

Naudascher M, Jaillon P, Lecocq B, Lecocq V, Ferry A, Hilaire J, Maria JF (1989) Effects of falipamil (AQ-A39) on heart rate and blood pressure in resting and exercising healthy volunteers. J Cardiovasc Pharmacol 14:1–5

Nayler WG (1988) Calcium Antagonists. Academic Press, London, United Kingdom, pp1–298

Nayler WG (1990) The Endothelins. Springer-Verlag, Berlin Heidelberg, Germany, pp1–183

Nayler WG (1991) The antiatherogenic effects of amlodipine: promise of preclinical data. Postgrad Med J. In Press

Nayler WG, Dillon JS, Elz J, McKelvie M (1985) An effect of ischemia on myocardial dihydropyridine binding sites. Eur J Pharmacol 115:81–89

Nayler WG, Elz JS, Buckley DJ (1988) The stunned myocardium: effect of electrical and mechanical arrest and osmolarity. Am J Physiol 255:H60–H69

Nayler WG, Gu XH (1991) (-)[^{3}H]Amlodipine binding to rat cardiac membranes. J Cardiovasc Pharmacol 17:587–592

Nayler WG, Buckley DJ, Leong J (1990a) Calcium antagonists and the 'stunned' myocardium. Cardioscience 1:61–64

Nayler WG, Liu J, Panagiotopoulos S (1990b) Nifedipine and experimental cardioprotection. Cardiovasc Drugs Ther 4 (Suppl 5):879–886

Nayler WG, Panagiotopoulos S (1986) Calcium antagonism. In: Kelly DT (ed) Proceedings of II Asian Pacific Adalat Symposium, Adis Press, New Zealand, pp3–11

Neil-Dwyer G, Mee E, Dorrance D, Lowe D (1987) Early intervention with nimodipine in subarachnoid haemorrhage. Eur Heart J 8:41–47

Nesto RW (1990) Rationale for treatment of silent myocardial ischaemia. Focus on nifedipine. Cardiovasc Drugs and Therapy 4 (Suppl5):929–934

Nesto RW, Cohn LH, Collins JJ Jr, Wynne J, Holman L, Cohn PF (1982) Inotropic contractile reserve: a useful predictor of increased 5-year survival and improved postoperative left ventricular function in patients with coronary artery disease and reduced ejection fraction. Am J Cardiol 50:39–44

Neuser D, Rosen B (1990) Calcium antagonist and the proliferation of vascular smooth muscle cells. Satellite Symposium "Antiatherosclerotic Potentials of Calcium Antagonists" at 13th ISH meeting. Montreal, 1990, pp9–10

Nicoll DA, Logoni S, Philipson KD (1990) Molecular cloning and functional expression of the cardiac sarcolemmal Na^+-Ca^+ exchanger. Science 250:562–565

Nilsson I, Sjolund M, Palmberg L, Von Euler AM, Jonzon B, Thyborg I (1985) The calcium antagonist nifedipine inhibits arterial smooth muscle cell proliferation. Atherosclerosis 58:109–112

Nixon JV, Brown CN, Smitherman TC (1982) Identification of transient and persistent segmental wall motion abnormalities in patients with unstable angina by two-dimensional echocardiography. Circulation 65:1497–1503

Noda M, Ikeda T, Kayano T, Suzuki H, Takeshima H, Kurasaki M, Takahashi H, Numa S (1986) Existence of distinct sodium channel messenger RNA's in rat brain. Nature 320:118-192

Noda M, Shimizu S, Tanabe T, Takai T, Kayano T, Ikeda T, Takahashi H, Nakayama H, Kanaoka Y, Minamino N (1984) Primary structure of Electrophorus Electricus sodium channel deduced from cDNA sequence. Nature 312:121–127

Nohl H (1987) A novel superoxide radical generator in heart mitochondria. FEBS Lett 214:269–273

Nomoto A, Hirosumi J, Sekiguchi C, Mutoh S, Yamaguchi I, Aoki H (1987) Antiatherogenic activity of FR34235 (Nilvadipine), a new potent calcium antagonist. Atherosclerosis 64:255–261

O'Dowd BF, Lefkowitz RJ, Caron MG (1989) Structure of the adrenergic and related receptors. Annu Rev Neurosci 12:67–83

Ohnishi A, Yamaguchi K, Kusuhara M, Abe K, Kimura S (1989) Mobilization of intracellular calcium by endothelin in Swiss 3T3 cells. Biochem Biophys Res Commun 161:489–495

Olivari MT, Bartorelli C, Polese A, Fiorentini C, Moruzzi P, Guazzi M (1979) Treatment of hypertension with nifedipine, a calcium antagonist agent. Circulation 59:1056–1062

Ondrias K, Misik V, Gergel D, Stasko A (1989) Lipid peroxidation of phosphatidylcholine liposomes depressed by the calcium channel blockers nifedipine and verapamil and by the antiarrhythmic-antihypoxic drug stobadine. Biochem Biophys Acta 1003:238-245

Ondrias K, Borgatta L, Kim DH, Ehrlich BE (1990) Biphasic effects of doxorubicin on the calcium release channel from sarcoplasmic reticulum of cardiac muscle. Circ Res 67:1167-1174

Opie LH (1990) Clinical Use of Calcium Channel Antagonist Drugs, 2nd edn. Kluwer Academic Press, Boston, USA, pp1-286

Orekhov AN (1990) In vitro models of antiatherosclerotic effects of cardiovascular drugs. Am J Cardiol 66:23I-28I

Orekhov AN, Tertov VU, Khashimov KA, Kudryashou SA, Smirnov VN (1986) Antiatherosclerotic effects of verapamil in primary culture of human aortic intimal cells. J Hypertens 4 (Suppl 6):S153-S155

Osterrieder W, Holck M (1989) In vitro pharmacologic profile of RO40-5967, a novel Ca^{2+} channel blocker with potent vasodilator but weak inotropic action. J Cardiovasc Pharmacol 13:754-759

Packer M (1988) Neurohormonal interactions and adaptations in congestive heart failure. Circulation 77:721-730

Packer M (1990) Calcium channel blockers in chronic heart failure. The risks of physiologically rational therapy. Circulation 82:2255-2257

Packer M, Kessler PD, Lee WH (1987) Calcium-channel blockade in the management of severe chronic congestive heart failure: a bridge too far. Circulation 75 (Suppl V):V-56-V-64

Packer M, Lee WH, Medina N, Yushak M (1985) Comparative negative inotropic effects of nifedipine and diltiazem in patients with severe left ventricular dysfunction. Circulation 72 (Suppl III):III-275 (abstract)

Packer M, Leon M, Bonow RO, Kieval J, Rosing DR, Subramanian VB (1982) Hemodynamic and clinical effects of combined verapamil and propranolol therapy in angina pectoris. Am J Cardiol 50:903-912

Packer M, Medina N, Medina M (1984) Adverse hemodynamic and clinical effects of calcium channel blockade in pulmonary hypertension secondary to obliterative pulmonary vascular disease. J Am Coll Cardiol 4:890-901

Page IH (1987) Hypertensive Mechanisms. Orlando, Grune Stratton

Page E, McCalister LP (1973) Quantitative electron microscopic description of heart muscle cells. Application to normal, hypertrophied and thyroxin-stimulated hearts. Am J Cardiol 31:172-181

Pang DC, Johns A, Patterson K, Parker-Bothelho LH, Rubanyi GM (1989) Endothelin-1 stimulates phosphatylinositol hydrolysis and calcium uptake in isolated canine coronary arteries. J Cardiovasc Pharmacol 13 (Suppl 5):S75-S79

Panza G, Grebb JA, Sanna E, Wright AG Jr, Hanbauer I (1985) Evidence for down-regulation of ^{3}H-nitrendipine recognition sites in mouse brain after long-term treatment with nifedipine or verapamil. Neuropharmacology 34:1113-1117

Panza JA, Quyyumi AA, Brush JE, Epstein SE (1990) Abnormal endothelium-dependent vascular relaxation in patients with essential hypertension. N Eng J Med 323:22-27

Papageorgiou P, Morgan KG (1990) Changes in [Ca^2]$_i$ following receptor-mediated activation of hypertrophic vascular smooth muscle. Biophys J 57 (2):158a (abstract)

Papageorgiou P, Morgan KG (1991) Increased Ca^{2+} signalling after α adrenoceptor activation in vascular hypertrophy. Circ Res 68:1080-1084

Parker JO, Enjalbert M, Bernstein V (1988) Efficacy of the calcium antagonist isradipine in angina pectoris. Cardiovasc Drug Ther 1:661-664

Parmley WW (1990) Vascular protection from atherosclerosis: potential of calcium antagonists. Am J Cardiol 66:16I-22I

Pasternac A (1989) Myocardial stunning in hypertrophic cardiomyopathy? J Am Coll Cardiol 13:1419-1421

Patel B, Kloner RA (1987) Analysis of reported randomized trials of streptokinase therapy for acute myocardial infarction in the 1980's. Am J Cardiol 59:501-504

Patel B, Kloner RA, Przyklenk K, Braunwald E (1988) Postischemic myocardial 'stunning': a clinically relevant phenomenon. Ann Int med 108:626-628

Pedersen OL (1981) Calcium blockade as a therapeutic principle in arterial hypertension. Acta Pharmacol Toxicol 49 (Suppl II):1–31

Pepine C (1989) Nicardipine, a new calcium channel blocker: role for vascular selectivity. Clin Cardiol 12:240–246

Perez-Reyes E, Kim HS, Lacerda AE, Horne W, Wei X, Rampe D, Campbell KP, Brown AM, Birnbaumer L (1989) Induction of calcium currents by the expression of the α_1-subunit of the dihydropyridine receptor from skeletal muscle. Nature 340:233–236

Persson B, Wysocki M, Andersson OK (1989) Long-term renal effects of isradipine, a calcium entry blocker, in essential hypertension. J Cardiovasc Pharmacol 14:22–24

Petruk KC, West M, Mohr G, Weir BKA, Benoit BG, Gentili F, Disney GS, Tucker WS, Purves GB, Miller JOR, Hunter KM, Richard MT, Durity FA, Chan R, Clein LJ, Maroun FB, Godon A (1988) Nimodipine treatment in poor-grade aneurysm patients. J Neurosurg 69:505–517

Philippon J, Grob R, Pagreon F, Gugiari M, Rivierez M, Viars P (1986) Prevention of vasospasm in subarachnoid haemorrhage: a controlled study with nimodipine. Acta Neurochir 82:110–114

Pickard JD, Murray GD, Illingworth R, Shaw MDM, Teasdale GM, Foy PM, Humphrey PRD, Lang DA, Nelson R, Richards P, Sinar J, Bailey S, Skene A (1989) Effect of oral nimodipine on cerebral infarction and outcome after subarachnoid haemorrhage. British Aneurysm Nimodipine Trial. Br Med J 298:633–642

Pillai NP, Ross DH (1987) Proceedings of International Symposium on Calcium Antagonists. New York City , Feb 10–13

Pincon-Raymond M, Rieger F, Fosset M, Lazdunski M (1985) Abnormal transverse tubule system and abnormal amount of receptors for Ca channel inhibitors of the dihydropyridine family in skeletal muscle from mice with embryonic muscular dysgenesis. Dev Biol 112:458–466

Pool PE, Spann JB, Buccino RA, Sonnenblick EH, Braunwald E (1967) Myocardial high energy phosphate stores in cardiac hypertrophy and heart failure. Circ Res 21:365–373

Przyklenk K, Ghafari GB, Eitzman DT, Kloner RA (1989) Nifedipine administered after reperfusion ablates systolic contractile dysfunction of postischemic 'stunned' myocardium. J Am Coll Cardiol 13:1176–1183

Przyklenk K, Kloner RA (1987a) Acute effects of hydralozine and enalapril on contractile function of postischemic 'stunned' myocardium. Am J Cardiol 60:934–936

Przyklenk K, Kloner RA (1987b) Nifedipine administered postreperfusion ablates the phenomenon of the stunned myocardium. Circulation 76 (Suppl IV):IV198 (abstract)

Przyklenk K, Kloner RA (1988) Effect of verapamil on postischemic 'stunned' myocardium: importance of timing of treatment. J Am Coll Cardiol 11:614–623

Przyklenk K, Whittaker P, Kloner RA (1990) In vivo infusion of oxygen free radical substrates caused myocardial systolic, but not diastolic dysfunction. Am Heart J 119:807–815

Puett DW, Forman MB, Cates CV, Wilson BH, Hande KR, Friesinger GC, Virmani R (1987) Oxypurinol limits myocardial stunning but does not reduce infarct size after reperfusion. Circulation 76:678–686

Quaife RA, Kohmoto O, Barry WH (1991) Mechanism of reoxygenation injury in cultured ventricular myocytes. Circulation 83:566–577

Quinn MT, Parthasarathy S, Fong LG, Steinberg D (1987) Oxidatively modified low density lipoproteins – a potential role in recruitment and retention of monocyte/macrophages during atherosclerosis. Proc Natl Acad Sci USA 84:2995–2998

Rahimtoola SH (1985) A perspective on the three large multicenter randomized clinical trials of coronary bypass surgery for chronic stable angina. Circulation 72 (Suppl 5):V125–V135

Rahimtoola SH (1989) The hibernating myocardium. Am Heart J 117:211–221

Ramkumar V, El-Fakahany EE (1984) Increase in [^{3}H]nitrendipine binding sites in the brain in morphine-tolerant mice. Eur J Pharmacol 102:371–372

Ramkumar V, El-Fakahany EE (1986) Selective reduction in the density of [^{3}H]nimodipine binding sites in rat ventricular tissue following reserpine treatment. Pharmacologist 28:113a

Ramkumar V, El-Fakahany EE (1988) Prolonged morphine treatment increases rat brain dihydropyridine binding sites: possible involvement in development of morphine dependence. Eur J Pharmacol 146:73–83

Rankin JS, Newman GE, Muhlbaier LN, Behar VS, Fedor JM, Sabiston DC Jr (1985) The effects of coronary revascularization on left ventricular function in ischemic heart disease. J Thorac Cardiovasc Surg 90:818–832

Rao PS, Cohen MV, Mueller HS (1983) Production of free radicals and lipid peroxides in early experimental myocardial ischaemia. J Mol Cell Cardiol 15:713–716

Rardon DP, Cefali DC, Mitchell RD, Seiler SM, Hathaway DR, Jones LR (1990) Digestion of cardiac and skeletal muscle junctional sarcoplasmic reticulum vesicles with Calpain II. Effects on Ca^{2+} release channel. Circ Res 67:84–96

Rardon DP, Cefali DC, Mitchell RD, Seiler SM, Jones LR (1989) High molecular weight proteins purified from cardiac junctional sarcoplasmic reticulum vesicles are ryanodine-sensitive calcium channels. Circ Res 64:779–789

Raschack M (1984) Prolonged cardioprotective effects of anipamil, a new calcium antagonist. Eur Heart J 5:10 (abstract)

Reduto LA, Freund GC, Gaeta JM, Smalling RW, Lewis B, Gould KL (1981) Coronary artery reperfusion in acute myocardial infarction: beneficial effects of intracoronary streptokinase on left ventricular salvage and performance. Am Heart J 102:1168–1177

Reeves JP, Bailey CA, Hale CC (1986) Redox modification of sodium-calcium exchange activity in cardiac sarcolemmal vesicles. J Biol Chem 261-4948–4955

Reicher-Reiss H, Vered Z, Goldbourt U, Neufeld HN (1987) Efficacy of nisoldipine compared with nifedipine in chronic stable angina pectoris. In: Hugenholtz PG, Meyer J (eds) Nisoldipine. Springer-Verlag, Berlin, pp233–237

Reimer KA, Murry CE, Yamasawa I, Hill ML, Jennings RB (1986) Four brief periods of myocardial ischemia cause no cumulative ATP loss or necrosis. Am J Physiol 251:H1306–H1315

Renaud JF, Kazazoglou T, Schmid A, Romey G, Lazdunski M (1984) Differentiation of receptor sites of [^{3}H]nitrendipine in chick hearts and physiological relation to the slow Ca^{2+} channel and to excitation-contraction coupling. Eur J Biochem 139:673–681

Ress D, Palmer RMJ, Hodson HF, Moncada S (1989) L-arginine is the physiological precursor for the formation of nitric oxide in endothelium-dependent relaxation. Br J Pharmacol 96:418–424

Reynolds EE, Mok LLS (1990) Role of thromboxane A_2/prostaglandin H_2 receptor in the vasoconstrictor response of rat aorta to endothelin. J Pharmacol Exp Ther 252:915–921

Rios E, Brum G (1987) Involvement of dihydropyridine receptors in excitation-contraction coupling in skeletal muscle. Nature 325:717–720

Rius RA, Govoni S, Trabucchi M (1986) Regional modification of brain calcium antagonist binding after in vivo chronic lead exposure. Toxicology 40:191–197

Rius RA, Lucchi L, Govoni S, Trabucchi M (1987a) In vivo chronic lead exposure alters [^{3}H]nitrendipine binding in rat striatum. Brain Res 322:180–183

Rius RA, Bergamaschi S, DiFonso F, Govoni S, Trabucchi M, Rossi F (1987b) Acute ethanol effect on calcium antagonist binding in rat brain. Brain Res 402:359–361

Robinson MJ, Teasdale GM (1990) Calcium antagonists in the management of subarachnoid haemorrhage. Cerebrovasc Brain Metabolism Rev 2:205–226

Rosemblat M, Hidalgo L, Vergaro C, Ikemoto N (1981) Immunological and biochemical properties of transverse tubular membranes isolated from rabbit skeletal muscle. J Biol Chem 256:8140–8148

Ross RN (1986) The pathogenesis of atherosclerosis. New Eng J Med 314:488–490

Rossouw JE, Lewis B, Rifkind BM (1990) The value of lowering cholesterol after myocardial infarction. New Eng J Med 323:1112–1119

Rouleau JL, Parmley WW, Stevens J, Wikman-Coffelt J, Sievers R, Mahley RW, Havel RJ, Brecht W (1983) Verapamil suppresses atherosclerosis in cholesterol-fed rabbits. J Am Coll Cardiol 1:1453–1460

Rousseau E, Smith JS, Henderson JS, Meissner G (1986) Single channel and $^{45}Ca^{2+}$ flux measurements of the cardiac sarcoplasmic reticulum calcium channel. Biophys J 50:1009–1014

Rousseau M, Hanet C, Desager J-P, Pouleur H (1987) Effects of long-term therapy with the association of nisoldipine and a beta-blocker on exercise tolerance and coronary hemodynamics in patients with stable angina: a comparison with monotherapy. In: Hugenholtz PG, Meyer J (eds) Nisoldipine. Springer-Verlag, Berlin, pp213–222

Rousseau MF, Gurné O, Benedict CR, Van Eyll C, Pouleur H (1990) Effects of nisoldipine on the time-dependent changes in left ventricular function and neurohumoral status in patients with ischemic heart disease. In: Litchlen PR, Krayenbuhl HP (eds) New Aspects on Nisoldipine. Schattauer, Stuttgart, pp 69–83

Rowe GT, Manson NH, Caplan M, Hess ML (1983) Hydrogen peroxide and hydroxyl radical mediation of activated leucocyte depression of cardiac sarcoplasmic reticulum. Participation of the cyclooxygenase pathway. Circ Res 53:584–591

Ruegg UT, Hof RP (1990) Pharmacology of the calcium antagonist isradipine. Drugs 40 (Suppl 2):3–9

Ruilope LM, Alcazar JM (1990) Renal effects of calcium entry blockers. Cardiovasc Drugs and Therapy 4:979–982

Rusch NJ, Hermsmeyer K (1988) Calcium currents are altered in the vascular muscle cell membranes of spontaneously hypertensive rats. Circ Res 63:997–1002

Ruth P, Rohrkasten A, Biel M, Bosse E, Regulla S, Meyer HE, Flockerzi V, Hofmann F (1989) Primary structure of the β subunit of the DHP-sensitive calcium channel from skeletal muscle. Science 245:1115–1118

Ryle PR (1984) Free radicals, lipid peroxidation and ethanol hepatotoxicity. Lancet ii:461

Sagie A, Sclarovsky S, Strasberg B, Agmon J (1988) Acute myocardial ischemia with prolonged left ventricular dyskinesia and mural thrombus formation in asymmetric septal hypertrophy. Chest 93:888–890

Saito T, Nakao K, Mukoyama M, Imura H (1990) Increased plasma endothelin level in patients with essential hypertension. N Eng J Med 322:205

Saito T, Yanagisawa M, Miyauchi T, Suzuki N, Matsumoto H, Fujino M, Masaki T (1989) Endothelin in human circulating blood: effects of major surgical stress. Jap J Pharmacol 49: (abstract 215P)

Sakurai T, Yanagisawa M, Takuwa Y, Miyazaki H, Kimura S, Goto K, Masaki T (1990) Cloning of a cDNA encoding a non-isopeptide-selective subtype of the endothelin receptor. Nature 348:732–735

Salmasi, A-M (1990) Nisoldipine in occult ischaemic heart disease. In: Lichtlen PR, Krayenbuhl HP (eds) New Aspects on Nisoldipine. Schattauer, Stuttgart, pp 29–38

Sanchez JA, Stefani E (1978) Inward calcium current in twitch muscle fibres of the frog. J Physiol 283:197–209

Sanna E, Head GA, Hanbauer I (1986) Evidence for a selective localization of voltage-sensitive Ca^{2+} channels in nerve cell bodies of corpus striatum. J Neurochem 47:1552–1557

Sauter A, Rudin M (1990a) Calcium antagonists for reduction of brain damage in stroke. J Cardiovasc Pharmacol 15 (Suppl 1): S43–S47

Sauter A, Rudin M (1990b) Experimental studies with isradipine in stroke. Drugs 40 (Suppl 2):44–51

Sauter A, Rudin M, Wiederhold KH (1989) Cytoprotective characteristics of dihydropyridine calcium antagonists in a rat model of stroke: implications for clinical trials. In: Hartmann A, Kuschinsky W (eds) Cerebral Ischemia and Calcium. Springer Verlag, Berlin-Heidelberg, pp 282–291

Schaper J, Froede R, St Hein TA, Buck A, Hashizume H, Speiser B, Friedl A, Bleese N (1991) Impairment of the myocardial ultrastructure and changes of the cytoskeleton in dilated cardiomyopathy. Circulation 83:504–514

Scheidt S, LeWinter MM, Hermanovich J, Venkataraman K, Freedman D (1986) Efficacy and safety of nicardipine for chronic, stable angina pectoris: a multicentre randomized trial. Am J Cardiol 58:715–721

Schmid A, Kazazoglou T, Renaud JF, Lazdunski M (1984) Comparative changes of levels of nitrendipine Ca^{2+} channels, of tetrodotoxin-sensitive Na^{2+} channels and of oubain-sensitive voltage-dependent $(Na^{+}+K^{+})$-ATPase following denervation of rat and chick skeletal muscle. FEBS Lett 172:113–118

Schneider MF, Chandler WK (1973) Voltage dependent charge movement in skeletal muscle: a possible step in excitation-contraction coupling. Nature 242:244–246

Schofer J, Hobuss M, Aschenberg W, Tews A (1990) Acute and long-term haemodynamic and neurohumoral response to nisoldipine vs captopril in patients with heart failure: a randomized double-blind study. Eur Heart J 11:712–721

Schomig A (1990) Catecholamines in myocardial ischemia. Systemic and cardiac release. Circulation 82 (Suppl II):II-13–II-22

Schuster EH, Bulkley BH (1981) Early post infarction angina. Ischemia at a distance and ischemia in the infarct zone. N Eng J Med 305:1101–1105

Schwartz A (1971) Calcium and the sarcoplasmic reticulum. In: Harris P, Opie L (eds) Calcium and the Heart. Academic Press, London, pp66–92

Schwartz A, McKenna E, Vaghy PL (1988) Receptors for calcium antagonists. Am J Cardiol 62:36–66

Schwartz JS, Bache RJ (1988) Combined effects of calcium antagonists and nitroglycerin on large arterial diameter. Am Heart J 115:964–969

Schwartz LM, McCleskey EW, Almers W (1985) Dihydropyridine receptors in muscle are voltage-dependent but most are not functional calcium channels. Nature 314:747–751

Schwenke DC, Carew TE (1989a) Initiation of atherosclerotic lesions in cholesterol-fed rabbits. I. Focal increases in arterial LDL concentration precede development of fatty streak lesion. Arteriosclerosis 9:895–907

Schwenke DC, Carew TE (1989b) Initiation of atherosclerotic lesions in cholesterol-fed rabbits. II. Selective retention of LDL vs. selective increases in LDL permeability in susceptible sites of arteries. Arteriosclerosis 9:908–918

Scriabine A, Schuurman T, Traber J (1989) Pharmacological basis for the use of nimodipine in central nervous system disorders. FASEB J 3:1799–1806

Seitelberger R, Zwolfer W, Huber S, Schwarzacher S, Binder TM, Peschl F, Spatt J, Holzinger C, Podesser B, Buxbaum P, Weber H, Wolner E (1991) Nifedipine reduces the incidence of myocardial infarction and transient ischemia in patients undergoing coronary bypass grafting. Circulation 83:460–468

Serruys PW, Suryapranata H, Planellas J, Wijns W, Vanhaleweyk CLJ, Soward AL, Jaski BE, Hugenholtz PG (1985) Acute effects of intravenous nisoldipine on left ventricular function and coronary hemodynamics. Am J Cardiol 56:140–146

Sharma RV, Butters CA, Bhalla RC (1986) Alterations in the plasma membrane properties of the myocardium of spontaneously hypertensive rats. Hypertension 8:583–591

Shattock MJ, Manning AS, Hearse DJ (1982) Effects of hydrogen peroxide on cardiac function and postischaemic functional recovery in the isolated 'working' rat heart. Pharmacology 24:118-122

Shaw S, Jayatilleke E, Ross WA, Gordon EF, Lieber CS (1981) Ethanol-induced lipid peroxidation by long-term alcohol feeding and attenuation by methionine. J Lab Clin Med 98:417–428

Shepherd JT (1990) Increased systemic vascular resistance and primary hypertension: the expanding complexity. J Hypertens 8 (Suppl 7):S15–S27

Shichiri M, Hirata Y, Ando K, Emori T, Ohta K, Kimoto S, Ogura M, Inoue A, Marumo F (1990) Plasma endothelin levels in hypertension and chronic renal failure. Hypertension 15 (Suppl 5):493–496

Shimokawa H, Tomoike H, Nabeyama S, Yamamoto H, Araki H, Nakamura M, Ishii Y, Tanaka K (1983) Coronary artery spasm induced in atherosclerotic miniature swine. Science 221:560–562

Shull GE, Schwartz A, Lingrei JB (1985) Amino acid sequence of the catalytic subunit of the (Na^+ and K^+) ATPase deduced from a complimentary DNA. Nature 316:691–695

Siesjo BK, Agardh CD, Bengtsson F (1989) Free radicals and brain damage. Cerebrovasc Brain Metabolism Rev 1:165–211

Siesjo BK, Bengtsson F (1989) Calcium fluxes, calcium antagonists, and calcium-related pathology in brain ischemia, hypoglycaemia, and spreading depression: a unifying hypothesis. J Cereb Blood Flow Metab 9:127–140

Sievers RE, Rashid T, Garrett J, Blumein S, Parmely WW (1987) Verapamil and diet holt progression of atherosclerosis in cholesterol-fed rabbits. Cardiovasc Drugs Ther 1:65–69

Simonson MS, Dunn MJ (1990) Endothelin: Pathways in transmembrane signalling. Hypertension 15 (Suppl I):I-5–I-12

Simpson PJ, Lucchesi BR (1987) Free radicals and myocardial ischemia and reperfusion injury. J Lab Clin Med 110:13–30

Singh S, Doherty J, Udhoji V, Smith K, Gorwit J, Bekheit S, Mather S, Stein W, Fellippo JS, Hearan P, Chen Y, Taylor C (1989) Amlodipine versus nadolol in patients with stable angina pectoris. Am Heart J 118 (Suppl 5):1137–1138

Sitsapesan R, Williams AJ (1990) Mechanisms of caffeine activation of single calcium-release channels of sheep cardiac sarcoplasmic reticulum. J Physiol 423:425–439

Skattebol A, Triggle DJ (1986) 6-Hydroxydopamine treatment increases β-adrenoceptors and Ca^{2+} channels in rat heart. Eur J Pharmacol 127:287–289

Slish DF, Engle DB, Varadi G, Lotan I, Singer D, Dascal N, Schwartz A (1989) Evidence for the existence of a cardiac specific isoform of the α_1 subunit of the voltage-dependent calcium channel. FEBS Lett 250:509–514

Smith, JS, Coronado R, Meissner G (1986) Single-channel measurements of the calcium release channel from skeletal muscle sarcoplasmic reticulum. Activation by calcium, ATP and modulation by Mg. J Gen Physiol 88:573–588

Smith JS, Rousseau E, Meissner G (1989) Calmodulin modulation of single sarcoplasmic reticulum Ca^{2+}-release channels from cardiac and skeletal muscle. Circ Res 64:352–359

Solomon RA, Correll JW (1988) Rupture of a previously documented asymptomatic aneurysm enhances the argument for prophylactic surgical intervention. Surg Neurol 30:321–331

Somlyo AV (1979) Bridging structures spanning the junctioning gap at the triad of skeletal muscle. J Cell Biol 80:743–750

Somlyo AV (1985) Excitation-contraction coupling and the ultrastructure of smooth muscle. Circulation 57:497–507

Southorn PA, Powis G (1988) Free radicals in medicine. II. Involvement in human disease. Mayo Clin Proc 63:390–408

Spetzler RF, Hadley MN (1989) Protection against cerebral ischemia: the role of barbiturates. Cerebrovasc Brain Metabolism Rev 1:212–229

Stack RS, Phillips HR , Grierson DS, Behar VS, Kong Y, Peter RH, Swain JL, Greenfield JC Jr (1983) Functional improvement of jeopardized myocardium following intracoronary streptokinase infusion in acute myocardial infarction. J Clin Invest 72:84–95

Stahl LD, Aversano TR, Becker LC (1986) Selective enhancement of function of stunned myocardium by increased flow. Circulation 74:843–851

Stahl LD, Weiss HR, Becker LC (1988) Myocardial oxygen consumption, oxygen supply/demand heterogeneity and microvascular patency in regionally stunned myocardium. Circulation 77:865–872

Stary HC (1987) Macrophages, macrophage foam cells, and eccentric intimal thickening in the coronary arteries of young children. Atherosclerosis 64:91–108

Stary HC (1989) Evolution and progression of atherosclerotic lesions in coronary arteries in children and young adults. Arteriosclerosis 9:119–132

Steen PA, Newberg LA, Milde JH, Michenfelder JD (1983) Nimodipine improves cerebral blood flow and neurological recovery after complete cerebral ischemia in the dog. J Cereb Blood Flow Metab 3:38–48

Steenbergen C, Murphy E, Levy L, London RE (1987) Elevation in cytosolic free calcium concentration early in myocardial ischaemia in perfused rat heart. Circ Res 60:700–707

Steinberg D, Parthasarathy S, Carew TE, Khoo JC, Witztum JL (1989) Beyond cholesterol: modification of low density lipoprotein that increase its atherogenicity. New Eng J Med 320:915–924

Strasser RH, Marquetant R, Kubler W (1990) Adrenergic receptors and sensitization of adenyl cyclase in acute myocardial ischemia. Circulation 82 (Suppl II):II23–II29

Strickberger SA, Russek LN, Phair RD (1988) Evidence for increased aortic plasma membrane calcium transport caused by experimental atherosclerosis in rabbits. Circ Res 62:75–80

Striessnig J, Knaus H-G, Glossmann H (1988) Photoaffinity-labelling of the calcium-channel-associated 1,4-dihydropyridine and phenylalkylamine receptor in guinea-pig hippocampus. Biochem J 253:39–47

Striessnig J, Scheffauer F, Mitterdorfer J, Schirmer M, Glossmann H (1990) Identification of the benzothiazepine-binding polypeptide of skeletal muscle calcium channels with (+)-cis azidodiltiazem and anti ligand antibodies. J Biol Chem 265:363–370

Struyker-Boudier HAJ, Smits JFM, De Mey JGR (1990) The pharmacology of calcium antagonists: a review. J Cardiovasc Pharmacol 15 (Suppl 4):S1–S10

Sugiyama T, Yoshisumi M, Takaku F, Urabe H, Tsukakoshi M, Kasuya T, Yazaki Y (1986) The elevation of the cytoplasmic calcium ions in vascular smooth muscle cells in SHR-measurement of the free calcium ions in single living cells by laser microfluorospectrometry. Biochem Biophys Res Comm 141:340–345

Sunkel CE, Fau de Casa-Juana M, Cillero FJ, Priego JG, Ortego MP (1988) Synthesis, platelet aggregation inhibitory activity, and in vivo antithrombotic activity of new 1,4-dihydropyridines. J Med Chem 31:1886–1890

Suzuki T, Kurosawa H, Naito K, Otsuka M, Ohashi M, Takaita O (1991) Binding characteristics of a new 1,5-benzothiazepine, clentiazem, to rat cerebral cortex and skeletal muscle membranes. Eur J Pharmacol 194:195–200

Swain JL, Sabina RL, Hines JJ, Greenfield JC, Holmes EW (1984) Repetitive episodes of brief ischaemia (12 min) do not produce a cumulative depletion of high energy phosphate compounds. Cardiovasc Res 18:264–269

Szabo L (1989) (S)-Emopamil, a novel calcium and serotonin antagonist for the treatment of cerebrovascular disorders. 2nd communication: Brain penetration, cerebral vascular and metabolic effects. Arzneimittelforschung 39:309–314

Tagawa H, Tomoike H, Nakamura M (1991) Putative mechanisms of the impairment of endothelium-dependent relaxation of the aorta with atheromatous plaque in heritable hyperlipidemic rabbits. Circ Res 68:330–337

Takahashi M, Catterall WA (1987) Identification of an α subunit of dihydropyridine-sensitive brain calcium channels. Science 236:88–92

Takahashi M, Seagar M, Jones J, Reber B, Catterall WA (1987) Subunit structure of dihydropyridine-sensitive calcium channels from skeletal muscle. Proc Natl Acad Sci USA 84:5478–5482

Takenaka T, Handa J (1979) Cerebrovascular effects of YC-93, a new vasodilator, in dogs, monkeys, and human patients. Int J Clin Pharmacol Biopharmacol 17:1–11

Takeshima H, Nishimura S, Matsumoto T, Ishida H, Kangawa K, Minamino N, Matsuo H, Ueda M, Hanaoka M, Hirose T, Numa S (1989) Primary structure and expression from complementary DNA of skeletal muscle ryanodine receptor. Nature 339:439–445

Talajic M, Nayebpour M, Jing W, Nattel S (1989) Frequency-dependent effects of diltiazem on the atrioventricular node during experimental atrial fibrillation. Circulation 80:380–389

Tanabe T, Beam KG, Adams BA, Niidome T, Numa S, (1990) Regions of the skeletal muscle dihydropyridine receptor critical for excitation-contraction coupling. Nature 346:567–569

Tanabe T, Beam KG, Powell JA, Numa S (1988) Restoration of excitation-contraction coupling and slow calcium current in dysgenic muscle by dihydropyridine receptor cDNA. Nature 336:134–139

Tanabe T, Takeshima H, Mikami A, Flockerzi V, Takahashi H, Kangawa K, Kojima M, Matsuo H, Hirose T, Numa S (1987) Primary structure of the receptor for calcium channel blockers from skeletal muscle. Nature 328:313–318

Taylor AL, Golino P, Buja LM, Eckels RM (1987) Is postischemic systolic dysfunction primarily caused by reperfusion. Circulation 76 (Suppl IV):IV228 (abstract)

Taylor SH (1989) The efficacy of amlodipine in myocardial ischaemia. Am Heart J 118:1123–1128

Taylor SH, Lee P, Jackson N, Cocco G (1989) A four-week double-blind, placebo-controlled, parallel dose-response study of amlodipine in patients with stable exertional angina pectoris. Am Heart J 118 (Suppl 5):1133–1134

Teasdale G, Mendelow AD, Graham DI, Harper AM, McCulloch J (1990) Efficacy of nimodipine in cerebral ischemia or hemorrhage. Stroke 21 (Suppl IV):IV-123–IV-125

Tettenborn D, Dycka J (1990) Prevention and treatment of delayed ischemic dysfunction in patients with aneurysmal subarachnoid hemorrhage. Stroke 21 (Suppl IV):IV-85–IV-89

Thadani U, the Amlodipine Study Group (1989) Amlodipine: A once-daily calcium antagonist in the treatment of angina pectoris – A parallel dose-response, placebo-controlled study. Am Heart J 118 (Suppl 5):1135

Thandroyen FT, Muntz KH, Buja LM, Willerson JT (1990) Alterations in β-adrenergic receptors, adenyl cyclase, and cyclic AMP concentrations during acute myocardial ischemia and reperfusion. Circulation 82 (Suppl II):II30–II37

Thaulow E, Goth BD, Heusch G, Gilpin E, Schulz R, Kroeger K, Ross J (1989) Characteristics of regional myocardial stunning after exercise in dogs with chronic coronary stenosis. Am J Physiol 257:H113–H119

The Danish Study Group on Verapamil in Myocardial Infarction (1990) Effect of verapamil on mortality and major events after acute myocardial infarction (The Danish Verapamil Infarction Trial II). Am J Cardiol 66:779–785

The Israeli SPRINT Study Group (1988) Secondary prevention reinfarction Israeli nifedipine trial (SPRINT). A randomized intervention trial of nifedipine in patients with acute myocardial infarction. Eur Heart J 9:354–364

Thomassen A, Bagger JP, Nielsen TT, Henningsen P (1987) Metabolic and hemodynamic effects of nicardipine during pacing-induced angina pectoris. Am J Cardiol 59:219–224

Thompson GR (1991) What should be done about asymptomatic hypercholesterolaemia? Br Med J 302:605–606

Thompson JA, Hess ML (1986) The oxygen free radical system: a fundamental mechanism in the production of myocardial necrosis. Prog Cardiovasc Dis 28:449–462

Tomita K, Ujiie K, Nakanishi T, Tomura S, Matsuda O, Ando K, Shichiri M, Hirata Y, Marumo F (1989) Plasma endothelin levels in patients with acute renal failure. New Eng J Med 321:1127

Towart R (1981) The selective inhibition of serotonin-induced contractions of rabbit cerebral vascular smooth muscle by calcium antagonist dihydropyridines. Circ Res 48:650–657

Towart R, Kazda S (1979) The cellular mechanism of action of nimodipine (Baye9736) a new calcium antagonist. Br J Pharmacol 67: 409–410

Toyo-Oka T, Aizawa T, Suzuki N, Hirata Y, Miyauchi T, Shin WS, Yanagisawa M, Masaki T, Sugimoto T (1991). Increased plasma level of endothelin-1 and coronary spasm induction in patients with vasospastic angina. Circulation 83:476–483

Triggle DJ (1990a) Calcium antagonist drug development. Curr Cardiovasc Patents 2:365–384

Triggle DJ (1990b) Calcium antagonists: history and perspective. Stroke 21 (Suppl IV):IV-49–IV-56

Triggle DJ, Langs DA, Janis RA (1989) Ca^{2+} channel ligands: structure-function relationships of the 1,4-dihydropyridines. Med Res Rev 9:123–180

Tseng-Crank JCL, Tseng GN, Schwartz A, Tanouye MA (1990) Molecular cloning and functional expression of a potassium channel cDNA isolated from a rat cardiac library. FEBS Lett 268:63–68

Tsuji K, Tsutsumi S, Ogawa K, Miyazaki Y, Satake T (1987) Cardiac $alpha_1$ and beta adrenoceptors in rabbits: effects of dietary sodium and cholesterol. Cardiovasc Res 21:39–44

Tzivoni D, Banai S, Benhorin J, Gavish A, Medina A, Stern S (1990) Effects of nisoldipine on exercise test parameters in patients with stable angina. In: Lichtlen PR, Krayenbuhl HP (eds) New Aspects on Nisoldipine. Schattauer, Stuttgart, pp21–27

Tzivoni D, Banai S, Botvin S, Zilberman A, Weiss TA, Gavish A, Medina A, Benhorin J, Rogel S, Caspi A, Stern S (1991) Effects of nisoldipine on myocardial ischemia during exercise and during daily activity. Am J Cardiol 67:559–564

Uematsu D, Greenberg JH, Hickey WF, Reivich M (1989) Nimodipine attenuates both increases in cytosolic free calcium and histologic damage following focal cerebral ischaemia and reperfusion in cats. Stroke 20:1531–1537

Vaghy PL, Striessnig J, Miwa K, Knaus HG, Itagaki K, McKenna E, Glossmann H, Schwartz A (1987a) Identification of a novel 1,4-dihydropyridine and phenylalkylamine-binding polypeptide in calcium channel preparations. J Biol Chem 262:14337–14342

Vaghy PL, Williams JS, Schwartz A (1987b) Receptor pharmacology of calcium entry blocking agents. Am J Cardiol 59:9A–17A

Valdeolmillos M, O'Neill SC, Smith GL, Eisner DA (1989) Calcium-induced calcium release activates contraction in intact cardiac cells. Pflugers Arch 413:676–678

Verheul HA, Moulizn AC, Hondema S, Schouwink M, Dunning AJ (1991) Late results of 200 repeat coronary artery bypass operations. Am J Cardiol 67:24–30

Von Arnim T, Reuschel-Janetschek E, Erath A (1987) Effects of oral nisoldipine on transient and exercise-induced ischaemia in patients with coronary heart disease. In: Hugenholtz PG, Meyer J (eds) Nisoldipine. Springer-Verlag, Berlin, pp288–295

Wagenknecht T, Grassuci R, Frank J, Saito A, Inui M, Fleischer S (1989) Three dimensional architecture of the calcium channel/foot structure of sarcoplasmic reticulum. Nature 338:167–170

Wagner JA, Reynolds IJ, Weisman HF, Dudeck P, Weisfeld ML, Synder SH (1986) Calcium antagonist receptors in cardiomyopathic hamster: selective increases in heart, muscle, brain. Science 232:515–518

Wagner JA, Sax FL, Weisman HF, Porterfield J, McIntosh C, Weisfeldt ML, Snyder SH, Epstein SE (1989) Calcium-antagonist receptors in the atrial tissue of patients with hypertrophic cardiomyopathy. N Engl J Med 320:755–761

Waller DG, Challenor VF (1990) The combination of slow-release nifedipine and atenolol for stable angina. Cardiovasc Drugs and Therapy 4 (Suppl 5):899–904

Walsh RA (1989) The effects of calcium entry blockade on normal and ischemic ventricular diastolic function. Circulation 80 (Suppl IV): IV-52–IV-58

Ware JA, Johnson PC, Smith M, Salzman EW (1986) Inhibition of human platelet aggregation and cytoplasmic calcium responses by calcium antagonists: studies with aequorin and quin-2. Circ Res 59:39–42

Warner TD, De Nucci G, Vane JR (1989) Rat endothelin is a vasodilator in the isolated perfused mesentary of the rat. Eur J Pharmacol 159:325–326

Wartman A, Lampe TL, McDann DS, Boyle AJ (1967) Plaque reversal with Mg EDTA in experimental atherosclerosis: elastin and collagen metabolism. J Atheroscler Res 7:331–341

Watanabe T, Kusumoto K, Kitayoshi T, Shimamoto N (1989) Positive inotropic and vasoconstrictive effects of endothelin–1 in in vivo and in vitro experiments: Characteristics and role of L-type calcium channels. J Cardiovasc Pharmacol 13 (Suppl 5):108–111

Waters D, Lesperance J, Francetich M, Causey D, Theroux P, Chiang Y-K, Hudon G, Lemarbre L, Reitman M, Joyal M, Grosselin G, Dyrda I, Macer J, Havel RJ (1990) A controlled clinical trial to assess the effect of a calcium channel blocker on the progression of coronary atherosclerosis. Circulation 82:1940–1953

Watts JA, Norris TA, London RE, Steenbergen C, Murphy E (1990) Effects of diltiazem on lactate, ATP, and cytosolic free calcium levels in ischemic hearts. J Cardiovasc Pharmacol 15:44–49

Weber KT, Janicki JS, Shroff SG, Pick R, Chen RM, Bashley RI (1988) Collagen remodelling of the pressure-overloaded, hypertrophied nonhuman primate myocardium. Circ Res 62:757–765

Weinstein DB, Heider JG (1988) Antiatherogenic properties of the calcium antagonists. Am J Med 86 (Suppl A):27–32

Weinstein DB, Heider JG (1989) Antiatherogenic properties of calcium channel blockers. Am J Med 84:102–108

Weisfeldt ML (1987) Reperfusion and reperfusion injury. Clin Res 35:13–20

Welsch M, Nuglisch J, Krieglstein J (1990) Neuroprotective effect of nimodipine is not mediated by increased cerebral blood flow after transient forebrain ischemia in rats. Stroke 21 (Suppl IV):IV-105–IV-107

Whiting RL (1987) Animal pharmacology of nicardipine and its clinical relevance. Am J Cardiol 59:3J–8J

Whorton AR, Montgomery ME, Kent RS (1985) Effect of hydrogen peroxide on prostaglandin production and cellular integrity in cultured porcine aortic endothelial cells. J Clin Invest 76:295–302

Wibo M, Bravo G, Godfraind T (1991) Postnatal maturation of excitation-contraction coupling in rat ventricle in relation to the subcellular localization and surface density of 1,4-dihydropyridine and ryanodine receptors. Circ Res 68:662–673

Wier WG, Yue DT (1985) The effects of 1,4-dihydropyridine type Ca^{2+}-channel antagonists and agonists on intracellular $[Ca^{2+}]_i$-transients accompanying twitch contraction of heart muscle. In: Fleckenstein A, Van Breemen C, Gross R, Hoffmeister F (eds) Cardiovascular Effect of Dihydropyridine-Type Calcium Antagonists and Agonists. Springer, Berlin, pp188–194

Williams AJ, Ashley RH (1989) Reconstitution of cardiac sarcoplasmic reticulum calcium channels. Ann NY Acad Sci 560:163–173

Willis AL, Nagel B, Churchill V, Whyte M, Smith DL, Mahmud I, Pappione DL (1985) Antiatherosclerotic effects of nicardipine and nifedipine in cholesterol-fed rabbits. Atherosclerosis 5:250–255

Wines PA, Schmitz JM, Pfister SL, Clubb FJ, Buja LM, Willerson JT, Campbell WB (1989) Augmented vasoconstrictor responses to serotonin precede development of atherosclerosis in aorta of WHHL rabbit. Arteriosclerosis 9:195–202

Webb RC,Bohr OF (1982) Reactivity of vascular smooth muscle in hypertension. Fed Proc 41:2387-2393

Witztum JL (1990) The role of monocytes and oxidized LDL in atherosclerosis. Atherosclerosis Rev 21:59-69

Xie Z, Wang Y, Askari A, Huang WG, Klaunig JE, Askari A (1990). Studies on the specificity of the effects of oxygen metabolites on cardiac sodium pump. J Mol Cell Cardiol 22:911-920

Yamada Y, Yokota M, Furumichi T, Furui H, Yamauchi K, Saito H (1990) Protective effects of calcium channel blockers on hydrogen peroxide induced increases in endothelial permeability. Cardiovasc Res 24:993-997

Yamamoto Y, Tomoike H, Egashira K, Nakamura M (1987) Attenuation of endothelium-related relaxation and enhanced responsiveness of vascular smooth muscle to histamine in spastic coronary arterial segments from miniature pigs. Circ Res 61:772-778

Yang Z, Bauer E, Von Segesser L, Stulz P, Turina M, Luscher TF (1990a) Different mobilization of calcium in endothelin-1 induced contractions in human arteries and veins. Effect of calcium antagonists. J Cardiovasc Pharmacol 16:654-660

Yang Z, Richard D, Von Segesser L, Bauer E, Stulz P, Turina M, Luscher TF (1990b) Threshold concentrations of endothelin-1 potentiate contractions to norepinephrine and serotoxin in human arteries: A new mechanism of vasospasm. Circulation 82:188-195

Yanagisawa M, Kurihara H, Kimura S, Tomobe Y, Kobayashi M, Mitsui Y, Yazaki Y, Goto K, Masaki T (1988) A novel potent constrictor peptide produced by vascular endothelial cells. Nature 332:411-415

Yanagisawa M, Masaki T (1989a) Endothelin, a novel endothelium-derived peptide. Biochem Pharmacol 38:1877-1883

Yanagisawa M, Masaki T (1989b) Molecular biology and biochemistry of the endothelins. Trends Pharmacol Sci 10:374-378

Yasue H, Morikami Y (1990) Efficacy of slow-release nifedipine on ischemic attacks in patients with variant angina. Cardiovasc Drugs and Therapy 4:915-918

Yasutomi N, Kogame T, Kawakami K, Komasa N, Iwasaki T (1989) Stunned myocardium in hypertrophic cardiomyopathy with normal coronary arteries. Am Heart J 118:1069-1073

Yool AJ, Schwartz TL (1991) Alteration of ionic selectivity of a K^+ channel by mutation of the H5 region. Nature 349:700-704

Yoshimoto S, Ishizaki Y, Sasaki T, Murota S (1991) Effect of carbon dioxide and oxygen on endothelin production by cultured porcine cerebral endothelial cells. Stroke 22:378-383

Zamora MR, O'Brien RF, Rutherford RB, Weil JV (1990) Serum endothelin-1 concentrations and cold provocation in primary Raynaud's phenomenon. Lancet 336:1144-1147

Zebra E, Komorowski TE, Faulkner JA (1990) Free radical injury to skeletal muscles of young, adult and old mice. Am J Physiol 258:C429-C435

Zeiher AM, Drexler H, Wollschlager H, Just H (1991) Modulation of coronary vasomotor tone in humans. Progressive endothelial dysfunction with different early stages of coronary atherosclerosis. Circulation 83:391-401

Zemel PC, Sowers JR (1990) Relation between lipids and atherosclerosis: epidemiological evidence and clinical implications. Am J Cardiol 66:7I-12I

Zernig G (1990) Widening potential for Ca^{2+} antagonists: non L-type Ca^{2+} channel interaction. Trends in Pharmacol Sci 11:38-44

Zhao M, Zhang H, Robinson TF, Factor SM, Sonnenblick EH, Eng C (1987) Profound structural alterations of the extracellular collagen matrix in postischemic dysfunctional ("stunned") but viable myocardium. J Am Coll Cardiol 10:1322-1334

Zorzato F, Fujii J, Otsu K, Phillips M, Green NM, Lai FA, Meissner G, MacLennan DH (1990) Molecular cloning of cDNA encoding human and rabbit forms of the Ca^{2+} release channel (ryanodine receptor) of skeletal muscle sarcoplasmic reticulum. J Biol Chem 265:2244-2256

Zweier JL, Flaherty JT, Weisfeldt ML (1987a) Direct measurement of free radical generation following reperfusion of ischaemic myocardium. Proc Natl Acad Sci USA 84:1404-1407

Zweier JL, Rayburn BK, Flaherty JT, Weisfeldt ML (1987b) Recombinant superoxide dismutase reduces oxygen free radical concentrations in reperfused myocardium. J Clin Invest 80:1728-1734